Beginner's Guide to Homeopathy

Know-how of Common Ailments and their Homeopathic Management

Arranged and Compiled by

T. S. Iyer

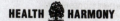

An imprint of
B. Jain Publishers (P) Ltd.
USA—EUROPE—INDIA

BEGINNER'S GUIDE TO HOMEOPATHY

Revised Enlarged Edition: 2007
12th Impression: 2014

All rights reserved. No part of this book may be reproduced, stored in a retrieval system or transmitted, in any form or by any means, mechanical, photocopying, recording or otherwise, without any prior written permission of the publisher.

© with the publisher

Published by Kuldeep Jain for

HEALTH HARMONY
An imprint of
B. JAIN PUBLISHERS (P) LTD.
1921/10, Chuna Mandi, Paharganj, New Delhi 110 055 (INDIA)
Tel.: +91-11-4567 1000 • Fax: +91-11-4567 1010
Email: info@bjain.com • Website: www.bjain.com

Printed in India at Amar Ujala Publications Ltd., Noida

ISBN: 978-81-319-0255-4

Dedicated to

The Memory of the late

Dr. W. Younan, M.B., C.M. (Edinburgh)

of

Calcutta

A Veteran Hahnemannian Homeopath

To *whom*

I am greatly indebted for all my knowledge
and experience of Homeopathy as taught
by Hahnemann—
the Great Founder.

CONTENTS

Foreword to the First Edition xvii
Foreword to the Second Edition xxi
Preface to the First Edition xxiii
Preface to the Second Edition xxvii
List of Medicines xxix

PART–I

INTRODUCTION

1. Introductory 1
2. The Organon (A Synopsis) 7
3. Hahnemann's 'Chronic Diseases' (A Synopsis) 27
4. Hahnemann's Nosology 42
5. Hahnemann's Philosophy 51
6. The Application of Homeopathy 57
   (a) The Examination of the Patient 57
   (b) The Selection of Similar Remedy 64
   (c) The Single Remedy 66
   (d) On the Administration of Medicines and the Repetition of Doses 75
   (e) General Hints on Health and Diet 82
   (f) Diet and Other Restrictions During Treatment 85
   (g) General Instructions About Diet 87
   (h) The Study of the Materia Medica 93

PART-II

TREATMENT OF DISEASES

CHAPTER I. *Affections of the Head* : 101
  1. Giddiness, Vertigo 101
  2. Headache 101
     (a) Congestive Headache 103
     (b) Catarrhal Headache 104
     (c) Rheumatic Headache 105
     (d) Bilious Headache 105
     (e) Nervous Headache or Neuralgic Headache 106

CHAPTER II. *Diseases of the Eyes* : 113
  1. General Remarks 113
  2. Sore Eyes of Young Infants 113
  3. Inflammation of the Eyes– Ophthalmia 114
  4. Chronic Inflammation of the Eyelids–Chronic
     Ophthalmia 115
  5. Stye on the Eyelids 115
  6. After Operations on the Eye 116

CHAPTER III. *Affections of the Ears* : 117
  1. Mumps 117
  2. Inflammation of the Ear– Earache 119
  3. Running of the Ears 120
  4. Hardness of Hearing 121

CHAPTER IV. *Affections of the Nose* 122
     Bleeding from the Noses– Epistaxis 122

CHAPTER V. *Diseases of the Organs of Respiration* : ... 124
  1. Catarrh or Common Cold 124
  2. Cough 126

CONTENTS

3. Croup 129
4. Bronchitis 131
5. Asthma 133
6. Whooping Cough 138
7. Pleurisy or Pleuritis 141
8. Pneumonia 143

CHAPTER VI. *Diseases of the Heart* : 147

CHAPTER VII. *Blood Pressure* 155
1. Hypertension–High Blood Pressure 155
2. Hypotension–Low Blood Pressure 166

CHAPTER VIII. *Affections of the Throat* : 174
1. Sore Throat 174
2. Tonsilitis or Inflammation of the Tonsils 177
   (a) Definition 177
   (b) Acute Tonsilitis 179
   (c) Chronic Enlargement of the Tonsils 180
3. Enlargement of the Uvula or Falling of the Palate 181
4. Diphtheria 181

CHAPTER IX. *Affections of the Teeth* : 185

CHAPTER X. *Affections of the Mouth* : 189
1. Gumboil, Sore Mouth 189
2. Inflammation and Swelling of the Tongue 189

CHAPTER XI. *Affections of the Stomach and Abdomen* : 191
1. Catarrh of the Stomach, Heartburn, Waterbrash, Sour–Stomach 191
2. Biliousness 192
3. Nausea and Vomiting 192

4.	Sea-Sickness or Vomiting from Travelling in a Carriage or Motor-Car or by Air	193
5.	Colic or Griping Pain in the Bowels	193
6.	Dyspepsia or Indigestion	194
7.	Constipation	199
8.	Piles of Hemorrhoids	202
9.	Worms and Itching of the Anus	204
10.	Prolapsus of the Anus	206
11.	Hernia or Rupture	207
12.	Diarrhea	211
13.	Dysentery	218
14.	Cholera :	220
	(a) Prophylactics	220
	(b) Chlorine	221
	(c) Cholera Proper	222
15.	Affections of the Liver	226
16.	Jaundice	229
17.	Affections of the Spleen	231
18.	Urinary Disorders	232
	(a) Retention of Urine in Infants	232
	(b) Difficult and Painful Urination in Children and Adults	233
	(c) Frequent Urination–Involuntary Urination–Wetting the Bed	234

CHAPTER XII. *Diabetes* : 235
    1. Diabetes Mellitus, Glycosuria 235
    2. Diabetes Insipidus, Polyuria 238

CHAPTER XIII. *Diseases of the Kidneys* : 239
    Nephritis–Inflammation of the Kidneys 239

CONTENTS

CHAPTER XIV. *Typhlitis, Perityphlitis and Appendicitis* . 248

CHAPTER XV. *Cancer–Carcinoma* : 255
1. Cancer of the Tongue 256
2. Cancer of the Lower Lip 258
3. Cancer of the Esophagus 260
4. Cancer of the Stomach 260
5. Cancer of the Intestines 266
6. Cancer of the Rectum 266
7. Cancer of the Breast 269
8. Cancer of the Womb 272

CHAPTER XVI. *Fevers* : 278
1. Ordinary Fevers 278
2. Influenza 279
3. Measles 281
4. Chicken-Pox 284
5. Small-Pox 285
6. Ague and Intermittent Fever–Malaria 288
7. Typhoid Fever 295
8. Rheumatic Fevers–Acute Rheumatism 299
9. Gastric and Bilious Fever 301
10. Filarial Fever–Filariasis 302

CHAPTER XVII. *Diseases of the Women* : 304
1. Delayed and Obstructed Menstruation 304
2. Suppression of the Menses 306
3. Menorrhagia–Profuse Menstruation 308
4. Dysmenorrhea–Painful Menstruation 310
5. Tardy and Scanty Menstruation 313
6. Chlorosis or Green Sickness 315
7. Change of Life–Cessation of Menses 317

8. Prolapsus of the Uterus or Falling of the Womb 319
9. Leucorrhea–Whites 321

CHAPTER XVIII. *Derangements during Pregnancy* : 325
1. General Remarks 325
2. Derangments during Pregnancy 326
    (a) Continued Menstruation 326
    (b) Headache and Vertigo during Pregnancy 326
    (c) Morning Sickness 328
    (d) Constipation during Pregnancy 330
    (e) Diarrhea 330
    (f) Itching–Pruritis 331
    (g) Hysterical Fits–Fainting 331
    (h) Palpitation of the Heart 335
    (i) Toothache 333
    (j) Neuralgia 334
    (k) Pains in the Back and Sides 334
    (l) Cramps 334
    (m) Varicose Veins or Swelling of the Veins 336
    (n) Hemorrhoids or Piles 337
    (o) Jaundice 339
    (p) Incontinence of Urine 339
    (q) Dysuria and Strangury 340
    (r) Depression of Spirits 340
3. Influence of Existing Diseases upon Pregnancy–
   Prophylactics Applied to Chronic and
   Hereditary Diseases 341
4. Miscarriage or Abortion 342
5. Flooding During Pregnancy or at Delivery 345
6. Preparation of the Breasts 347
7. Easy Delivery 347
8. False Pains 347

CONTENTS

Chapter XIX. *Treatment after Delivery* : 350
1. Labour–Child-birth 350
2. Treatment after Delivery 352
   (a) Flooding after Delivery 353
   (b) After Pains 353
   (c) Duration of Confinement 353
   (d) Diseases following Parturition–The Lochia 354
   (e) Milk Fever 355
   (f) Suppressed Secretion of Milk 356
   (g) Excessive or Involuntary Secretion of Milk 357
   (h) Diarrhea after Confinement 357
   (i) Constipation after Confinement 357
   (j) Retention of Urine or Painful Urination 350
   (k) Sore Nipples 359
   (l) Gathered Breasts 359
   (m) Child-bed Fever or Puerperal Peritonitis 361
   (n) Milk Leg or Crural Phlebitis 362
   (o) Nursing Sore Mouth 363
   (p) Perspiration after Delivery 364
   (q) Excessive Perspiration after Delivery 365
   (r) Weakness from Nursing 366
   (s) Falling off of the Hair 366

Chapter XX. *Treatment of Infants* : 367
1. Antipsoric Prophylactics 367
2. Ecchymosis on the surface of the Skull 367
3. Deformities, Monstrosities 368
4. Marks 368
5. Cyanosis–Blue Discoloration 368
6. Swelling and Elongation of the Head 369
7. The Meconium or First Discharge from the Bowels ... 369

8.	Sore Eyes	369
9.	Congenital Hernia	370
10.	Hardening of the Cellular Tissue	370
11.	Swelling of the Infant's Breasts	370
12.	Hiccough	371
13.	Obstruction of the Nose– 'Snuffles'	371
14.	Sore Mouth–Thrush	372
15.	Sore-Throat	372
16.	Jaundice	372
17.	Excoriation or Raw Surface	373
18.	The "Gum" or "Red Gum"	373
19.	Retention of Urine	373
20.	Constipation	373
21.	Diarrhea	374
22.	Colic	374
23.	Continual Crying of Infants without apparent cause	375
24.	Restlessness and Wakefulness	375
25.	Scurf on the Head	375
26.	Milk-Crust	376
27.	Scald Head–Ringworm of the Scalp	376
28.	Spasms or Convulsions	378
29.	Teething–Dentition	378
30.	Summer Complaint	379
31.	Heat Spots–Prickly Heat	381
32.	Discharge from the Ears	381
33.	Leucorrhea or Whites of Children	382
34.	Weaning	382
35.	Stuttering	382
36.	Wetting the bed	382
37.	Oldish Appearance of Suckling	383

CONTENTS

CHAPTER XXI. *Diseases of Children* : 384
1. Rickets–Rachitis 386
2. Scurvy 388
3. Malnutrition, Wasting, Marasmus 388
4. Tuberculosis (Disease of Glands and Bones) 392
5. Epidemic Diarrhea of Children 396
6. Severe Urgent Cases with Collapse 397

CHAPTER XXII. *General dyscrasias and constitutional treatment* : 399
1. Scrofulosis 399
2. Tuberculosis 404
3. Glandular Affections 406
4. Diseases of the Bones 407
5. Advantages of Constitutional Treatment 408

CHAPTER XXIII. *Diseases of the Aged* 411

CHAPTER XXIV. *Diseases of the Brain and Nervous System* :
1. Inflammation of the Brain 417
2. Convulsions, Spasms or Fits 422
3. Hysteria 428
4. Epilepsy 429
5. Chorea-St. Vitus' Dance 432

CHAPTER XXV. *Paralysis* 435

CHAPTER XXVI. *Anterior Poliomyelitis* 444

CHAPTER XXVII. *Neuritis* 448

CHAPTER XXVIII. *Diseases of the Skin* : 453
1. Itching of the Skin 453
2. Itch, Scabies 453
3. Eczema 455

4.	Nettle-Rash–Urticaria	462
5.	Erysipelas : St. Anthony's Fire	465
6.	Herpes Zoster or Shingles, Herpes Circinatus or Ringworm	467
7.	Whitlow–Felon	469
8.	Pimples on the Face–Acne	470
9.	Abscesses	470
10.	Boils	472
11.	Carbuncle	473
12.	Chilblain–Frostbite	473
13.	Corns	475
14.	Warts	475
15.	Falling out of the Hair	476
16.	Affections of the Nails	477
17.	Bed Sores	478
18.	Leucoderma	478

CHAPTER XXIX. *Some General Diseases* : 480

1.	Chronic Rheumatism	480
2.	Lumbag–Pain in the Loins and Back	485
3.	Sciatica	486
4.	Sleeplessness	487
5.	Sunstroke	490
6.	Convalescence	493
7.	Emergencies–Euthanasia (Easy Death)	495
8.	Collapse	496
9.	Homeopathic Prophylaxis	499
10.	Vaccination	500

CHAPTER XXX. *External Injuries, Burns and Scalds* : 502

| 1. | Injuries | 502 |
| 2. | Burns and Scalds | 504 |

CONTENTS

3. External Remedies 505
4. Stings 505
5. Foreign Substances in the Eye, Ear, Nose and Throat 505

CHAPTER XXXI. *Consequences of Spirituous Liquors, Coffee, Tea, Tobacco, Acids, etc.*: 507
1. Drunkenness 507
2. Effects of Drunkenness 507
3. Bad Effects of Coffee 508
4. Bad Effects of Tea 508
5. Tobacco 508
6. Spices 508
7. Sour Things 508

CHAPTER XXXII. *Effects of Injurious Drugs in General Use* : 510
1. Opium of Ganja 510
2. Hydrate of Chloral 510
3. Quinine 510
4. Digitalis 511
5. Magnesia Salts or Epsom Salts 511
6. Castor Oil 512
7. Sulphur, Iodine and Iodide of Potassium 512
8. Mercury 512
9. Lead 513
10. Arsenic 513
11. Iron 514

CHAPTER XXXIII. *Poisoning* : 515
1. *Poisons* : 515
   (a) Gases 515
   (b) Acids 515

	(c)	Alkaline Poisons	516
	(d)	Metallic Substances	516
	(e)	Vegetable Poisons	516
2.	*Poisoned wounds–Stings and Bites of Animals* :		
	(a)	Stings of Bees, etc.	517
	(b)	Bites of Snakes	517
	(c)	Bites of Mad Dogs	517

PART–III

BIBLIOGRAPHY 521

APPENDIX   I. Therapeutic Index 523
             II. Materia Medica (In Brief) 544
             III. Glossary 607

INDEX 639

FOREWORD TO THE FIRST EDITION

"Healing" is an Art and not a mechanical routine. It is only he who has the capacity to apply his fine intellect, to unravel the various causes that bring about a diseased condition in an individual, assess their correct values and apply the simplest means to bring the individual easily, speedily and permanently to his normal condition, can be called a True Physician. Each individual is a separate entity and different individuals react to the same causes differently. So, it is the individual and not the cause, that has to be studied carefully, though, the cause has to be taken into account. It is the individual that has to be treated and not the cause. This is the correct way of treatment. Any treatment that takes into account only the cause and prescribes a routine treatment for all individuals affected by that cause is a very crude form of treatment and is liable to cause the individual great harm.

Most diseases, except accidents and malformations which cannot be really called diseased though they have to be treated, have their origin in some faulty conditions in which the individual lives, such as faulty food, bad habits, unhealthy surroundings, etc. So long as these faulty conditions persist, any form of treatment can give only temporary benefit. To give permanent relief, the faulty conditions must be removed and treatment given to correct the harm already done by the faulty conditions. Unless the causes that were responsible for the unhealthy state are removed, the diseased conditions are always liable to recur and form the basis for chronic diseases. It is the first duty of a true physician to try his best to find out the faulty condition that caused the disease in his patient and advise him to rectify the faulty condition. Giving a few doses of medicine without such advice, is a great negligence on the part of the physician.

Nature produces certain symptoms, such as fever, vomiting, diarrhea, pains, etc., in the course of a disease. These symptoms are the reactions of the individual's vitality to cure himself of that disease. Thus, fever is produced to inhibit the growth of any germs that might be responsible for the disease, as they cannot grow at high temperatures, vomiting or diarrhea is produced to empty and clean the bowels, pain to give rest to the affected part etc. Thus, all symptoms are the curative reactions of the individual's vitality, and the correct method of treatment is to follow the path of Nature, which is the individual's vitality, and give medicines that work in the same way, that is, that produce symptoms which are found in the patient. In this way we will be helping nature and the cure will be easy, speedy and permanent. The other method of treatment, that is, giving medicines which have contrary effect, which is greatly followed by other schools, especially Allopathy, is very harmful and in most cases suppresses, without curing, the disease. This is another cause for many chronic diseases.

It is an individual's vitality that really conquers and cures his disease. A physician with his medicines can only help the vitality to affect the cure. Medicines as such, cannot cure diseases. They can only suppress the symptoms and give a false impression of a cure, when given for their contrary effects. Sometimes it may happen that the vitality has become so weakened in an individual that it cannot be roused to sufficient strength to cure the disease, and this is how that some cases become fatal. (I do not mean those that die on account of faulty treatment.)

To acquire and practise this Fine Art of Healing, a vast study, keen intellect and great experience are required. It is only people with these attributes that can become really successful Homeopathic

FOREWORD TO THE FIRST EDITION

Physicians. A conscientious physician must be a student all his life. But one's life is not long enough to acquire all the knowledge required. So one must draw upon the experience and knowledge of others and supplement it with one's own knowledge and experience. So it becomes the bounden duty of every successful and intelligent practitioner to put down in writing his experiences and knowledge for the benefit of others, and for the good of Humanity. Moreover, the experiences and their interpretation by some, will be different from those of others. The study of the experiences and the methods of approach of different physicians, will greatly enhance the knowledge of even an experience physician.

We are greatly indebted to Mr. T. S. Iyer for the trouble he has taken in putting down his experiences, and methods of approach for the benefit of posterity. He is a man of large experience, keen intellect and great industry. Though he has had no regular medical education, being a mathematician and an economist, he made an intelligent study of Hahnemann's law of Cure for nearly 40 years, improved his knowledge by travel and study of the work in various institutions in America, and has acquired great experience. He devoted his life for the good of humanity and has acquired great fame by many miraculous cures he has effected. He is widely known in South India as one of the greatest physicians of the day. His philanthropy has become a byeword. Real worth and philanthropy in a physician is a rare combination.

He has expounded the Law of Cure of Hahnemann very clearly in his Introduction, and dealt concisely and lucidly with the conception of how acute and chronic diseases are caused and should be treated by the Homeopathic law of Cure. The section dealing with "Diet" is very important, because about 75% of our diseases are directly or indirectly attributable to faulty dieting. In the same section he deals with general habits, exercise, etc. If diet, exercise and habits are properly regulated, more than half the battle is won and the path for a complete cure is made smoother and shorter.

Regulation of diet in various diseases is one of the most important points of treatment and not many physicians are well informed in this subject. This section should be carefully studied.

Then comes the important section on "Medicine", which is very comprehensive. The most common diseases which are met with in practice, their causation, prevention and cure are briefly but very instructively dealt with, and this section will be of great practical use to every practitioner, young or old. As has been already stated, the name (cause) of a disease is not so important as the individual's reaction to it, but for easy reference, some comprehensive name should be given to a group of symptoms and the common name of diseases in use are as good as any other. This important section deals, briefly with definition, causation, prophylaxis and treatment. Of course the treatment portion cannot be exhaustive, as different individuals react differently. But the most common reactions with their remedies are clearly indicated. The preventive (prophylaxis) aspect of certain diseases is very instructive.

For individuals who react in a way different to what was indicated in the above section, a brief section on general Materia Medica has been included. And a Therapeutic Index is also given for easy reference. Though poisoning is more an accident than a disease, it is the doctor's duty to treat poisonings and accidents, and so a section on the this subject also has been introduced.

Mr. T. S. Iyer has very modestly designated his compilation as a "Beginner's Guide". I am sure even experienced practitioners will find some very useful matter in it and it is a very good reference book for acute and chronic cases. Beginners will find it very useful to understand, learn and practise Homeopathy. I am quite confident that this book will become very popular and will be greatly in demand.

Col. K. V. Ramana Rao,

I.M.S. (Retd.)

FOREWORD TO THE SECOND EDITION

Sri T. S. Iyer has again yielded to the popular demand that he should give instruction on additional subjects in his "Beginner's Guide to Homeopathy" and has taken great pains in making many useful additions to his already popular Guide, which required a second edition in such a short time. His new Chapters on:

1. Diseases of the Heart
2. Blood Pressure
3. Diabetes
4. Diseases of the Kidneys
5. Intestinal Disorders
6. Cancer
7. Diseases of the Children
8. General Discrasias and Constitutional treatment
9. Diseases of the Aged
10. Paralysis
11. Anterior Poliomyelitis
12. Neuritis etc.

and many additions to the existing chapters, are of very great value and are worth careful study by all doctors, especially beginners.

The most commonly used drugs are included in the Therapeutics of all diseases. Though particular individuals might require other drugs, the commonly used drugs should be studied first before discarding them, always keeping in mind the rule that only that drug which corresponds to be Totality of the symptoms of the patient, is indicated, especially if there are any outstanding uncommon symptoms and not any other drug though it is reputed to give excellent result in any particular disease.

Shri T. S. Iyer has dealt clearly with the causation, symptoms, diagnosis, prognosis etc., of diseases and the student will do well to study them carefully to distinguish the various diseases and determine their seriousness. Though the symptoms and not the pathological changes in a patient, guide the selection of the proper drug, administration of drugs only does not complete the whole treatment and other aids such as surgical interference, proper dieting, rest, exercise etc., will be urgently required in some conditions, such as Ruptured Extra-uterine pregnancy, Duodenal ulcer or Appendicular Abscess etc., and unless these aids are resorted to, the case may end fatally. A clear understanding of the pathological changes that might be taking place in any case, is very important to determine the aids that are required for proper treatment. If the beginner or any physician who has not got such clear knowledge of the pathological changes, has any doubt in any particular case, he is strongly advised to consult a senior physician to avoid fatal mistakes.

We are greatly indebted to Sri. T. S. Iyer for the great trouble he has taken in his advanced age, to give such clear and useful instruction to the beginners and laymen who are anxious to treat others or themselves and their families (I would advise them to start treating themselves and then their families and lastly others and not begin with others) in the clear and simple Homeopathic way. And we hope that this second edition of the "Beginner's Guide to Homeopathy" will be as enthusiastically received by the public as the first edition was, for their own great advantage.

Col. K. V. Ramana Rao,
I.M.S. (Retd.)

PRRFACE TO THE FIRST EDITION

This is a small handbook intended for the use of beginners in Homeopathy and families who may wish to utilish Homeopathic remedies for ordinary ailments in their initial stages, and also for allopathic physicians who may be interested in Homeopathy and may wish to try these remedies. I am not a Graduate in Medicine but am only a layman who became interested in Homeopathy on accounts of its special advantages and thought that it was possible to study the subject with the help of the many classical works available, and to obtain the necessary experience for practice with the guidance of experienced physicians of the school. I was able to procure a large library of all important books on the subject and a large number of journals from the U.S.A., and to make an intensive study over thirty-eight years ago and had the help of an experienced Homeopathic Physician in the beginning, and later I was able to get into intimate touch with the late Dr. W. Younan. M.B., of Calcutta, a veteran Hahnemannian Homeopath of over forty years standing who was very much interested in me and helped and guided me in all possible ways in obtaining a sound knowledge of the subject, both in theory and in practice, particularly because I was an earnest student who was intent on gaining all possible knowledge and experience with a view to do social service and help the poor after my retirement from Government service. During my stay of seven years in Calcutta, I was able to attend Dr. Younan's clinic and to get valuable experience from the numerous difficult cases he was treating. My object in collecting a large number of books was to popularise Homeopathy in South India where it was not sufficiently well-known, and to make these valuable books available to all those who might become interested in Homeopathy.

My object in compiling this handbook is to get more people interested in the subject, and to present the subject in a practical way which could be easily understood by all and to embody the experience gained by me during all these years which could be made use of by others.

As the system of treatment and the selection of remedies are primarily based on the symptoms of patients, it may be possible for beginners to utilise the system for the treatment of ordinary cases of every day ailments if they have a fair knowledge of Anatomy, Physiology and Materia Medica. But to do justice to Homeopathy and to obtain the best advantage of the system in treating difficult and complicated cases, a good knowledge of Anatomy, Physiology, Pathology, Surgery, Botany, Chemistry and Materia Medica is absolutely necessary, as one must know clearly the true nature, condition and progress of the disease in a patient before he will be able to apply the most appropriate remedy suitable to the case. I would, therefore, advise beginners to obtain a fair working knowledge of these subjects in order to get good results from the cases they may treat. Graduates in Allopathic medicine can be easily trained in the system and can become successful practitioners if they can get the necessary training and experience from a Homeopathic Medical College or a experienced Homeopathic Physician for some time.

Homeopathy as a system of medicine has got numerous advantages over every other system. They are :

1. Homeopathic medicines have been standardised and are prepared according to the methods prescribed in the American Pharmacopoeia by reputed firms of over a century's standing in U. S. A.
2. They are the *cheapest* of all the medicines prepared under every other known system of Medicine.
3. They are most suitable for domestic practice and can be

easily handled and administered by any one, as they are readily available for use in the form of globules which are the minimum doses required.

4. As the doses administered are very small, there is no danger of over-dosing and no harm will result form the administration of wrong remedies. The medicines administered are *single* remedies and there is no compounding or ad-mixture of different medicines, and so there can be no mistake in administering remedies.

5. As the choice of remedies is based on the symptoms presented by the patient and detailed by him, and the symptoms really represent what the patient *feels* in his inner being, they are a far better and safer guide in ascertaining the nature of his real ailment than all the elaborate analysis and examination which the physician may conduct on his person and which really amount to a pure guess or opinion or diagnosis of the patient's complaint. The Allopathic physician has to give a name to the disease before he can prescribe any medicine, and if the diagnosis proves wrong, he has to change the medicine after some time. On the other hand, the Homeopathic system of case-taking coupled with the physical examination of the patient gives a true picture of the case which enables the physician to prescribe a suitable remedy. If two or three doses of a remedy so selected, do not help, another medicine can be chosen without loss of time and with no bad effects from the previous doses. The great advantage of Homeopathic remedies is that there is absolutely no bad effect left in the patient as a result of excessive medication.

6. The medicines are highly efficient in their action, even one or two doses of a correctly chosen remedy produce remarkable effects and in extreme cases work a wonderful

change in the condition of the patient at a critical stage.

7. As the Homeopathic treatment is purely constitutional based on the symptoms of the patient., it covers all stages and is both preventive in the initial stage and also curative when it develops into a full-fledged disease. Thus, most diseases can be aborted by proper medicines in the initial stages, before they develop into complicated ones.

8. As the medicines are very cheap and at the same time quite efficient, they are the most suitable for a poor country like India. As no elaborate equipment in the form of numerous medicines and other paraphernalia for compounding medicines are required, it is possible to extend necessary medical help to the poor people even in the remotest parts of the country without much trouble and expense if qualified doctors can be trained for the purpose and sent out.

If Homeopathy is recognised as a superior system of Medicine and becomes popular throughout of the country, and if more people avail themselves of its supreme advantages and are benefited thereby, I shall not have laboured in vain for all these years.

MAYAVA RAM,
December, 1948.   T. S. IYER.

PREFACE TO THE SECOND EDITION

I am grateful for the very good response for this Beginner's attempt of mine to write a Handbook for the use of Beginners on this important system of medicine, and I am glad that a larger number of people are becoming interested and are willing to give it a fair trial. It is encouraging that a second edition is called for within such a short time, and so, as desired by several of my allopathic friends who have now taken to Homeopathy and are practising it with confidence, I take this opportunity of enlarging the scope of this Beginner's Guide in order to include the treatment of a larger number of diseases which come before the regular practitioner, and so make the book useful for a larger number of people. I have dealt in greater detail about 'Preventive treatment, and constitutional treatment' because they are much more vital and important for the *preservation* of normal health than the actual treatment of diseases for the *restoration* of normal health, and Homeopathy lays much greater stress on this aspect of human welfare than any other system and shows the way. I have also added chapters relating to the treatment of Poliomyelitis and Cancer, two of the much dreaded diseases of the present day, and have shown that while vast sums of money are being spent both in the U.S.A. and Great Britain for the investigation of the etiology of these diseases and in discovering new remedies for a cure, eminent Homeopathic Physicians in both these countries have been doing silent work and treating and curing a large number of these cases in different stages of development with great success, with the help of a number of remedies proved and worked out by Hahnemann and his followers.

I hope that this edition will prove useful for all who are interested in Homeopathy, and that a larger number of people will benefit by this highly scientific system of medicine.

MAYAVA RAM,
December, 1952.   T. S. IYER.

LIST OF MEDICINES

A. Medicines Most Commonly Used

Aconite Nap. 30
Antimonium Tart. 30
Apis Mell. 30
Argentum Nitricum 30
Arnica Mont. 30
Arsenicum Album 30
Baryta Carbonica 30, 200
Bryonia 30
Calcarea Carbonica 30, 200
Calcarea Phosphorica 6, 30
Cantharis Vesi. 30
Causticum 30
Chamomilla 30
China 30
Cina 200
Cuprum Metallicum 30
Drosera Rot. 30
Dulcamara 30
Euphrasia off 30

Gelsemium 30
Hepar Sulphur 6, 30
Ignatia Amara 30, 200
Ipecacuanha 30
Lycopodium Clav. 30, 200
Mercurium Corrosivus 30
Mercurius Solublis 30
Natrium Muriaticum 30
Nux Vomica 30
Opium 30
Phosphorus 30
Pulsatilla Pratensis 30, 200
Rhus Tox. 30
Secale Cor. 30
Sepia off. 30
Silicea Terra 30
Sulphur 30, 200
Variolinum 30, 200
Veratrum Album 30

B. Medicines Less Commonly Used

Allium Cepa 30
Aloes Soc. 30
Antimonium Crudum 30
Aurum Metallicum 30
Baptisia Tinct. 30
Calcarea Fluorica 30

Carbo Vegetablis 30
Caulophyllum 30
Chelidonium Majus 30
Cimicifuga 30
Cocculus Indicus 30
Coffee Cruda 30

Camphora 6	Colocynthis 30
Conium Mac. 30	Petroleum 30
Corallium Rubrum 30	Phosphoricum Acid 30
Eupatorium Perfoliatum 30	Plumbum Met. 30
Glonoinum 30	Podophyllum Pellatum 30
Graphites 30	Psorinum 30, 200
Hamamelis Vir. 30	Rheum Palnatum 30
Hyoscyamus Niger 30	Ruta Grav. 30
Hypericum Perf. 30	Sabina 30
Kali Bichromicum 30	Sanguinaria 30
Kali Carbonicum 30	Spigelia Anth. 30
Lachesis Mutus 30	Spongia Tosta 30
Ledum Pal. 30	Stannum Met. 30
Mercurius Sulphuricus 30, 200	Staphysagria 30
Mezereum 30	Stramonium Off. 30
Natrium Sulphuricum 6 x (trit) 30, 200	Symphytum 30
	Tabacum 30
Nitricum Acidum 30	Thuja Occ. 30

Tinctures For External Use

Arnica Mont. Q	Apis Mel. Q	Hypericum Q
Cantharides Q	Calendula Q	Ruta Grav. Q

The medicines should be kept in a dry place not exposed to the heat or light of the sun, free from odours and excluded as far as possible from bright light

Numerous new medicines have been added in the second revised edition but these have not been included in the above list.

PART – I
INTRODUCTION

INTRODUCTORY

Homeopathy

Homeopathy may be defined as the *therapeutic method of symptom–similarity*. In the field of Medicine, therefore, Homeopathy deals only with therapeutics, i.e., treatment of disease. This Homeopathy treatment of disease is further limited to the use of certain pharmacologic preparations prepared according to certain well-defined principles laid down by the founder.

This law of Homeopathy relationship is two-fold, viz., (a) we have a group of symptoms expressing the disease, and (b) we have a group of symptoms caused by the effect of some drug on the healthy human body. In applying this law in practice, if a disease is curable and if a medicine which has the same group of symptoms corresponding to the disease is given in conformity with the homeopathic rules of practice, a cure is bound to follow.

Homeopathy is therefore, a special form of using drugs, and the practice of this system is not in conflict with the great field of modern medicine. The main points of advantage which homeopathy has over the other systems of medicine are: (a) greater attention paid to the study of the scope and usefulness of drugs in the treatment of disease; (b) the use of single remedies whose effects are well known and the laws for their administration which are based on certain well-defined principles; and (c) the absence of possibility of any danger to the patient by their wrong or excessive administration. Briefly, homeopathy is a practical method of using drugs backed up by the experience of over two centuries, which will hold good for all time, because symptoms of disease and symptoms of drugs do not change and that is the rock on which the foundation of homeopathy rests.

Hahnemann and the New Law of Cure

The great founder Samuel Hahnemann was born at Meissen, near Dresden in Germany on the tenth day of April, 1755. Early in 1775, he went to Leipsic where he supported himself by giving instructions in German and French and by translating English books. After many hardships he received a Degree of M.D. in 1779. He practised Medicine in different towns. He was acquainted with almost every ancient and modern language, with the literature of the medical profession of his own and of ancient times. He was also a great chemist, a good mineralogist and botainst, a sanitarian and an experienced practical physician, in fact an all-round scientific man.

Similia Similibus Curentur

The first promulgation of this principle on which the homeopathic rule of practice is based was made by Hahnmann in 1796 in an essay published in Hufeland's Journal entitled, "On a New Principle for Ascertaining the Curative Properties of Drugs". The occasion publishing this essay was the experience gained from six years' work along certain lines. Six years before he had made some tests of the effects of Peruvian bark on himself, having been led thereto by translating Cullen's 'Materia Medica' and was not satisfied with the explanation given regarding its action. He knew, of course, the power of cinchona bark to cure ague malaria, but he could not understand how it could produce this beneficial effect. Eager to elucidate the matter, he decided to test the drug on a healthy person–himself. He took the usual dose and it produced all the symptoms of an attack of ague malaria, not only the chill, heat and sweating, but several of the minor symptoms usually accompanying an attack. After the attack had passed off, he waited

INTRODUCTORY

a while and on repeating the dose, he repeated the experience. In other words, he found that the drug which he knew to be the best agent to cure ague malaria, produced upon him an attack very similar to ague–an unexpected, and a surprising result. Could this indicate existence of a general law applicable to other drugs as well– or all drugs in general? Hahnemann determined to investigate the matter further. His object was to verify this intuition by the inductive method of research and see for himself the action of drugs in health and disease. Two lines of research were open to him to examine the records of the past (his vast linguistic attainments and knowledge of medical practice fitted him especially for such a task) or he could in actual practice treat diseases with similar remedies and note the results. He pursued with the aid of a few friendly physicians both lines of research and for six years, before he ventured to publish anything about the matter. He experimented patiently and painstakingly, a fitting foundation untainted by current theories and free from dogmatic assertions. Further zealous pursuit along these lines of experimentation and drug application finally established to his satisfaction at least the belief in a law of drug action which he expressed in latin as *Similia Similibus Curentur*, "let likes be cured by likes." It does not state a law of Nature. His appeal then to actual experience guided by principle and the elimination of all mere theories, however alluring, as a basis for therapeutic action, was the first great step towards modernism in medical thought and practice. Hahnemann by introducing into medicine the training drug action, founded the Science of Pharmacology. Nine years of further investigation into this new field enabled Hahnemann to prepare and publish a work in Latin, "On the Positive Effects of Medicines," and at the same time, declare the principle of similars as a law of general application. Five year more of further reflection and experiment enabled him to perfect his system, and embody its principles in this great book, the "Organon of Rational Medicine." The following year he published volume one of his "Materia Medica Pura" containig original proving made by himself and members of his family and assisted later by some enthusiastic physicians the gathered around him at the University of Leipsic. In 1821, he published the final sixth volume containing the positive effects of sixty-four medicines. With the publication of these two great works, Hahnemann provided both the theoretical and practical requirements of homeopathy as a distinct method of therapeutics. He was the first to apply the inductive method of research to thereapeutics. We see, then that homeopathy supplies us with a law resting upon natural facts and free from all speculations and follows a strictly scientific method which is the curative method of scientific medicinal therapeutics. In 1822, appeared a second edition of this work, with considerable additions to the symptomatology of all the remedies and some new medicines besides. A third and a fourth edition were published after some years.

In 1828, Hahnemann published his, 'Chronic Diseases' containing the symptomatology of a completely new series of medicines – a series of deeply acting drugs, like *Calcarea*, Sulphur etc., the so–called anti-psoric remedies. The symptomatology of these remedies was not wholly pathogenetic, but included observations at the bed side, or what were called *clinical symptoms*.

A second edition, greatly enlarged and now containing the symptomatology of twenty-five remedies besides the twenty-two of the first edition, appeared between 1834 and 1838. A peculiar feature of the provings in this work is that the bulk of these must have been obtained with the thirtieth potency, and often are observation when given to the sick, differing entirely therefore, from the pathogenetic effects of the Materia Medica Pura.

Besides Hahnemann and his immediate workers, Constantine Hering of Philadelphia, contributed the best provings to the 'Homeopathic Materia Medica,' some of his drugs ranking in importance with Hahnemann's own. Of these, *Lachesis, Glonoine,* and *Apis mel.* take first rank.

A Synopsis of the main principles in the 'Organon' and 'Chronic Diseases' will be useful to beginners and has been adapted, with suitable modifications from, 'A Compend of the Principles of Homeopathy by Wm. Boericke, M.D.'

THE ORGANON (A Synopsis)

1. The physician's highest and only duty is to restore health to the sick, which is called healing. Healing ought to be accompanied in the most speedy, most gentle, and most reliable manner. To do this, he must know the ailment of the patient, select the remedy, the dose and its repetition according to each individual case. Sanitation and hygiene are studies in which every physician must be well versed.
2. Constitution of the patient, his mind and temperament, occupation, mode of living and habits, social and domestic relations, age and sexual functions, etc. give us the individuality of the patient.
3. Deviations from the normal state show themselves by morbid signs or symptoms. The totality of these symptoms, this outwardly reflected image of the inner nature of the diseased state i.e., of suffering dynamic, or living force, is the principal and only condition to be recognised in order that they may be removed and health restored.
4. Life, a dynamic principle, animates the material body and this material body passes away as soon as it is bereft of this life-force. In health, harmonious vital force becomes deranged by the dynamic influence of some morbific agency inimical to life, hence, abnormal functional activity, manifesting itself by morbid sensations and functions, by morbid symptoms. This morbidly changed life-force can only be restored to its normal state by a similarly acting dynamic power of the appropriate remedy, acting on the omnipresent susceptibility of the nerves of the organism.

The total removal of all symptoms is health restored, and therefore, the totality of symptoms observed in each individual case can be the only indication to guide us in the selection of a remedy. These aberrations from the state of health can only be removed by the curative power inherent in medicine to turn the sensorial condition of the body again into its normal state.

5. Experiments on animals, vinesection (scientific dissection or experiment) and autopsy (post-mortem examination) can never reveal the inherent power of medicine, the healthy human body alone is the appropriate subject for such experiments, where they excite numerous definite morbid symptoms, and it follows that if drugs act as curative remedies, they exercise this curative power only by virtue of altering bodily feelings through the production of peculiar symptoms, which then they are able to remove from the sick, in other words, the remedy must be able to produce an artificial morbid condition similar to that of the natural disease.

6. Experience teaches that all drugs will, without exception, cure diseases, the symptoms of which are as similar as possible to those of the drugs, and leave none uncured.

Natural diseases are removed by proper medicines, because the normal state is more readily affected by the right dose of a drug than by natural morbific agencies.

Physical and partly physical terestrial forces show their greatest power where this life-power is below par, hence they do not affect everybody nor do they do so at all times. We may, therefore, assert that extraneous, noxious agencies possess only a subordinate and conditional power, while drug potencies have an absolute unconditional power.

Drug disease is substituted for the natural disease, when the drug causes symptoms most similar to that which is to

INTRODUCTORY

be cured, and it is hardly possible to perform a cure by means of drugs incapable of producing in the organism a diseased condition similar to that which is to be cured.

Palliation of prominent symptoms should be ignored, as it provides only in part for a single symptom, it may bring partial relief but this is soon followed by a perceptible aggravation of the entire disease.

Primary and after or counter effect of drugs

7. During the primary effect of a drug, the vital force receives the impression made upon it by the drug and allows the state of health to be altered by it. The vital force then rallies and either calls forth the exact opposite state of feeling or neutralises the impression made upon it by the drug, thereby establishing the normal state of health. The former, a *counter effect* and the latter a *curative effect*.

8. Diseases peculiar to mankind are of two classes:
   (1) *Acute diseases* rapid, morbid processes caused by abnormal states and derangements of the vital force.
   (2) *Chronic diseases*, originating by infection with a chronic miasm, acting deleteriously upon the living organism and undermining health to such a degree that the vital force can only make imperfect and ineffectual resistance, which may result in the final destruction of the organism.

Acute diseases may be sporadic, endemic or epidemic. Allopathy is responsible for many an incurable disease. Owing to the use of several drugs, the organism becomes gradually and abnormally deranged according to the character of the drug used.

True chronic diseases arise mostly from Syphilis, Sycosis and Psora. The latter (Psora) is often fundamental cause and source of countless forms of diseases, figuring as peculiar and definite diseases in our text books on Pathology.

9. Individualisation in the investigation of a case of disease, demands unbiassed judgment, sound common sense, attentive observation and carefulness and accuracy in noting down the image of the disease.

Directions are then given for noting down all the symptoms of the patient both in acute and chronic diseases (vide paras. 84 to 104).

The physician is then required to select the corresponding drug which in its effects on healthy persons produces symptoms strikingly similar to those of the disease. Upon subsequent enquiry regarding the effects of the remedy, the physician should then take into account the remaining symptoms, or new symptoms which may have appeared, for selecting another remedy.

The physician should be acquainted with the full range of disease-producing power of each drug, that is, all morbid symptoms and changes of the state of health which each drug is capable of producing by itself in healthy persons, in order to discover what elements of disease each is able to produce and inclined to excite by itself in the condition of mind and body. Thus, the disease-producing power of drugs can be made available homeopathically in the case of all diseases.

10. Instructions are then given in regard to the mode of administering drugs for proving, the conditions which should be observed by the provers, viz., about diet, dosage, record of their symptoms, etc. (vide paras. 118 to 145)

Thus, a collection of genuine, pure and undeceptive effects of simple drugs should be accumulated and a Materia Medica of that kind should contain and represent in similitude the elements of numerous natural diseases hereafter to be cured by these means, and should exclude every supposition, every mere assertion or fiction. A drug fully tested with regard to its power of altering human health, and whose symptoms represent the greatest degree of similitude with the totality of symptoms of a given natural disease, will be the most suitable and reliable homeopathic remedy for that particular disease, its specific curative agent.

A medicine possessing the power to produce an artificial disease most similar to the natural disease to be cured, exerts its dynamic influence upon the morbidly disturbed vital force and in the right dose will affect the parts of the organism where the natural disease is located and will excite in them an artificial disease.

A well-selected homeopathic drug will remove a natural acute disease of recent origin, even if severe and painful, an older affection will disappear in a few days, and recovery progress to full restoration of health. Old, complicated diseases demand longer time for their removal. Chronic drug diseases, complicating an uncured natural disease, yield only after great length of time, if they have not become quite incurable.

11. For a few insignificant symptoms of recent origin, no medical treatment is needed, a slight change of diet and habits of living suffice for their removal.

In searching for the homeopathic specific remedy, the more prominent, uncommon and peculiar (characteristic) symptoms of the case should bear the closest possible similitude to the symptoms of the drug. The more general symptoms deserve less notice, as generalities are common to every disease and almost to every drug.

12. Although a well-selected remedy quietly extinguishes an analogous disease without exciting additional sensations, it may produce a slight aggravation resembling the original disease, so closely that the patient considers it as such. Aggravations caused by larger doses may last for several hours, but in reality these are only drug effects somewhat superior in intensity and very similar to the original disease. The smaller the dose of the drug, so much smaller and shorter is the apparent aggravation of the disease during the first hours. Even in chronic cases, after the days of aggravation have passed, the convalescence will progress almost uninterruptedly for days.

13. If in acute cases the remedy was not properly selected, we must examine the case more thoroughly for the purpose of constructing a new picture of the disease. Cases may occur where the first examination of the disease and the first selection of the remedy prove that the totality of the symptoms of the disease is not sufficiently covered by the symptoms of a single remedy; and when we are obliged to choose between two medicines which seem to be equally well-suited to the case, we must prescribe one of these medicines, and it is not advisable to administer the remedy of our second choice without a renewed examination of the patient, because it may no longer correspond to the symptoms which remain after the case has undergone a change and often a different remedy will be indicated. If the medicine of our second choice is still suited to the remnant of the morbid condition, it would now deserve much more confidence and should be employed in preference to others.

14. Diseases presenting only a few symptoms may be called partial (one-sided) diseases; their chief symptoms indicating either an internal affection, or headache, or diarrhea, or

only a local one. A more careful examination often reveals more occult symptoms, and if this fails, we must make the best of these few prominent symptoms as guides in the selection of the medicine. As for such partial disease, the selected remedy may also be only partially adapted, it may excite necessary symptoms, and symptoms of the disease will be developed which the patient had not previously perceived at all or only imperfectly, thus facilitating the task of selecting a more accurate homeopathic remedy.

15. After the completion of the effect of each dose of medicine, the case should be re-examined, in order to ascertain what symptoms remain and the corresponding remedy then selected, and so on till normal health is restored.

16. Local diseases are those affections which are of recent origin and caused by external injury. Affections of external parts requiring mechanical skill, belong to surgery alone, but often the entire organism is affected to such an extent by injuries as to require dynamic treatment in order that it may be placed in the proper condition for the performance of the curative operation.

17. Affections of external parts, not caused by external inujuries, proceed from an internal morbid state and all curative measures must be taken with reference to the state of the whole system, in order to effect the obliteration and cure of the general disease by internal remedies.

In examining such a case, the record of the exact state of the local disease is added to the summary of all symptoms, and other peculiarities to be observed in the general condition of the patient, in order to get the totality of the symptoms and to select the corresponding remedy which removes the local as well as the general symptoms. Not withstanding the well-regulated habits of the patient, a remnant of the disease may still be left in the affected part, or in the system at large, which the vital force is unable to restore to its normal state; in that case the actual local disease frequently proves to be the product of psora, which has remained dormant in the system, where it is now about to become developed into an actual chronic disease. Anti-psoric treatment will be necessary to remove this remainder and to relieve the habitual symptoms peculiar to the patient previous to the acute attack.

18. It is not advisable to combine the local application of a medicine simultaneously with its internal use, for the disappearance of the local symptom renders it nearly impossible to determine whether the disease has also been terminated by the internal remedy. Relying on the internal remedy alone, the removal of the local disease proves the achievement of a radical cure, and of complete recovery from the general disease.

19. When the system is affected with some chronic disease which threatens to destroy vital organs or life itself and which does not yield to the spontaneous efforts of the vital force, the latter endeavours to substitute a local disease on some external part of the body, whether the internal disease is transferred by derivation, in order to lessen the internal morbid process. But still the internal disease may increase constantly and their nature will be compelled to enlarge and aggravate the local symptoms in order to make it a sufficient substitute for, and to subdue the internal disease.

20. Most chronic diseases originate from three chronic miasms; internal syphilis, internal sycosis, and particularly from internal psora. Each of these must have pervaded the whole organism and penetrated all its parts before the primary representative local symptom makes its appearance for the prevention of the internal disease. The suppression of the local symptom may be followed by innumerable chronic

diseases, the true physician cures the great fundamental miasm together with which its primary as well as its secondary symptoms disappear.

21. Before beginning the treatment of a chronic disease we must find out whether the patient ever had been infected by syphilis or by gonorrhea although it is rare to meet with uncomplicated cases of these affections, as we usually find them often complicated with psora, the most frequent and fundamental cause of chronic diseases. It will be necessary to inquire into all former treatment and what mineral waters have been employed and with what results, in order to understand the deviations which the treatment had produced in the original disease, to convert this artificial deterioration and to determine the course now to be pursued.

22. A full anamnesis of the case ought now to be recorded, also the state of mind and temperament of the patient, as it may be useful to direct or modify the mental condition by psychical means. Guided by the most conspicuous and characteristic symptoms, the physician will be enabled to select the first anti-psoric, anti-syphylitic or anti-sycotic remedy for the beginning of the cure.

23. The state of the patient's mind and temperament if often of most decisive importance in the selection of the remedy, as each medical substance affects also the mind in a different manner. Mental diseases must only be treated like all other affections and they are curable only by remedies similar to the disease.

24. Most mental alienations are in reality bodily diseases, only these mental and emotional symptoms develop in some cases more or less rapidly, assume a state of most conspicuous one-sidedness, are finally transferred like a

local disease into the invisibly fine organs of the mind, where they seem to obscure the bodily symptoms; in short, the disorder of the coarser bodily organs are transferred, as it were, to the almost spiritual organs of the mind, where the dissecting knife will search in vain for their cause.

25. In recording the totality of symptoms of such a case, we must obtain an accurate description of all physical symptoms which prevailed before the disease degenerated into a one-sided mental disorder. We compare then, these early symptoms with their present indistinct remnants, which occasionally appear during lucid intervals, and add the symptoms of the mental state as observed by the physician and attendants of the patient.

26. Though a patient may be relieved of an acute mental disorder by non-anti-psoric medicine, no time must be lost in perfecting the cure by continued anti-psoric treatment, so that the disease may not break out a new, which will be prevented by strict adherence to well-regulated diet and habits. If neglected, psora will be usually developed during the second attack, and may assume a form, periodical or continuous, and much more difficult to cure.

27. Mental diseases, not the result of physical or bodily affections, of recent date, and which have not yet under mind the physical health too seriously, admit of the speedy cure by physical treatment, while careful regulations of habits will re-establish the health of the body, but as a measure of precaution, a course of anti-psoric treatment is advisable, in order to prevent a recurrence of the attack of mental aberration. Proper hygiene and physical regimen of the mind must be strictly enforced by the physician and attendants. *The treatment of insane persons should be conducted with a view to the absolute avoidance of corporal punishment or torture. Physicians and*

INTRODUCTORY

attendants should always treat such patients as if they regarded them as rational beings.

28. Intermittent diseases also claim our attention. Some return at a certain period, and there are others, apparently non-febrib affections, resembling intermittents by their peculiar recurrences. There are also affections characterised by the appearance of certain morbid conditions, alternating at uncertain periods with morbid conditions of a different kind. Such alternating diseases are mostly chronic and a product of developed psora, in rare instances they are complicated with syphilitic miasms. The first needs purely anti-psoric treatment, the lattter an alternation of anti-psoric with anti-syphilitics.

29. Typical intermittents recur after a certain period of apparent health, and vanish after an equally definite period. Apparently non-febrile morbid conditions, recurring at certain periods are not of sporadic or epidemic nature, they belong to a class of chronic, mostly genuine psoric diseases. Sometimes an intercurrent dose of highly potentized Peruvian bark extinguishes the intermittent type of the disease.

30. In sporadic or epidemic intermittents, not prevalent endemically in marshy districts, each attack is mostly composed of two distinct stages, chill and heat, or heat and then chill; still more frequently they consist of three stages, chill, heat and finally sweat. The remedy, usually a non-anti-psoric, must have the power to produce in healthy persons the several successive stages similar to the natural disease, and should correspond as closely as possible with the most prominent and peculiar stage of the disease, but the *symptoms which mark the condition of the patient during the apyrexia, should chiefly be taken for guides, in selecting the most striking homeopathic remedy. The*

best time to administer the remedy is a short time after the termination of the paroxysm, when the medicine has time to devlope its curatue effect without violent action or disturbance and the vital force is then in the most favourable condition to be gently modifed by the medicine and restored to healthy action. If the apyrexia is very brief, or if it is distrubed by the after effects of the preceding paroxysm, the dose of the medicine should be administered when the sweating stage diminished or when the subsequent stages of the paroxysm decline.

31. One dose may suffice to restore health, but when a new attack threatens, the same remedy should be repeated provided the complex of symptoms remains the same; but the intermittent is apt to recur, when the noxious influences, which first orginated the disease, continue to act upon the convalescent patient as would be the case in marshy localities, and to eradicate the tendency to relapses, the patient ought to be removed to a mountainous region. When this suitable remedy fails to break up the paroxysms, unless continued exposure to marsh miasma is at fault, we may blame the latent psora for it, and anti-psoric remedies are needed for a cure.

32. Epidemics of intermittents in non-malarial districts partake of the nature of chronic diseases; each epidemic possesses a peculiar uniform character, common to all individuals attacked by the epidemic and this uniform character points out the homeopathic remedy for all cases in general. This remedy usually also relieves patients, who, previous to this epidemic had enjoyed good health, and who were free from developed psora.

33. In such epidemic intermittents our anti-psorics fail, but a few does of *Sulphur* or *Hepar sulphur,* repeated at long intervals, will aid in their cure. Malignant intermittents,

attacking single persons not residing in marshy districts, need in the beginning a non-anti-psoric remedy which should be continued for several days, for the purpose of reducing the disease as far as possible.

Where this fails, psora is sure in the act of development and anti-psoric alone will give relief.

34. Intermittent fevers, indigenous to marshy countries, or places subject to inundations, will hardly affect young and healthy people, if their habits are temperate, and if they are not weakened by want, fatigue, or excesses. Endemics are apt to attack new comers, but a few doses of high potencies of *China off.* will easily rid them of the fever, provided their mode of life is very simple, and if there is no latent psora in them, which, where such is the case, necessitates anti-psoric treatment.

Mode of application of curative remedies.

35. Perceptible or continued improvement in acute or chronic diseases invariably counter-indicates the repetition of any medicine whatever, for every new dose would disturb the process of recovery. A very minute dose of the similimum, if uninterrupted in its action, will gradually accomplish all the curative effects it is capable of producing, in a period varying from forty to one hundred days. Yet the physician and the patient will like to reduce this period. This is possible under three essential conditions; firstly, if the medicine selected with the utmost care was perfectly homeopathic, secondly, if it was given in the minutest dose, so as to produce the least possible excitation of the vital force, and yet sufficient to effect the necessary change in it, and thirdly, if this minutest, yet powerful dose of the best selected medicine *be repeated at suitable intervals*; and if these conditions are observed, we might repeat this potency in

fourteen, twelve, ten, eight or seven days, in chronic cases assuming an acute form, and demanding greater haste, these intervals may be reduced still more, but in acute disease, the remedies may be repeated at much shorter intervals, for instance twenty-four, twelve, eight, or four hours, and in most acute cases, at intervals varying from one hour to five minutes.

36. The dose of the same remedy is to be repeated until recovery follows, or untill the remedy ceases to produce improvement; and with the change of symptoms a fresh examination may indicate another remedy.

37. Every medicine which produces new and troublesome symptoms not peculiar to the disease to be cured, is not homeopathic to the case. An antidote must be given, selected with great care in regard to the similitude of the case, or if the accessory symptoms are not too violent, the next remedy should be given at once, in order to replace the inappropriate one. If in urgent cases, we see after a few hours that the selection of the remedy was faulty and the patient fails to improve, or new symptoms are discovered, we must select with greater care another remedy which is more accurately adapted to the new state of the case.

38. There are some remedies, as *Ignatia, Bryonia Alba, Rhus Rad*, in some respects, *Belladonna*, which show alternating effects on the state of the health, composed of partly opposite primary effects, if after the exhibition of one of these remedies, no improvement follows, we must in a few hours, in acute cases, give a new potency of the same remedy.

If in a chronic psoric case, the anti-psoric fails to relieve, there must be some irregularity of regimen or some other vigorous influence acting upon the patient, which must be removed before a permanent cure can be accomplished.

Incipient improvement, however slight, is indicated by increased sensation of comfort, greater tranquility and ease of the mind and return of naturalness in the feelling of the patient. To find out improvement or aggravation, the physician must examine the patient closely upon every symptom contained in the record of the case. If these show that neither new nor unusual symptoms have appeared and that none of the old ones have increased, and especially if the state of mind and disposition is found to be improved, the medicine must also have produced an essential and general improvement in the disease, or at all events, it may soon be expected. Where delay occurs beyond expectation, there must be some fault in the regimen of the patient or the protracted homeopathic aggravation produced by the medicine must be attributed to the insufficient reduction of the dose.

39. New and important symptoms, mentioned by the patient, indicate that the medicine was not well selected, though the patient may think he is improving, his condition may even be worse, which will soon make itself apparent.

40. No physician should have favourites among drugs nor should he disregard medicines on account of their failure. Very often the fault is the physician's or the supposition a wrong one, his only duty is to select the similimum in every case.

41. On account of the minuteness of the homeopathic doses, great care must be taken in the diet and regimen of the patient and especially in chronic cases, we have to search carefully for such impediments to a cure, because these diseases are often aggravated by obscure, noxious influences of that kind as well as by errors in regimen, which, being frequently overlooked, exercise a noxious

influence. Daily walks, light manual labour, proper nutritious food and drink, unadulterated with medicinal substances are to be recommended. In acute cases, we have only to advise the family to obey the voice of nature by gratifying the patient's ardent desires, without offering or urging him to accept hurtful things. In acute cases, the temperature of the bedroom and the quantity of the covering should be regulated entirely according to the wishes of the patient, while every kind of mental exertion and emotional disturbance is to be avoided.

Medicines

42. Detail instructions are given for the selection of the substances belonging to the animal and vegetable kingdom and the preparation of medicines from them. The more relevant paragraphs which are important are quoted in full. (vide paras. 264 to 292)

Para. 269 (*Sixth Edition*) : The homeopathic system of medicines develops for its special use to a hitherto unheard of degree, the inner medicinal power of the crude substances by means of a process peculiar to it and which has hitherto never been tried, whereby only they all become immeasurably and penetratingly efficacious and remedial, even those that in the crude state give no evidence of the slightest medicinal power on the human body. This remarkable change in the qualities of natural bodies develops the latent, hitherto unperceived, as if slumbering hidden, dynamic powers which influence the life principle, change the well-being of animal life. This is effected by the mechanical action upon their smallest particles by means of rubbing and shaking, and *through the addition of an indifferent substance, dry or fluid, are separated from each other*. This process is called dynamizing, potentizing (development of medicinal power) and products are dynamizations of potencies in different degrees.

INTRODUCTORY

Para. 270 (*Fifth Edition*) : Thus, two drops of the fresh vegetable juice mingled with equal parts of alcohol are diluted with ninety-eight drops of alcohol and potentized by means of two successions, whereby the first development of power is formed, and this process is repeated through twenty-nine more phials, each of which is filled three quarters full with ninety-nine drops of alcohol, and each succeeding phial is to be provided with one drop from the preceding phial (which has already been shaken twice) and is in its turn twice shaken and in the same manner at last the 30th development of power which is the one most generally used.

Para. 270 (*Sixth Edition*) : In order to best obtain this development of power, a small part of the substance to be dynamized, say one grain, is triturated for three hours, with three times one hundred grain sugar of milk according to the method described below up to the one-millionth part in powder form. For reasons given below, one grain of this powder is dissolved in 500 drops of a mixture of one part of alcohol and four parts of distilled water, of which one-drop is put in a vial. To this are added one hundred drops of pure alcohol and given one hundred strong successions with the hand against a hard but elastic body (perhaps on a leather bound book).

This is the medicine in the first *degree* of dynamization with which small sugar globules (of which 100 will weigh one grain) may then be moistened and quickly spread on blotting paper to dry and kept in a well-corked vial with the sign of (I) degree of potency. Only one globule of this is taken for further dynamization, put in a second new vial (with a drop of water in order to dissolve it) and then with 100 drops of good alcohol and dynamized in the same way with 100 powerful successions.

With this alcoholic medicinal fluid, globules are again moistened, spread upon blotting paper and dried quickly, put into a well-stoppered vial and protected from heat and sunlight and given the sign (II) of the second potency. And in this way the process is continued till the twenty-ninth is reached. Then with 100 drops of alcohol by means of 100 successions, an alcoholic medicinal fluid is formed with which the 30th dynamization degree is given to properly moistened and dried sugar globules.

By means of this mechanical procedure, provided it is carried out regularly according to the above teaching, a change is effected in the given drug, which in its crude state shows itself only as a material, at times as unmedicinal material but by means of such higher and higher dynamization, it is changed and subtilized at last into spirit-like medicinal power, which, indeed, in itself does not fall within our senses, but for which the medicinally prepared globule, dry, but more so when dissolved in water, becomes the carrier and in this condition, manifests the healing power of this invisible force in the sick body.

Note 155 to para. 270 (Sixth Edition) : According to first directions (as in para. 270 of the fifth edition quoted above), one drop of the liquid of a lower potency was to be taken to 100 drops of alcohol for higher potentization. This proportion of the medicine of attenuation to the medicine that is to be dynamized (100 : 1) was found altogether too limited to develop thoroghly and to a high degree the power of the medicine by means of a number of such successions without specially using great force of which wearisome experiments have convinced me.

But if only one such globule be taken, of which 100 weigh one grain, and dynamize it with 100 drops of alcohol, the proportion of 1 to 50,000 and even greater will be had, for 500 such globules can hardly absorb one drop for their saturation. With this disproportionate higher ratio between medicine and diluting medium, many succussive strokes of the vial filled two-thirds with alcohol can produce a much greater development of power. But with so small a diluting medium as 100 to 1 of the medicine, if many successions by means of a powerful machine are forced into it, medicines are then developed, which especially in the higher degree of dynamization, act almost immediately, but with furious, even dangerous, violence, especially in weak patients, without having a lasting, mild reaction of the vital principle. But the method described by me, on the contrary, produces medicines of highest development of power and mildest action, which, however, if well chosen, touches all suffering parts curatively. In acute fevers, the small doses of the lowest dynamization degrees of these thus perfected medicinal preparations, even of medicines of long continued action (for instance, *Belladonna*) may be repeated in short intervals. In the treatment of chronic diseases, it is best to begin with the lowest degrees of dynamization and when necessary advance to higher, ever more powerful but mildly acting degree.

Para. 285 (Fifth Edition) : The diminution of the dose essential for homeopathic use, will also be promoted by diminishing its volume, so that, if, instead of a drop of a medicinal dilution, we take, but quite a small part of such a drop of a dose, the object of diminishing the effect still further will be very effectually attained, and that this will be the case may be readily conceived for this reason, because with the smaller volume of the dose but few nerves of the living organism, can be touched, whereby the power of the medicine is certainly also communicated to the whole organism but in a weaker power.

Note 2 to the above : For the purpose of sub-dividing a drop, it is most convenient to employ fine sugar globules of the size of poppy seeds, one of which imbibed with the medicine, and put into the dispensing vehicle, constitutes a medicinal dose, which contains about the three-hundredth part of a drop, for three hundred such small globules will be adequately moistened by one drop of alcohol. The dose is vastly diminished by laying one such globule alone upon the tongue and giving nothing to drink. If it be necessary, in the case of a very sensitive patient, to employ the smallest possible dose and to bring about the most rapid result, one single olfaction merely will suffice.

Note 2 to para. 288 : A globule of which ten, twenty, or one hundred weigh one grain, impregnated with the 30th potentized dilution, and then dried, retains for this purpose all its power undiminished for at least eighteen or twenty years (my experience extends this length of time) even though the phial be opened a thousand times during the period, if it be but protected from heat and the sun's light.

Para. 272 (Sixth Edition) : Such a globule (of the size of a poppy seed saturated with the thirtieth dilution prepared as indicated in para. 270) placed dry upon the tongue, is one of the smallest doses for a moderate recent case of illness. Here, but few nerves are touched by the medicine. A similar globule, crushed with some sugar of milk and dissolved in a good deal of water and stirred well before every administration will produce a far more powerful medicine for the use of several days. Every dose, no matter, how minute, touches, on the contrary, many nerves.

43. Genuine and unadulterated medicines, retaining their full virtues are the first requisites of a physician and in the treatment of disease only one single medicine should be used at one time; which will give relief in diseases where of the total symptoms are accurately known. Too strong a dose, of even a well-selected drug, will produce an unnecessary surplus of effect upon the over-excited vital force, and will be injurious, while the same similar drug-disease, if exerted within proper limits, would have gently effected a cure.

44. Experience proves that the dose of a homeopathically selected remedy cannot be reduced so far as to be inferior in strength to the natural disease, and to lose its power of extinguishing and curing at least a portion of the same, provided that this dose, immediately after having been taken, is capable of causing a slight intensification of symptoms

of the similar natural disease though this homeopathic aggravation is very often almost imperceptible.

45. The homeopathic similimum will operate chiefly upon the diseased parts of the body, which have become extremely susceptible to a stimulus so similar to their own disease. The smaller dose will change the vital action of those parts into an artificial drug-disease, and the organism be freed from the morbid process.

46. In homeopathic practice, the diminution to the dose and its effect is conveniently accomplished by lessening the volume of the dose. In using a solution of this kind a much greater surface supplied with sensitive nerves, susceptible of medicinal influence is brought in contact with the medicine, and we must take care that the medicine is equally and intimately imparted to every particle of solvent fluid. The effect of medicines in liquid forms penetrates and spreads through all parts of the organism, with such inconceivable rapidity from the point of contact with the sensitive nerves supplying the tissues, that this effect may, with propriety, be defined spirit-like of dynamic.

47. Remedies in their dynamic dose, may be given by the mouth and tongue, by olfaction or by external application over parts avoiding those subject to pain or spasms or skin eruption.

3. HAHNEMANN'S CHRONIC DISEASES.
(A Synopsis)

(Theoretical part)

1. All chronic diseases are so inveterate immediately after they have become developed in the system that unless they are throughly cured by art, they continue to increase in

intensity until the moment of death. They never disappear of themselves, nor can they be diminished, much less conquered or extinguished, by the most vigorous constitution or the most regular mode of life and even strictest diet.

2. Psora is the oldest, most universal and most pernicious chronic miasmatic disease. Existing for many thousands of years, its morbid symptoms have increased to such an extent that its secondary symptoms have become inumerable.

3. The ancient nations designated psora as leprosy by which the external parts of the body became variously disfigured, and during the middle ages the Crusaders spread it over Europe. Cleanliness, increased refinement and more select nourishment succeeded in diminishing the disgusting appearance of psora so as to reduce the disease, towards the end of the fifteenth century, to the ordinary eruption of an itch. But about this time, 1493, the second contagious chronic disease, syphilis began to raise its fearful head.

4. During the first centuries of leprosy, the patients, though they suffered much in consequence of lancinating pains in the tumors and scabs, and the vehement itching all round, enjoyed nevertheless a fair share of general health, for one obstinately lasting eruption upon the skin served as a substitute for the internal psora, and further more the leprous patients were kept apart from human society and thus the contagion remained limited and rate.

5. But the milder form of psora, in the shape of an itch, infected a far greater number of people, and the itch vesicles being constantly ruptured by scratching and their contents spread over the skin, and those things which had been touched by such patients, psora became the most contagious and most universal of the chronic poisons. Though this eruption by its easier concealment may attack

INTRODUCTORY

many persons, still the essence of this reduced psora remains unchanged, and being more easily repelled from the skin, it appears so much more imperceptibly upon the inner surface producing severe secondary ailments.

6. At the time before leprosy was reduced, there were much less nervous affections, painful ailments, spasms, cancerous ulcers, adventitious formations, weaknesses, paralysis, consumptions and degenerations of either mind or body, than there are now, aided probably by universal use of coffee and tea for the last two centuries.

7. The most universal of external means has done an immense amount of mischief, for secondary ailments will sooner or later manifest themselves as results of the psoric reaction.

8. Many cases from ancient and recent writers can be cited to convince the observer that the itch with its varieties, tinea capitis, crusta lactea, herpes, etc. are the external vicarious symptoms of an internal disease affecting the whole organism and that psora is the most pernicious of all chronic poisons. It is well-known that all infections first attack the whole organism internally before the vicarious affection manifests itself.

9. In acute diseases, the local symptoms, together with the disease, leave the system as soon as they have run through their regular course. In chronic diseases, the local affection may either be removed or disappear by itself, when at the same time the internal disease may increase, unless it is cured by art.

10. In considering the formation of the three chronic maladies, psora, sycosis, syphilis, as well as that of the acute infectious diseases, three cardinal points must be noticed; (a) the period when the infection took place; (b) the period when the whole organism began to be tainted with the infectious poison, until it became a complete internal disease; (c) the

manifestation of the external symptoms, by which nature indicates the complete development of the infectious disease in the internal organism.

11. The infection in acute as well as in chronic diseases, takes place in a moment, provided this moment is favourable to the contagious influence, the whole nervous system becomes infected in a moment. The human small-pox, measles, etc. will run through this course, and the fever which is peculiar to each of these different forms of infection, together with the cutaneous eruption, will break out a few days after the internal disease has completed its development.

12. The mode of contagion in chronic contagious diseases is the same, but after the internal disease is completed, there is this difference, that the chronic poison continues in the organism, and even develops itself from year to year, unless it is extinguished and thoroughly cured by art.

13. Syphilitic contagion happens at those places which come in contact with the syphilitic virus and receives it into themselves by friction; the internal organism is roused in a moment by this infection, and not until the internal disease is completely developed, does nature try to form at the spot where the contagion took place, a local symptom as a substitute for the internal disease. By extinguishing the internal disease with an internal remedy, the chancre becomes also cured without any external application.

14. Psora is the most contagious of all chronic diseases, as it taints the system, especially that of children, by simply touching the skin. Not till the whole orgnism has been adapted to the nature of the chronic contagious disease, do the morbidly affected vital powers try to alleviate the internal disease by local symptoms and the eruption is merely the ultimate boundary of the psoric development, a

substitute for the internal disease, which together with its secondary ailments, remains in a latent condition. External applications may check the local symptoms, but too often the internal psora is thus aggravated.

15. There are many symptoms which reveal the existence of psora, but they cannot all be found upon one person, one has more, the other less, in one they come out progressively, in another they remain suppressed, this depends greatly upon the constitution and the external circumstances of the patient. These affections do not prevent him from leading a tolerably comfortable existence, provided he is young and robust, is not obliged to fatigue himself, has all his wants provided for, is not exposed to chagrin or grief and has a cheerful, calm, patient and contented temper. In this case, psora may continue slumbering for years without becoming developed into a permanent chronic disease.

16. However, a trivial cause, an ordinary vexation, a cold, an irregularity in the diet, etc. may in a more advanced age, cause a violent though short attack of disease, out of proportion with the moderately exciting cause, especially during the fall, winter and early spring.

17. But whenever the vital power has been reduced by some mental ailments or by a bodily affection, the latent psora becomes aroused and develops a host of inveterate symptoms; some one of the psoric chronic diseases breaks form, unless more favourable circumstances set in diminishing the intensity of the disease and making its development more moderate (here follow the symptoms of the aroused psora, differing according to the individuality of the patient and the extent of the psoric intoxication).

18. Sycotic excrescences are often accompanied with a sort of gonorrhea from the urethra, are sometimes dry and in

the form of warts, but more frequently soft, spongy, emitting a fetid fluid, of a sweetish taste, bleeding readily and having the form of a coxcomb or a cauliflower. In man, they appear upon the glans around or beneathe the prepuce, in woman they surround the pudenda. Surgery and Mercury are still much abused in sycosis, the expiration of the excerscences only lead to their appearance at some other place and the internal use of mercurials rouses a latent psora and we deal with a combination of psora and sycosis. Our duty then is to annihilate the psoric miasm by the indicated antipsoric and then we use the remedies indicated for sycosis (*Thuja, Nitric acid*), and for syphilitic complications, Mercury remain the remedy.

19. The syphilitic contagion is more general than the poison of sycosis. The treatment of syphilis is only difficult when complicated with the psoric poison. The former is rarely complicated with sycosis, but whenever it exists we meet psora as an additional complication.

20. Chancre and bubo are the original representations or syphilis, and if not interfered with, they might remain during life and no secondary symptoms will appear. By considering the chancre a mere local ulcer and by removing it by external means, the disease is forced to manifest itself throughout the organism with all the secondary symptoms of a fully developed syphilis; hence it is that the internal disease is more permanently cured, while the chancre or the bubo are yet existing as its vicarious types, especially in young persons of a cheerful temper, where often one single minute dose of Mercury suffices, and Hahnemann prefers that preparation which goes by his name. If more than one dose should be required, the lower potencies may then be employed.

21. The second stage sets in when the chancre has been especially removed by external means, but even then provided there is no latent psora, the secondary symptoms may be prevented by the soluble Mercury, and the original spot of the chancre can no more be traced, while without that internal treatment a reddish morbid-looking red or bluish scar remains. Bubo, when not complicated with psora, only needs the same treatment.

22. In the third state we find syphilis complicated with psora and the patient suffered already from psora when the syphilitic infection took place or false internal and external treatment caused a combination of the psoric with the syphilitic element and it takes then more than one remedy to remove the evil consequences. It may be here observed that it is the nature of the psoric poison to break forth in consequence of great concussions of the system and violent in roads upon the general health.

23. In order to reach this marked syphilis (pseudosyphilis), we must remove from the patient all hurtful external influences and put him on an easily and vigorously nourishing diet and regulate his general mode of life. The most appropriate anti-psoric according to the new symptoms, and when the latter has accomplished its action, the single dose of Mercury must be allowed to act as long as it is capable of exercising a curative influence.

24. In old difficult cases, ailments remain which are neither purely psoric or syphilitic. Here several courses of anti-psoric are needed, until the last trace of all provocation has ceased. After this we give a lower potency of Mercury and allow it to act until the skin has recovered its healthy color at the spot where the venereal chancre stood.

25. A complication of the three chance poisons must be treated on the same principles. Anti-psoric first and then that poison

whose symptoms are most prominent. Afterwards the remaining portion of the psoric symptoms must be removed and then the last races of syphilis and sycosis by other adequate remedies. A return of a healthy color of the skin on places which had been affected is the surest sign of a perfect restoration.

26. As long as the psora eruption is yet existing upon the skin, psora exhibits itself in its simple and most natural integrity, and may be cured in the easiest, quickest and safest manner, but when the internal disease is deprived of its vicarious symptoms, the psoric poison is forced to spread over the most delicate parts of the internal organism and to develop its secondary symptoms.

27. The psoric poison having prevaded millions of organisms for thousands of years, has gradually developed out of itself an endless number of symptoms, varied according to differences of constitution, climate, residence, education, habits, occupation, mode of life, diet and various other bodily and mental influences; herein different anti-psoric remedies will be required for the eradication of the psoric poison.

28. Only the recent itch with the eruption still existing upon the skin, can be completely cured by the dose of *Sulphur*, but such a speedy cure is not always possible, as the age of the patient has great influence upon the result of the treatment. In eruptions which have existed for some time on the skin, it ceases to be a vicarious symptom for the internal disease, and secondary psoric affections will manifest themselves; in such a case, *Sulphur* does not suffice, and it requires several anti-psorics for a cure.

29. With reference to diet and mode of life, whatever is injurious to the action of the remedies must be avoided, and with lingering diseases we must consider the age, occupation and social conditions of the patient. Strict diet

INTRODUCTORY

alone will hardly ever cure a disease, and it is unreasonable to insist upon a mode of life which is impossible for a patient to follow; only that which is generally injurious to health, ought to be carefully avoided.

30. Rich patients must walk more than they usually do, moderate dancing, rural entertainments, music and amusing lectures, theatres once in a while, are allowable, but they must never play cards, riding on horse-back or in a carriage ought to be restricted. All amorous intercourse and sexual excitement, reading lewd novels, supertitious and exciting books are to be carefully avoided.

31. The literary man should take much exercise in the open air, in bad weather do some light mechanical work in the house. During treatment, he ought to limit his literary work and in mental diseases reading must be positively forbidden.

32. Chronic patients must avoid domestic medicines and abstain from perfumes. Those who are accustomed to wear wool may continue to do so, but as the case progresses and the weather becomes warmer, cotton or linen ought to be substituted. Daily ablutions are often more advisable than baths.

33. In regard to eating, one should consent to restrictions in order to be freed from a troublesome chronic disease and only in abdominal affections restrictions are more necessary. As regards beverages, coffee has pernicious effects upon the mind and body. Young people do not need it, and older persons should wean themselves generally from its use, and be satisfied with roast rye or wheat, whose smell and taste is very much like coffee. Tea ought to be entirely avoided during treatment of chronic diseases. Old people cannot be suddenly deprived of their wine, but by mixing it with water and sugar, they can gradually reduce its strength, in fact, the patient cannot be too abstemious in

relation to alcoholic beverages, it is a law of nature that the apparent increase of strength and animal heat consequent upon the use of ardent spirits will be followed by a state of depression and diminution of heat.

34. Beer is so much adulterated, that it becomes injurious to health, vinegar and lemon juice are especially hurtful to those who are affected with nervous and abdominal complaints, sweet fruits may be used moderately, beef, wheat, or rye-bread, cow's milk and fresh butter are the most natural food, hence also for chronic patients. Next to beef comes mutton, old chickens, young pigeons. Goose, duck or pork are less admissible. Salt and smoked meats are to be used in great moderation. Fish ought to be boiled and eaten without any spiced sauces, herrings and sardines in moderate quantities. Moderation in both eating and drinking is a sacred duty for all chronic patients.

35. Restriction in the use of tobacco is especially necessary when the intellectual functions are affected, when the patient does not keep well, is dyspeptic and constipated.

36. Excessive fatigue, working in marshy regions, injuries and wounds, excessive heat or cold, starvation, poverty, unwholesome food are less capable of rousing latent psora or aggravating a manifested psoric disease than an unhappy marriage or a gnawing conscience. Grief and sorrow are the chief cause which either develop latent psora or aggravate an already existing secondary psoric affection.

37. Mineral springs and all medicinal influences ought to be avoided and when the patient used them he ought to abstain for some time from all medicines and follow a strict diet in the country.

38. All excesses injure mind and body; by vicious practices the most robust bodies often fail and the latent psora entering in combination with a badly managed syphylitic poison gives

rise to most distressing diseases. We must then remove first the psoric poison and thus prevent all secondary chronic affections.

39. The physician must never interrupt the action of an antipsoric remedy nor exhibit an intermediate remedy on account of every trifling ailment, a carefully selected remedy should act till it has completed its effect.

40. Suppose the remedy calls out symptoms which have existed before, this apparent aggravation and the development of new symptoms show that the remedy has attacked the disease in its inmost nature, and it must be left undisturbed.

41. Should the remedy cause new symptoms, which may be supposed to be inherent to the medicine, the remedy should be permitted to act for a while and generally these symptoms will disappear, but if they are troublesome, they show that the remedy was not properly chosen, and an antidote, if known, must be given, or another suitable antipsoric selected.

42. A homeopathic aggravation is a proof that a cure may be anticipated with certainty; but if the original symptoms continue with the same intensity, it shows that too large a dose made the cure impossible, neutralising its genuine homeopathic effects and causing a medicinal disease by the side of the natural disturbances. We then select an anti-psoric which corresponds to the symptoms of the natural and of the artificial disease. Should the same anti-psoric be still indicated, we must give it in a much higher potency and in a more minute dose. The doses can scarcely be too much reduced, provided the effects of the remedy are not disturbed by improper food, and of the artificial disease. Should the same anti-psoric be still indicated, we must give it in a much higher potency and in a more minute dose.

43. The physician should avoid three mistakes, that the dose an be too small, the improper use of the remedy, and in not letting the remedy act a sufficient length of time. The surest and safest way of hastening a cure is to let the medicine act as long as the improvement of the patient continues.

44. Psora is troublesome thing to deal with, exacerbations show only that the disease is writhing under the action of the remedy, but they will progressively diminish in frequecy and intensity if not interfered with by a new remedy, for the benign action of the former remedy, which was manifesting itself, is thus probably lost.

45. A second dose of the selected remedy is only indicated when the improvement which the first dose had produced, by causing the morbid symptoms gradually to become less frequent and less intense, ceases to continue after the lapse of fourteen, ten, or seven days, when it is evident that the medicine has ceased to act, the condition of the mind is the same as before, and no new or troublesome symptoms have made their appearance. It may be expedient to give this second minute dose in a somewhat lower potency.

46. *Sulphur, Hepar Sulph.* and *Sepia* excepted, the other anti-psorics, seldom admit of a favourable repetition of the same drug. One anti-psoric having fulfilled its object the modified series of symptoms generally requires another remedy. In cases treated by the old school it may be necessary to interpolate, once in a while, a dose of *Sulphur,* or *Hepar Sulph.* according to indications.

47. Alternating remedies in rapid succession is a sure sign that the right remedy was not selected, or that the symptoms were only carelessly studied. By such mismanagement, remedial agents seem to lose all their power, and mesmeric

action may succeed in calming the system. Let the palms of both your hands rest for about a minute upon the vertex, then move slowly down the body, across the neck, shoulders, arms, hands, knees, legs, feet and toes, this pass may be repeated.

48. The irritability of the patient may also be calmed by directing him to smell a globule moistened with the highest potency of the homeopathic medicine. By smelling of the medicine, its influence may be communicated to the patient in any degree. By increasing the number of inspirations the power of the medicine steadily increases.

49. Globules, kept in corked vials, protected from heat and sunshine preserve their medicinal powers for years.

50. Placebos may be used when the patient wishes to take medicine every day.

51. The cure of a chronic disease may be often retarded by bodily or mental accidents, or intercurrent diseases, due to malaria, or meteoric influences may set in, interrupting the anti-psoric treatment sometimes for several weeks, and olfaction of the non-anti-psoric remedy may suffice for the removal of the intermediate disease.

52. After the intercurrent disease is removed, the symptoms of the original chronic disease may be modified, or morbid symptoms may manifest themselves in other parts of the body. The patient must be throughly re-examined, so that the appropriate remedy may be chosen.

53. Great epidemic diseases, improperly treated and permitted to complete their course, arouse the latent psoric poison often to a high degree of intensity, manifesting itself in innumerable forms, anti-psoric treatment is the only safeguard.

54. The obstinate character of endemic disease is due to some psoric complication or the action of the psoric poison modified by the peculiar influence of the locality and peculiar mode of life of its inhabitants. The marshy exhaltions, especially of hot countries, appear, on account of their paralyzing influence over the vital forces, to be one of the most powerful excitants of the psoric poison, which can only be calmed by anti-psoric treatment. Recently developed symptoms are the first to yield to the action of anti-psorics, the older symptoms, which have permanently existed, are the last to disappear, hence local symptoms only pass off after the general health has been completely restored, and we must not be contented till the last vestige of psora is removed.

55. A great chronic disease may be cured in the space of one or two years, provided it was not mismanaged to the extent of having become incurable. In young robust persons half this space of time is sufficient. If we consider that the psoric poison has gradually ramified into the inmost recesses of the organism, patient and physician understand why much time must be necessary to master this parasitical enemy that has assailed the most delicate roots of the tree of life.

56. Where anti-psoric treatment is properly conducted, the strength of the patient increases from the start and this increase in strength continues during the whole treatment until the organism unfolds anew its regenerate life.

57. The best time for taking an anti-psoric is in the morning before breakfast. The patient ought then to wait about an hour before eating or drinking anything.

58. Anti-psoric should neither be taken immediately before nor during menstruation. If the menses appear too soon, too abundant, and last too long, she may smell on the fourth

INTRODUCTORY

day of a globule of a high potency of *Nux vomica*, and several days after, the anti-psoric may be taken. *Nux vom.* restores the harmony of the nervous functions and calms that irritability which inhibits the action of the anti-psoric.

59. Pregnancy offers a brilliant sphere of action to anti-psoric remedies, but only the highest potencies ought to be employed. Nursing ought to get their medicine through the milk of the mother or wet nurse.

60. The vital force, if left to itself, tries to palliate by producing secretions and evacuations, or diarrheas, vomiting, seats, ulcers, hemorrhages, etc., but they produce only an apparent alleviation of the primitive disease and in fact increase it on account of the great loss of nutritious pabulum which the patient has suffered.

61. At the beginning of anti-psoric treatment, constipation is often the great bugbear of the patient and an injection of pure tepid water may be allowed, which may be several times repeated, until the anti-psoric remedies succeed in regulating the proofs of the intestinal evacuations. *Sulphur* and *Lycopodium clav.* act most favourably under those circumstances. Hot baths interfere with the effect of anti-psoric treatment.

62. In the first edition, at the end of the directions for treating chronic diseases, Hahnemann had recommended the lightest electric sparks as an adjuvant for quickening parts that have been for a long time paralysed and without sensation, these to be used besides the anti-psoric treatment. This recommendation has now been withdrawn as it was found that this advice was not strictly followed in practice and that longer sparks have always been used to the detriment of patients. It has been found that there is an efficient Homeopathic local assistance for paralysed parts of such as are without sensation. This is found in *cold*

spring water from deep wells. The water may either be poured on these parts for one, two or three minutes or by douche-baths over the whole body of one to five minutes duration, either daily or an often as may be required, according to the circumstances, together with the appropriate internal, anti-psoric treatment, sufficient exercise in the open air and judicious diet.

4. HAHNEMANN'S NOSOLOGY

Chronic Diseases–Further explanation

The classification of diseases adopted by Hahnemann inclues two types, *acute* and *chronic.*

Acute diseases: Originate from defective hygiene, errors in diet, physical agents, cold, heat and other atmospheric changes, mental moral influences.

Again, telluric and meteoric and bacterial influences give rise to acute diseases, attacking a number of individuals, at the same time giving rise to epidemic and contagious diseases. Besides these general causes, there are types of acute disease which are transient activities of the hitherto dormant psoric miasm, rendered so from some cause or other. .

Chronic diseases: They are produced by infection from a chronic miasm, and which the vital powers of the organism, aided my hygienic and dietetic and sanitary measures are not able to extinguish. The chronic miasms giving rise to all forms of chronic diseases are *psora, syphilis* and *sycosis.* Hahnemann does not classify among these chronic diseases, such as result from living under unhygienic and insanitary influences, or trying mental conditions, dietetic errors, excesses of all kinds, etc. as those diseases disappear of themselves by mere change of regimen and surroundings and removing the cause, provided, however, there is not present one of the three chronic miasms, which are the lead causes of all chronic diseases.

Drug diseases: On the other hand prolonged drug use in heroic doses does produce a species of chronic disease which is most difficult to cure, and when such have attained a considerable hold, it would seem as if no remedy could be discovered for their radical cure.

Organon, paras. 74 *and* 75 : "It is a matter of regret that we are still obliged to count among chronic diseases very common affections which are to be regarded as the result of allopathic treatment and the continual use of violent, heroic medicine in large and increasing doses. Examples of that kind, are, the abuse of calomel, corrosive sublimate, mercurial ointment, nitrate of silver, iodine and its ointments, opium, valerian, quinine, digitalis etc. The use of purgatives persisted in for years etc." To which might be added the modern abuse of coal tar products, patent medicines. Such wanton treatment weakens the organism, abnormally deranged and wholly altered. Irritability and sensibility are increased or decreased, hypertrophy and atrophy, softening and indurations in certain organs and organic lesions are produced. Such are some of the results of nature's efforts to protect the organism against complete destruction by aggressive treatment with pernicious drugs.

The evolution of Hahnemann's doctrine of Chronic Diseases

After Hahemann's discovery of the Law of Cure in 1790, he worked incessantly investigating the action of drugs on the healthy, and practised according to the newly discovered law and by the light and aid the new Materia Medica was able to give. The success of this practical application of the Law of Cure was striking in the extreme, especially in the treatment of acute diseases and epidemics. As regards chronic diseases, Homeopathy was able to improve or ameliorate the conditions in a very short time. But though the patients were often very much relieved, they were not cured, for their complaints would return more or less by many unfavourable circumstances, such as errors of diet, unfavourable weather, mental emotions etc. Their return, under these circumstances, was generally attended with the appearance of news symptoms, often more troublesome and more difficult of removal than before. Through the treatment of these chronic diseases was conducted strictly according to the doctrines of the homeopathic art. Hahnemann was unable to discover the real cause of his failure to cure these chronic diseases. After hard labour and patient study and observation for ten years, he was able to discover his new theory in 1827.

Cause of Recurrence of Chronic Diseases.

His researches and reflection led him to the conclusion that the cause of the constant recurrence of chronic diseases after their apparent or partial removal by the homeopathic remedy, and their recurrence with new and grave symptoms, was that the symptoms manifesting themselves at any one time were *only a portion* of the deeply seated fundamental malady, whose great extent was shown by the new symptoms that appeared from time to time. He believed it to be a *chronic miasm*, which the body could not throw off spontaneously and unaided, not even by careful diet or regimen, but that it rather increased in intensity and extent from year to year.

"The most robust constitution, the best regulated life, and the greatest energy of the vital powers, are insufficient to extinguish them." Organon-para 78.

The Skin Phase of Chronic Diseases

His further research showed that the obstacle to the cure seemed to lie in a previous scabious eruption, which the patient frequently acknowledged having had, and from which he often dated all his sufferings. He believed that chronic diseases occurred on the suppression artificially, or disappearance from any cause, of a scabious itching eruption from the skin in otherwise healthy persons. This itch dyscrasia he called *psora*, meaning thereby the internal itch disease, with or without any present skin symptoms. It is the source of all varieties of skin disease, abnormal growths, tumors, deformity, mental diseases etc. In short, it is the parent of all chronic diseases with the exception of venereal diseases. It is the oldest, most universal and obstinate of all miasmatic diseases. The readiness with which these are suppressed and the immense development of local treatment has driven this psora within to more vital regions, and thus has led to the great increase of chronic maladies that afflict mankind.

The appearance of skin symptoms, or discharge from a mucus surface, shows that nature is making an effort to localise on the outskirts of the body the morbid process, removed as far as possible from the more vital parts of the organism, where it would be much more mischievous. Therefore, forcing it back into the interior by strong local treatment must necessarily work detrimentally to a radical and permanent cure (Para 203, Organon).

The Underlying Facts of the Psoric Theory

Though the psoric theory may not be accepted as a whole, it contains certain facts which are undeniable and go to establish *the essential truth* of the doctrine. These are the following:

(*a*) In many patients, the even and regular clinical course of disease is from some cause or other within themselves interfered with.

(*b*) Remedies apparently indicated and chosen according to the law of similars, fail to accomplish what, as a rule, they ought.

(*c*) This is especially true of most chronic diseases.

(*d*) It is a further fact that frequently the suppression or disappearance of a skin disease is followed by serious mischief in more vital organs such as, respiratory affections (asthma), after eczema on the head, etc. showing a reciprocal relation between the skin and internal organs. It is the presence of *this unseen but nevertheless very active and perturbing factor* that accounts for these conditions. The Hahnemannian conception of Psora is a very real thing and *that* is its passport to the general practitioner whose aim is to cure permanently rather than palliate and relieve for the time being. We may not know what Psora is, except that it consists of the sum of all the biological obstacles which resist, deface, complicate and alter the natural course of diseases and interfere with the action of the apparently well selected homeopathic remedy. In this wider sense, as indicating *cachexia* or *dyscrasia*, the Psora is founded in nature and truth. Though Hahnemann's theory is not proved, it is a most admirable working theory, a stepping stone by means of which we attain remarkable results in the treatment of diseases.

For the treatment of psoric diseases, what are known as *anti-psoric remedies* are required. Anti-psoric remedies are such as show in their pathogenis a tendency to act from within outwards, from above downwards, which abound in skin symptoms, and are deep and long-acting remedies, hence they are of special value in the treatment of chronic disease and for the eradication of inherited and constitutional disease tendencies. They show their *greatest medicinal power in highly attenuated form and do not bear* frequent repetition. Many of them are wholly inert in their crude state and require the pharmaceutical process of homeopathy to develop their latent medicinal force.

The principal anti-psoric remedies are *Sulphur, Calcarea Carb., Lycopodium clav., Sepia, Silicea, Natrium mur., Graphites, Arsenic Alb., Alumina* and many others. (For full list see 'Chronic Diseases.')

Besides *psora,* Hahnemann has included *sycosis* and *syphilis* as the two other miasms which from the basis of chronic diseases.

Sycosis is the suppression of the gonorrheal poison in the system. Its main local manifestation is the production of figwarts around the genital region, but its later constitutional symptoms are not confined to any part of the organism, but are a general deviation of health.

Hahnemann distinguishes two kinds of gonorrhea-one comparatively innocent-a urethral, catarrhal inflammation, and the other the sycotic form. In regard to the more common and comparatively innocent form, he says in his "Chronic Diseases".

"The miasm of the other common gonorrheas seems not to penetrate the whole organism, but only to locally stimulate the urinary organs. They yield either to a dose of one drop of *fresh parsley-juice* when this is indicated by a frequent urgency to urinate, or a small dose of *Cannabis ind.* or *Cantharis,* or *Copaiva* according to their different constitution, and the other ailments attending it. These should, however, be always used in the higher and highest dynamizations, unless a psora, slumbering in the body of the patient has been developed by means of a strongly affecting, irritating or weakening old-school treatment. In such a case, frequently, secondary gonorrhea, remain which can only be cured by anti-psoric treatment."

The *sycotic form of gonorrhea* differs in being a much more serious matter. Hahnemann describes it as follows:

"The discharge is from the beginning thickish, like pus, micturition is less difficult but the body of the penis swollen somewhat hard, the penis is also, in some cases, covered on the back with glandular tubercles, and very painful to the touch."

The characteristic features of sycosis are the wart-like cauliflower excrescences around the genitals, soft, spongy, bleeding, easily recurring when violently removed, frequently emitting a specific fetid fluid.

All heroic external treatment is forbidden, tending to produce the sycotic diathesis, only the external use of *Thuja* is permitted. For internal treatment, *Thuja* is the great anti-sycotic and may be followed by *Nitricum acidum*.

The violent suppression of a sycotic urethral discharge is often followed by chronic suffering, which if characterised by peculiar symptoms and conditions, among which the following have frequently been observed.

Symptoms of Suppressed Gonorrhea

Greater muscular debility is the most characteristic physical sign, anxiety, anguish, fear of associating with strangers, going into a crowd, great irriability, dysmenorrhea, before during and after flow with great debility, sterility, inflammation of the fallopian tubes, ovaries, neurasthenia, asthma, bronchial affection, distorted fingernails, eruption in the palms of the hands, dryness of the hair, etc. rheumatism setting in shortly after the suppression of the discharge or removal of the warts, ankle and knee are especially affected, pains worse before a storm and during the day.

Syphilis

The second chronic miasms, which is more widely spread than the fig-wart disease and which for four centuries (before Hahnemann's time) had been the source of many other chronic diseases, is the miasm of the venereal disease proper, the chancre-disease (syphilis). The treatment for this simple form as well as

INTRODUCTORY

those complicated with the two other miasms are mentioned in paras. 10 to 28 of the symopsis of 'Hahnemann's Chronic Diseases' given earlier.

Drug Diseases

Chronic diseases due to heavy drugging with allopathic medicines should be treated with suitable antidotes in continuous doses till the effects are removed.

(See the chapter relating to 'Drug effects etc.')

Eradicative Possibilities of Anti-psoric treatment

The greater evil of these miasms, is that they are made organic and rendered permanent by heredity. It is this fact of heredity and the pollution of the vital fluid entailed thereby that modifies not only the course of acute diseases, but establishes and makes a permanent field for chronic diseases. This hereditary gift and this organised field give rise to certain bodily constitutions and certain dyscrasic conditions. Acute diseases and possibly the action of remedies *run their course in the track marked out by these bodily constitutions,* which again are largely modified by the latent psoric taint.

In order to get a true and practical understanding of diseases, the physician has to ascertain whether the patient has inherited any of these miasms which form the ground for the invasion and development of acute and chronic diseases, and to treat him with suitable remedies.

Pre-natal treatment by means of Anti-psoric remedies

This is a peculiar field for homeopathy. By means of the deeply-acting anti-psoric remedies, the lower strata of perverted life where it first establishes itself in the finest fibre and cellular structures, can be restored. Medicines chosen wisely and given to the expectant mother, can benefit the coming child. Frequently with the indicated remedy, anatomical and structural deficiencies such as cleft-palate, hare-lip, eczema, epileptic fits, tuberculosis etc., can be prevented in families where such have appeared, because the taint that gave rise to them in former pregnancies may be neutralised by the timely administration of the homeopathic anti-psoric remedies.

Mental Diseases and their Treatment

Most mental diseases are in reality bodily diseases. Certain mental and emotional symptoms are peculiar to every bodily disease, these symptoms develop more or less rapidly and become predominant over all other symptoms, and are finally transferred, like a local disease, into the invisibly fine organs of the mind, where, by their presence, they see to obscure the bodily symptoms.

In regard to the totality of symptoms of a case of this kind, *all physical symptoms which prevailed before* the disease assumed the mental form are very essential. Comparison between these early symptoms and their present indistinct remnants, which may occasionally appear during intervals, or during transient amelioration of the mental disease, will show the continuance of the physical disease, although obscured.

(Study paras 214-220, Organon.)

Acute Insanity

Acute insanity, even though due to latent psora, should not be treated with anti-psoric remedies to start with but met with remedies like *Aconite nap., Belladonna* etc. in highly attenuated doses. After such treatment, anti-psoric remedies with well-regulated diet and habits, will do the rest. In the treatment of insanity, the medicines may be given mixed with the patient's usual drink, without his knowledge, thus obviating every kind of compulsion.

(Study paras 221-231, Organon, in this connection.)

Intermittent and Alternating Diseases

These are such as return at certain periods, or where certain morbid conditions alternate with each other. Such are mostly a product of developed psora.

The symptoms which mark the condition of the patient during the period of intermission should chiefly be taken as guides in selecting the most striking homeopathic remedy.

In intermittents, besides the importance of the apyrexia as offering most guiding symptoms for the selection of the remedy, the stage which is most prominent and peculiar should next be considered. The best time to administer the remedy is a short time after the termination of the paroxysm, when the patient has partially recovered from it. The vital force is then in the most favourable condition to be modified by medicine and restored to healthy action. Anti-psoric remedies will generally be required after other remedies corresponding to the special type of fever have failed to bring about a perfect cure.

(Study para 231-244, Organon.)

5. HAHNEMANN'S PHILOSOPHY

(*a*) Hahnemann was a vitalist. His philosophical conceptions were quite against the current materialistic pathological, bacterial, antitoxic theories, discoveries and facts *as a basis for therapeutics*. He thought that all these were insecure foundations on which to build a true science of therapeutics. His teachings in regard to disease and their cure are based on his conception of the existence of a vital principle animating the human body, and at the same time a similar vital principle or force embodied in every medicinal substance. Hahnemann saw in the body but an organism made up of material particles in themselves having no life, but vivified and embodied and adapted to the real, living man, the spirit within. The connection between the immaterial, spiritual and immortal being, and the body is supposed by him to be effected by means of the vital force, which he designates *dynamis*. We have then, in Hahnemann's physiology, (*i*) the spirit, the true man, (*ii*) the material body, receiving its life and health through, (*iii*) the vivifying vital force, the *dynamis*. From this conception follows the pathological deduction that the distrubance of the harmonius play of life, manifesting itself in symptoms affecting the functions and sensations we call disease, is a disturbance of this same vital force or *dynamis*. This *dynamis* differs from the material body in being of a more subtle quality and Hahnemann defines it, in contra-distinction of the material grossness of the body, as 'spirit-like'. The vital force is active throughout the body and is the immediate cause of every functional activity of all bodily growth. It is the *formative* force of the organism, is in fact the inner form which controls the molecular, chemical and mechanical processes, and used them for its own purposes, immaterial, hence beyond the penetration of the keenest sense or most powerful microscope, or the X-ray. *The vital force is the intermediate agent between the spirit and body*, enabling the spirit to dwell for a time in its material bodily clothing. Hahnemann's *dynamis or vital force* is not therefore the very seat of life, but only the *connecting medium between the rational spirit*, the true living man, and the *outer material covering by which man takes cognizance of this material world and its plane of external life*. It is not necesary to suppose this vital force to be an organised entity, but rather the first ultimation on the plane of matter by means of the finest degrees of that plane, of the moulding, organising and maintaining activity of the spirit within. In scientific language it may be called a kind of *molecular motion* guided for a definite end in view.

(*b*) In disease, the vimtal principle is first disturbed, its disturbance precedes functional and organic changes. Hence *disease is of dynamic origin* and the true causes of disease are such as affect the vital force, dynamic agents, mental conditions, passions, moral deteriorations in the individual or in the race. So called causes or immediate causes of disease can act only as secondary causes when the vital force has become weakened in its resisting power and allows untoward influences to affect the organism. The following paras of the Organon clearly teach this, paras 9, 10, 11, 12, 15, 16, 29.

"During health, the immaterial vital principle which animates the material body, rules absolutely. By it all its parts are maintained in admirable, harmonious vital operation, as regards both sensations and functions, so that our indwelling rational spirit can freely employ this living, healthy instrument for the higher purposes of our existence."

"The material organism, without the vital force, is incapable of sensation, function or self-preservation, it is dead and subject only to the physical laws of the external world, it decays and is again resolved into its chemical constituents, it is the immaterial, vital principle only, animating the material organism in health and disease, that imparts to it all sensation and enables it to perform its functions."

"In disease, it is only this immaterial automatic vital force, pervading the entire organism, that is primarily deranged by the dynamic influence upon it of a morbific agent inimical to life. Only the vital principle, thus deranged, can furnish the organism its abnormal sensations and set up the irregular processes we call disease, for, as a power invisible in itself, and only known by its effects on the organism, its morbid derangement only makes itself known by the manifestations of disease in the sensations and functions of those parts of the organism exposed to the senses of the observer and physician that is by *morbid symptoms* and in no other way can it make itself known."

"How the vital force causes the organism to display morbid phenomena that is *how* it produces disease, it would be no practical utility to know, and therefore, it will for ever remain concealed from the physician."

In the preface to the second volume of the "Materia Medica Pura", Hahnemann says, "Life is in no respect governed by any physical laws which govern only inorganic substances. The material substances comprising the human organism are not governed in their living composition, by the same laws to which inorganic substances are subjected, but follow laws peculiar to their vitality, they themselves are animated and vivified. As the organism, in its normal condition, depends only on the state of the vitality, it follows that the changed conditiion which we call disease or sickness, must likewise depend, not on the operation of physical or chemical principles, but on originally vital sensations and actions that is to say, a dynamically changed state of man a changed existence through which, eventually, the constituent parts of the body become altered in their character, as is rendered necessary in each individual case through the changed condition of the living organism."

Need of the Dynamized Remedy to affect changes in the Disturbed Vital Force

(c) Now the next step was almost inevitable. If disease is but a disturbed condition of the vital force, and this far removed from the grossness of matter, so fine as to be almost spirit-like, surely crude drugs cannot possibly affect it curatively and hence the need, for purposes affecting this disturbed dynamis, of the *dynamized* drug, of the potentized remedy, one from which all crude, grossly material parts have been eliminated. The following quotation from Paracelsus is interesting in this connection and may possibly serve as a clue to explain the action of the attenuated homeopathic medicines.

"Matter is connected with spirit by an intermediate principle which it receives from the spirit. This intermediate link between matter and spirit belongs to all three kingdoms of nature– and it forms, in connection with the vital force of the vegetable kingdom, the *'Primum Ens'*, which possesses the highest medicinal properties."

Such a preparation alone would approach in character and fineness that of the dynamis, hence the teaching in 'Organon', paras 16, 269, 275, 288, where it is said that it is only by means of the spirit-like influence of a morbific agent that our vital power can be diseased, and in like manner, only by spirit-like (dynamic) operation of medicine that health can be restored.

"The homeopathic system of medicine develops for its use, to a hitherto unhear of degree, the spirit-like medicinal powers of the crude substances by means of a process peculiar to it and which has hitherto never been tried, whereby only they all become penetratingly effficacious and remedial, even those that in their crude state give no evidence of the slightest medicinal power on the human body." (Para 256, Organon.)

Hahnemann discovered the fact that there existed a dynamic, vital principle in all drugs, a curative force, peculiar and individual and distinctive of each drug, that could be *practically* transferred to some medicinally inert substance and preserved indefinitely. This is not saying that it becomes separated from its material basis, but the particles of this material envelope, if present at all, must be capable of a sub-division infinitely beyond that accepted by modern science.

A drug, as we perceive it, is the *ultimate embodiment* of a medicinal force, differing in kind and degree in every drug, and Hahnemann devised or accidentally hit upon a method, probably the only practical method of securing this inner, living, medicinal force for therapeutic purposes.

(*d*) The keynote to homeopathy is the Hahnemannian teaching of the *Dynamis* or vital force. Homeopathy eliminates material causes of most diseases, material dosage of medicine and looks to the *real* cause of all diseases in the *disturbed vital force* and selects a *curative remedy corresponding to all the symptoms expressing the disturbance*, and administers it in a *dynamized* form, one in which the drug is free to all outward appearance of its proper material envelope. This view of disease does not countenance, therefore, a removal of the products of a disease as a cure of the disease itself, any more than blowing and cleaning of the nose is a cure for coryza. Hence, the mere excision of tumours is no permanent cure of the tumour disease. We must go behind the local *manifestation* and cure the *condition which produced the tumour*. Local astringent injections do not cure a leuorrhea, although the discharge is made to disappear, cauterizing a chancre will not cure the syphilitic cause of that outward manifestation of a general infection, a sulphur or zinc ointment applied to a skin disease, or a corrosive sublimate wash does not *cure,* although the skin itself may be freed. These measures merely *suppress* the local and ultimate manifestation of the disease. Metastases (change in the seat of the disease) are sure to appear sooner or later and invariably more serious than the primary disorder. To be sure, the physician pronounces these, *new* diseases, and the patient submits to further suppression and palliation, but a *cure*, is further off than ever. It must be borne in mind, that it is a fallacy to believe that diseases can be cured by the *expulsion* of material morbific matters. They cannot be permanently cured in that way, though of course, the immediate symptoms of discomfort of the patient may be thereby removed. The physician's duty, therefore, is more than of a medical scavenger, expelling supposed or real morbific matter. There is no question that the loathsome, vile or impure discharges in diseases are effete *products* of the disease itself, symptoms of the dynamic disturbances within and as such guides to the selection of the remedy not to be carelessly suppressed, for frequently they are a relief of the inner more dangerous evil. By suppressing these outer manifestations, curative efforts of nature, possibly, metastases towards other and more vital parts are likely to take place.

6. THE APPLICATION OF HOMEOPATHY

Homeopathy consists essentially in the application of the principles of similars and the selection of suitable drugs based on those principles. The homeopathic physician has to deal with two sets of phenomena in treating diseases. On the one hand the patient, with a certain train of morbid symptoms, and on the other, similar symptoms known to be produced in the healthy by some drug. The closer this correspondence in its essential features, the more certain and speedy the cure, on the principle that two like and similar forces when brought together may neutralise each other. This necessitates the consideration of the following points:

(*a*) The examination of the patient and the record of the symptoms,
(*b*) The selection of the remedy corresponding to this totality of symptoms,
(*c*) The administration of the single remedy,
(*d*) The dose and its repetition.

(a) The Examination of the Patient

The first duty of the homeopathic prescriber is clearly to understand the nature of the disturbed functions of the patient, to get at the full facts of the case so far as they are expressed by symptoms. The examination that elicits them must be thorough and complete, and will yield satisfactory results according to the perfection of the physician's general medical knowledge. The *subjective symptoms*, that is, a description by the patient of his feeling as they appear to him or his sensations, are of paramount importance in deciding between drugs that are capable of producing a similar change in the organism and serve to determine the one most nearly indicated remedy from among a group of more or less related remedies.

The totality of the symptoms must be the sole indication to determine the choice of the remedy

The totality of the symptoms consists in the systematic ascertaining of all the symptomatic facts necessary to determine the curative remedy. The totality of symptoms include every state of body and mind that we can discover, or have observed, or that have been reported to the physician, thus, every deviation from health. It includes every *subjective* symptom which the patient can describe correctly and every *objective* symptom the physician can discover by his senses, or with the help of the patient's attendants. In mental diseases and in the case of children and old people who are unable to express their symptoms clearly, objective symptoms are of special value.

Hahnemann's teaching on this point is expressed in paras 18 and 70 of the Organon as follows:

"It is then unquestionably true that, besides the totality of symptoms, it is impossible to discover any other manifestation by which disease could express their need of relief, hence, it undeniably follows that the totality of symptoms observed in each individual case of disease, can be the *only indication* to guide us in the selection of a remedy."

"All that a physician may regard as curable in diseases, consists entirely in the complaints of the patient and the morbid changes of his health perceptible to the senses–that is to say, it consists entirely in the totality of symptoms, through which the disease expresses its demand for the appropriate remedy, while on the other hand, every fictitious or obscure, internal cause and condition, or imaginary, material, morbific matter are not objects of treatment."

Acute Disease

In the treatment of acute diseases, it is much easier to ascertain the characteristic symptoms more readily as they are easily observed, and to select the corresponding remedies applicable to the case. During the prevalence of epidemic diseases, colds, grippe, eruptive diseases, etc., it is often the case that two or three remedies will cover the field. It is unnecessary to go into every detail of the symptomatology, since the epidemic remedies, when found, correspond to the *collective totality* of numerous cases and types of the epidemic disese, each single case of an epidemic disease presenting only a partial picture of the true totality of the epidemic.

The following particulars should, however, be ascertained in every case:

(*i*) The immediate cause of the disease is the most important and should be taken into account, as this is responsible for the change in the condition of the patient, such as, exposure to cold or heat, or getting over-heated, or wet in rain, over-exertion (mental or physical) or great exhaustion due to loss of vital fluids,

(*ii*) Affections of the mind brought about by sudden emotions, such as fright, grief and sorrow, vexation, anger, sensitiveness or irritability,

(*iii*) Result of over-eating or eating of wrong foods,

(*iv*) Consequences of spirituous liquors, coffee, tea, tobacco, acids, injurious drugs in general use, such as opium, ganja, chloral, quinine, mercurial preparations etc.,

(*v*) Adulterations and poisons by medications, inhaling gases and introduction of foreign substances into the stomach,

(*vi*) External injuries such as concussion, bruises, sprains, fractures, burns and scalds, etc.

The remedy most appropriate to the complaint according to the symptoms bearing a direct relation to the *last* cause should be chosen.

In choosing the remedy, the attending circumstances should also be taken into account :

(*i*) The nature of the constitution of the patient,

(*ii*) The temperament of the patient,

(*iii*) Locality of the trouble,

(*iv*) The sensations felt by the patient, i.e., if it is a pain, whether it is tearing, cutting, beating or throbbing,

(*v*) The occasion of the trouble getting better or worse, according to the time of day-morning, evening or night, to the state of the weather, whether damp, cold or dry, to the position of the body, whether when quiet or in motion, whether before or after eating, after sleep, when touched, pressed, etc.

(*vi*) Note the combination of symptoms, if for instance, when coughing is accompanied with headache, or headache with inclination to vomit, or with this inclination, shivering, etc.

Next in importance to the *cause* which is the first, the conditions of increase (aggravation) or decrease (amelioration) of the trouble, and the temperament of the patient have a high place in the selection of the suitable remedy.

Chronic Diseases : In getting at the symptoms, especially in chronic diseases, the following special precautions should be observed:

(*i*) The patient should be carefully questioned so as to ascertain all important and outstanding symptoms.

(*ii*) Leading questions should not be asked so as to make the patient answer 'yes' or 'no'.

- (*iii*) It is necessary to pay special attention to the mental condition of the patient and his intellectual functions.
- (*iv*) The modalities, especially the influence of the times of day, weather, season, position of body, exercise, sleep, etc.
- (*v*) The apparent immediate *cause of his sickness–the first indication of a departure from health is most important for selecting the remedy*, even at a later stage.
- (*vi*) The family history of the patient, including heredity, is a potent factor in determining disease.
- (*vii*) The history of the patient's previous diseases, particularly eruptions of any kind that may have been treated with strong local remedies, and so suppressed, also to all forms of local treatment generally, and the patient's medical habits, the use of patent medicines, purgatives, mineral waters, etc.
- (*viii*) Any alteration of groups of symptoms, such as gastric and rheumatic symptoms, rheumatic and catarrhal, bronchial and skin affections, etc., should be noted.
- (*ix*) Remember that, when a certain train of symptoms are present in some organ of the body, there are almost sure to be present, certain other symptoms, objective and subjective, in other organs often, anatomically, quite remote, and of which the patient may not probably be aware until his attention is drawn to them by the physician. For example, certain pains in the head co-exist with certain uterine affections, or anamolies of vision, etc.
- (*x*) Functional symptoms of an affected organ are of much less value than symptoms which occur in other parts during the exercise of the function of that organ. Burning pain in the urethra, during or after micturition, is of little value in gonorrhea, for it is usually present, but pain in the testicles, thighs, or abdomen during or after micturition, or symptoms of some other part not immediately concerned in that

function would be more important. So also, pain in the stomach after eating in indigestion, is not of as much value as vertigo or headache after eating would be in the same attack. Therefore, *symptoms that affect the general organism are of more value than those that are functionally related to the organ affected.*

(xi) Some symptoms are primary, others reflex. After an organic disease has become established, secondary modification of health take place, which do not offer valuable symptoms for purposes of prescribing the curative remedy. *Really valuable guiding symptoms, if found at all, will be in the earlier state of the patient before the organic changes have taken place,* thus in the treatment of an organic kidney disease, a curative remedy would be more likely to be found in the earlier symptoms that preceded the development of the dropsy, anemia, etc. characteristic of the later stages.

(xii) *General* or *absolute* symptoms are those which are common to all patients suffering from the same disease and they are essential for purposes of diagnosis. Thus, the fever, physical signs and bloody sputa are general or absolute symptoms of pneumonia.

Contingent or *peculiar symptoms* are those which vary with the individual and are not essentially pathognomonic of the disease, *but alway of the individual ptient. They are, therefore, the characteristic symptoms of the patient's totality of symptoms and hence most essential in selecting the remedy.* Hence, the rule.

.-The greater the value of a symptom for purchase of diagnosis, the less its value for the selection of the homeopathic remedy and vice versa.

The seemingly unimportant, peculiar, contingent symptoms of the patient, though valueless for purposes of diagnosis, are

INTRODUCTORY

the chief guiding symptoms for the selection of the homeopathic remedy.

(*xiii*) ***Totality of quality*** rather than of quantity is the basis for homeopathic prescribing. In any caase of disease, it is necessary to discover in what way, that is, *by what peculiar symptoms, does one case of illness differ from every other of the same disease.* How does the patient's typhoid or rheumatism differ from the typhoid or rheumatism of every other patient? This *special totality of quality, or of characteristics will unerringly lead to the curative homeopathic remedy. This is the Hahnemannian similarity.* It exists between the *characteristic* symptoms of the *patient* and the *characterisic* symptoms of the *drug, and we must* individualise *each case* in order to arrive at this desirable goal, for the selection of the homeopathic remedy. This differs from the mere *pathological similarity* which consists in matching diseased conditions or pathological processes as determined by pathological anatomy. It adapts the remedy to a *disease* rather than to the *individual patient.*

(*xiv*) **Partial or One-sided Diseases:** The best rule is to be most painstaking in eliciting symptoms, and then make the best use of the few symptoms to serve as guides in the selection of the remedy. Although the remedy may be but imperfectly adapted, it will serve the purpose of bringing to light the symptoms belonging to the disease, thus facilitating the choice of the next remedy. Organon, paras 173 to 184.

Diagnositc symptoms of a disease, although of the least importance for the selection of the remedy, may be all we have in a given case for guidance. If so, the remedy corresponding to them can be chosen by paying *special attention to their modalities, i.e., conditions of aggravation, concomitants, etc.* For example, in dysentery, the tenesmus is an important, diagnostic symptom, but no guiding one to any remedy, since many medicines has this general symptom, but it attended with any modalisties or concomitants it may become a leading indication, for example, *Nux vom.*, the tenesmus and pain in the back cease with the stool, *in Mercurius Sol., they continue after it.* In this way, *a general symptom may become a characteristic one*, leading to the choice of the curative drug.

(*b*) The Selection of the Similar Remedy (The Similimum)

The Interpretation of the Totality

Having taken a full stock of the case and thereby obtained the totality of the symptoms, before prescribing the homeopathically indicated remedy, correct all hygienic, dietetic and sanitary errors. Often a change in the mode of life or abstinence from some hurtful article of diet will be all that is necessary. But after these things have been attended to, whatever symptoms remain will call for medical treatment.

Having obtained a record of the totality of symptoms, a winnowing process must be instituted by eliminating the *general* symptoms and interpreting the totality according to the relative value of the symptoms, and thus *individualising* the case under treatment.

In para 83, Organon, Hahnemann says :

"Individualization in the investigation of a case of disease demands on the part of the physician, principally unbiassed judgement and sound sense, attentive observation and fidelity in noting down the image of the disease."

Hahnemann's first rule here is that the characteristics of the case must be similar to the characteristics of the drug.

Para 153. "The more prominent, uncommon and peculiar features of the case are specially and almost exclusively considered and noted *for these in particular should bear the closest similitude to the symptoms of the desired medicine,* if that is to accomplish the cure. By this individualisation then we eliminate the general symptoms common to similar pathological conditions, and present to view the individual patient as the pathological process affects him. The morbid forces of the disease tendencies, hereditary or acquired of the individual, give us his peculiar and therefore characteristic symptoms."

The indicated remedy in any case is the remedy that corresponds to the totality of symptoms, as interpreted according to the relative rank of symptoms, and not one covering merely some isolated characteristic or keynote symptoms, or on the other hand, one that corresponds merely to the pathological lesion. The objections to the key-note system of selecting the remedy are its disregard for the full study of the remedy and elevation, insted of some minor often clinical symptom, yielding at best only palliative results, while the objection to the pathological basis is its incompleteness, being only a partial picture of the totality of symptoms and therefore and unreliable basis for curative prescribing.

The similimum is the most similar remedy corresponsing to a case, one covering the true totality of symptoms, and when found is always curative, and in incurable cases, it is the best palliative remedy.

Unfortunately in the present state of our Materia Medica, and other limitations or our art, the exact *similimum* in any case of illness, is not always discoverable. While this is the ideal to be taught, the prescriber must more frequently be satisfied with the selection of a mere *similar* instead. The experience and practice of the homeopathic school teaches that any one of several more or less similar remedies may be used with like good results, that is, it may be sufficiently similar to bring about nature's reaction. The merely *similar* remedy though falling short of the dignity of *similimum* is not thereby removed from the capacity of curative service, but the curative response is not as direct and prompt as the results *from the administration of the similimum* which must ever *be the ideal to be sought in every homeopathic prescription.*

(c) The Single Remedy

The *single remedy* is the necessary corollary to the similar remedy. It is to be given alone, and not alternated or mixed with any other. Only then can its pure effects be evolved and estimated, and the single remedy must be given in the *smallest dose* that will bring about nature's reaction. The single remedy includes all chemical salts which are composite substances *which have been proved upon the healthy* and an entity and whose pathogenesis is knows, and which can be administered, but unmixed with any other medicinal substance, so as to obtain its own peculiar drug force unmodified by any other,

The *smallest dose* prescribed by Hahnemann for acute as well as chronic disease was a single globule (of the size of poppy seed) of the 30th potency, given dry on the tongue, or dissolved in water and repeated in small doses according to circumstances.

Posology (Potencies)

By *Posology (posos-how much)* is meant the science of dosage. By doses are meant the quantitites of drugs that are required to produce effects on the body whether the body is in a state of disease or normal health. In order to produce the *direct* effects of drugs, a definite quantity within a certain range is requisite. This can only be determined by experiments and state of health of the subject. It is known as the *physiological* dose. Homeopathy discovered the fact that there is an oppostion in effects between very large and small doses. A teaspoonful of wine of *Ipecac.*, causes sickness and vomiting, while drop doses cure the same. This physiological antagonism between large and small doses of drugs is one explanation made use of in regard to the Homeopathics Law. The *Homeopathic dose* is, therefore, necessarily *smaller* than the physiological dose, because the disease having already overtaken the body and rendered the affected parts very sensitive to outside influence, the curative dose has to be *smaller* in order to produce a beneficial influence.

Historical Development of the Homeopathic Dose

At first Hahnemann prescribed the usual full doses of medicine (*Ipecac.*, five grains, *Nux vom.*, four grains, *Cinchona Bark*, one to two drams), but soon found that aggravation would follow such dosage, if they were chosen according to the similar relationship to the diseased process. This led him naturally to a reduction of dosage, and as he obtained equally good or better result be kept on decreasing the amount. Finally, he hit upon the process of 'Dynamization' which he considered as "among the greatest discoveries of the age." In this connection, Hahnemann distinguishes carefully between *dilutions or attenuations and homeopathic dynamizations,* while the former are mere solutions retaining less and less of the distinctive *physical* properties, in the proportion in which they are mixed with the diluting vehicle, the latter is a real *potentization* of the medicinal force inherent in drugs. This he clearly teaches in the ' Preface to the fifth volume of his 'Chronic Diseases', as follows:

"Homeopathic *dynamizations* are processes by which the medicinal properties, which are latent in natural substances while in their crude state, become aroused and then become enabled to act in an almost *spiritual* manner on our life i.e., on our sensible and irritable fibre. This development of the properties of crude, natural substance (Dynamization) takes place as I have before taught, in the case of dry substances, by means of trituration in a mortal, but in the case of fluid substances, by means of shaking or succussion which is also a trituration. These preparations cannot be simply designated as solutions, although every preparation of this kind in order that it may be raised to a higher potency i.e., in order that the medicinal properties still latent within may be yet further awakened and developed, *must first undergo a further attenuation, in order that the trituration or succussion may enter still jurther into the very essence of the medicinal substance, and may thus also liberate and expose the more subtle part of the medicinal powers that lie hidden more deeply,* which could not be effected by any amount of trituration and succussion of the substances in their concentrated form."

For a quarter of a century, Hahnemann gave his remedies in varying potencies from the first to the 12th potency and finally fixed upon the 30th potency as the uniform standard for the dose of all remedies, and to be given in single globules saturated and subsequently dried.

Hahnemann's Latest Method

Hahnemann advised that a single dose of a well-selected homeopathic medicine should always be allowed first fully to expend its action, before a new medicine is given or the same one repeated. As the single dose required a long time to effect a cure, especially in more chronic cases, he thought it necessary to reduce this period and so during the last years of his life, he devised a new method by which this difficulty could be overcome. In para 246, Organon (*Sixth Edition*) he says, "and this may be very happily affected as recent and aftrepeated observations have taught me under the following condition: firstly, if the medicine selected with the utmost care was perfectly homeopathic, secondly, if it is highly potentized, dissolved in water and given in proper small dose, that experience has taught as the most suitable in definite intervals for the quickest accomplishment of the cure but with the precaution, *that the degree of every dose deviates somewhat from the preceding and following* in order that the vital principle which is to be altered to a similar medicinal disease be not aroused to untoward reactions and revolt as is always the case with unmodified and especially rapidly repeated doses."

Note 133 to para 247 (Sixth Edition)

We ought not even with the best chosen homeopathic medicine, for instance, one pellet of the same potency that was beneficial at first, to let the patient have a second or third dose, taken dry. In the same way, if the medicine was dissolved in water, and the first dose proved beneficial, a second or third and even smaller dose from the bottle *standing undisturbed* even in intervals of a few days, would prove no longer beneficial even though the original preparation had been potentized with ten successions, or as I suggtested later with this according to above reasons. *But through modification of every dose in its dynamization degree,* as I herewith teach, there exists no offence even if the doses he repeated more frequently even if the medicine be ever so highly potentized with ever so may succussions."

Para 248 (Sixth Edition)

"For this purpose, we potentize a new the medicinal solution (the solution of one globule of a throughly potentized medicine in 7 to 8 tablespoonfuls of water, with 8, 10, 12 succession) from which we give the patient one or (increasingly) several teaspoonful doses, in long lasting diseases, daily or every second day, in acute disease every two to six hours, and in very urgent cases every hour or oftener. Thus, in chronic disease, every correctly chosen homeoathic medicine, even those whose action is of long duration, may be repeated daily for months with ever increasing success. If the solution is used up (in seven to fifteen days) it is necessary to add to the next solution of the same medicine, if still indicated, one or (though rarely) several pellets of a higher potency with which we continue, so long as the patient experiences continued improvement without encountering one or another complaint that he never had before in his life. For this happens, if the balance of the disease appears in a group of *altered* symptoms then *another, one more homeopathically related medicine must be chosen in place of the last and administered in the same repeated doses, mindful,* however, of modifying the solution of every dose, with thorough vigorous succussions, thus changing its degree of potency and increasing it somewhat. On the other hand, should these appear during almost daily repetition of the well-indicated homeopathic remedy, towards the end of the treatment of a chronic disease, *so-called Homeopathic Aggravations* by which the balance of the morbid symptoms seem to again increase some what (the medicinal disease, similar to the original, now alonge persistently manifests itself). The doses in that case must then be reduced still further and repeated in longer intervals and possibly stopped several days, in order to see if the convalescence need no further medicinal aid. The apparent symptoms caused by the excess of the homeopathic medicine will soon disappear and leave undisturbed health in its wake.

See also paras 269, 270 and 272 (*Sixth Edition*) and note 155 thereto, reproduced on pages 17 to 20 cont.

Adaptation of the latest method to Higher Potencies

The procedure prescribed by Hahnemann, as detailed above, was with reference to the potencies developed and used by him and his followers, the highest being the 200th potency according to the old method, and 30th potency according to the latest method, which is said to be several thousand times stronger than the old medicines. Although medicines continued to be prepared according to the old method, as subsequent to Hahnemann's time and during the past fifty years and more, most medicines have been potentized

INTRODUCTORY

to the highest degrees and are being used by physicians, the question naturally arises for consideration whether a change is not called for in the method of administration in order to attain the same results. Keeping in mind the main principles laid down by Hahnemann, viz., (a) that the medicine selected with the utmost care should be strictly homeopathic, (b) that the medicine should be highly potentized, dissolved in water and given in proper small dose, (c) that the subsequent dose, if the same medicine is repeated, should be in a higher potency than the preceding one, (4) that the dose should be allowed to act undisturbed so long as there is improvement in the general condition of the patient, it has been found from experience that instead of starting a medicine from a certain lower potency, and giving the same with modified potency daily after succussing the solution a certain number of times and continuing this process *for a long time* till some change takes place, and then using a *higher* potency in the same manner for some more time, it will be much simpler if the medicine is given in *three distinative* potencies, in the ascending order in the general series, on three consecutive days, as in that case, the combined action of the three dises is very effective and continues for a long time. Thus, in *chronic cases,* if a certain medicine in chosen, it may be given in a small minute dose in watery solution, as three doses, in three different potencies, viz., (a) in the *30th potency,* (b) the *200th potency and (c)* the *1000th* potency on *three successive* days in the mornings and these may be allowed to act for a long time till some change is produced. This procedure has been tried and found to be much more effective than the single dose in a high potency, or the daily repeated doses as recommended by Hahnemann, and is therefore recommended for adoption. The procedure is as follows:

For acute diseases, the potencies to be used are 6 (or 12), 30, 200 and in some cases 1M according to the age, susceptibility of the patient and nature of the disease. The 30th potency is suitable in a majority of cases and the 200th in sensitive patients. One or two globules of the size of a poppy seed (or No.10 as supplied y commercial firms) of the potency selected may be dissolved in one or two ounces of water and *after the solution is well stirred, teaspoon* doses may be given at intervals of two to six hours according to the nature of the complaint, *care being taken to stir the solution each time vigorously for about a minute before each dose is given in order to raise its potency somewhat on each occasion.* When the solution is exhausted and further quantity has to be prepared, it may be prepared in the same way with one or two globules of the same potency if the progress is satisfactory, and dissolved in one or two ounces of water and the *solution well stirred for a few minutes so as to bring it up to the same level of potency as it was when the last dose was used,* and further doses may be continued *with the precaution of stirring it up well on each occasion.* If the progress is slow, globules of the next higher potency may be used for preparing the subsequent solutions and the teaspoon doses may be continued in the same way *but at longer intervals and with the precaution of stirring the solution being observed continuously."*

For chronic cases, the potencies to be used are of the series 30, 200, 1M, 10M, 50M, C.M., D.M. and M.M.

To start with, one dose each of 30, 200 and 1M potencies may be given on three successive days in the mornings. One or two globules No. 10 may be dissolved in about an ounce of water and given as one dose after the solution is well stirred. It will be necessary *to wait on this as long as there is imporvement* and when the next dose is called for, it may be commened with the next higher potency, viz., the 3 doses will be in 200, 1M and 10M potencies.

In *chronic* cases of some years' standing, it may be necessary to commence with the 1M potency to start with. Longer intervals should be allowed between doses as the higher potencies in the scale are used.

Note: Medicines are now being prepared according the latest method advocated in para 270 (*Sixth Edition*) by the Sewa Bhaban Pharmacy, Midnapaore, West Bengal, from I to XXX Potency. I have had occasion to try some of these remedies in different potencies and have found them very useful. Those who wish to utilise the latest method with these new medicines are advised to obtain them for trial. One principal advantage with these medicines is that they can be repeated daily daily or on alternate days in small doses in chronic cases without causing undue aggravation of symptoms and steady progressive improvement is noticed in the general condition of the patient after using the medicines for some time.

(d) On the Administration of Medicines and the
Repetition of Doses

Homeopathic medicines are prepared in the form of tinctures, triturations, dilutions and globules. The globules are the most convenient form for administering the *minimum* dose as recommended by Hahnemann. He advises the use of "one or two globules of the size of a poppy seed" (which corresponds to globules No.10 as supplied by commercial firms) and his immediate disciples and followers were using two globules No.10 for a dose for adults. He advised the use of the medicine in watery solution during his last days as being most effective, two globules No.10 (or one globule No.20) may be dissolved in one ounce of pure distilled water (or pure spring water boiled and cooled) and may be given in repeated doses as directed. When *trituration* is used, the quantity required is half a grain or as much as could be placed on the point of a pen knife, which could be dissolved in an ounce of water. *One important precaution of be observed is that the solution in which the globules are dissolved should be well stirred before use, and should be similarly stirred vigorously for about a minute before each dose is administered.*

(a) *For adults,* in *acute* diseases, the doses will be one or two teasopoons of the solution, at intervals of two to six hours according to the nature of the disease, and in emergencies, at shorter intervals ranging from fifteen munutes to half an hour.

For very sensitive persons, one teaspoon of the solution may be mixed with a glass of plain water, and after it is well stirred teaspoon doses may be given from the *second* glass. Subsequent doses may be given from the same glass after the solution is *well stirred.*

In *chronic* diseases, one or two globules No.10 may be dissolved in about an ounce of water and after the solution is well stirred, the whold may be given as one dose. The three consecutive doses on three successive days should be given in the same way. In the case of sensitive persons, *one globule No.*10 may be disolved in about an ounce of water and the solution may be given in three doses at intervals of three to six hours apart to avoid aggravation. In their case, the second and third doses may also be given after an interval of three to seven days between each, according to their sensitiveness to the action of remedies.

(b) *For children suffering chronic diseases,* the doses need not be given in theree different potencies as in the case of adults. The indicated remedy may be given in single doses in watery solution and repeated at intervals of a forthnight to two months according to the potency used.

The 200 and 1M potencies will be more useful in their case. One globule No.10 may be dissolved in one ounce of water and after the solution is well sitrred, *one teaspoon* or less as indicated below, according to their age, may be given at one time as *one dose.*

INTRODUCTORY

For children between 4 and 12 years– Half a teaspoon to one teaspoon.

For children between 1 and 3 years– Quarter of a teaspoon.

For new-born babies of one or two months– *one drop of the solution.*

For babies of 3 and 4 months– Two drops of the solution.

for 5 and 6 months– Three drops of the solution.

For 7 to 12 motnhs– Four to eight drops.

In the case of babies up to one year, the doses should be regulated according to the sensitiveness of the patient, the quantities being reduced in the case of sensitive babies and increased for those not so sensitive. The medicine may be used in the 30th potency, except where any other potency is specified and if these don't help, the 200th potency may be used. One globule No.10 may be dissolved in one ounce of water, *and after the solution is well stirred* doses may be given as prescribed above, and repeated at intervals of two to six hours according to the nature of the trouble, *and the solution should be wellstirred every time the dose is administered.*

The doses prescribed above should not be considered too small as the effect of the homeopathic remedies does not depend upon the *material* quantity of the medicine administered but on its *dynamic or spirit like* action, and as children are very sensitive to the action of these remedies, the minimum doses required in their case should be in *drops of the solution* according to age.

As most cases that will come to us for treatment will have been treated with allopathic or other systems of medicine, it will be necessary to ascertain what medicines were given last and to antidote the effects of these medicines by suitable remedies before a true picture of the real ilness of the patient could be made out and a suitable homeopathic remedy could be prescribed. Moreover, as the patient's immediate troubles may be due to over-drugging with strong medicaments, the effects of these should be neutralised before the homeopathic remedies can have any effect. A suitable *antidote* should therefore be prescribed to start with, and should be given in *one or more* repeated doses in watery solution. After the effects pass away, the symptoms which then present themselves should be taken into account in prescribing the appropriate remedy.

In acute diseases such as asthma, diarrhea or inflammatory fevers, it is necessary to administer the medicine in *teaspoon doses* at intervals of one, two or three hours according to the severity of the symptoms and in cases of cholera, every fifteen minutes or half an hour, till there is a change for the better. Otherwise two doses per day (morning and evening) will ordinarily be enough.

In chronic diseases, in the case of adults, the indicated remedy may be given in three different potencies in the ascending order as explained above on *three successive* mornings, one globule No.10 being dissolved in about an ounce of water and given as a single dose. In the case of very sensitive ptients in order to avoid sudden aggravation, the *one* dose may be given as three doses with some hours' interval between each, and the three separate doses may also be given with an interval of 3 to 7 days between each. *The solution should be well stirred before each dose is given.*

After the first dose of every medicine it is necessary to observe closely what changes, if any, take place in the patient. In very dangerous and painful cases, we need only ten to thirty minutes, in other serious complaints one to two hours, and in chronic cases, from threee days to a week. The patient is then either better, worse, or the same. If better, nothing more should be given as long as the improvement lasts. In acute disease, it is favourable symptom if the patient *falls asleep* soon after taking the remedy, also if he feels *generally better*, though the local symptoms may not show any improvement. The improvement here is largely psychical, and will soon be followed by the necessarily slower improvement on

INTRODUCTORY

the physical plane. The mental condition and general behaviour of the patient, if more tranquil and natural, are among the most certain and intelligble signs of incipient improvement, especially in acute diseases. If a sudden improvement ceases as suddenly and the patient gets worse, then another dose should be given, the second dose may in some cases be followed at first by an increase of the complaint, but in a short time by a more decided and lasting improvement. If a complaint has improved from a remedy given for some particular cause, but if the same cause occasions the old trouble a second time, then *another* suitable remedy should be chosen for the recurrence of the same trouble.

When the patient after having taken the medicine once or oftener, begins to feel better even to a small extent, it is better to stop the medicine lest it interfers with the improvement, but when the improvement stops, the same medicine should be repeated but in *smaller doses*. In case the symptoms have changed, another more appropriate medicine should be chose.

A *medicinal aggravation* may be known by the symptoms becoming *suddenly* worse after the administration of a remedy. The *aggravation of the disease is general* and *progressive*, manifesting such symptoms as belong to the advanced stage of the malady. Should a medicinal *aggravation* be severe, it may be necessary to counteract it by giving an antidote.

Sometimes during the course of a disease, the action of remedies is interrupted by some extraneous circumstance, such as, errors in diet, taking cold and so forth. Whenever this happens, the interruption should be removed by appropriate treatment, after which the previous remedies should be resumed.

Another wrong and dangerous practice which obtains among laymen and beginners in homeopathy is the frequent changing from one remedy to another. If a remedy is hastily and wrongly chosen and two or three doses are given in quick succession, and if as a result the patient does not improve, that remedy is given up, and some other which has also no resemblance to the case is chosen and produces no effect. Thus, both the prescriber and the patient are disappointed by such hasty action.

It may, therefore, be laid down as a *general rule* that great care should, in the first place, be exercised in selecting an appropriate remedy, and after it is judiciously selected and administered according to directions already given, *it should not be changed as long as benefit results from its employment, or until a reasonable lenght of time has been allowed for its action.*

In the treatment of *chronic* diseases, the following additional precautions are necessary. Hahnemann's instructions are that the symptoms should be *written out* and arranged according to the rules given in order to obtain accurate knowledge of the possible indicated remedies and the selection of the most similar among them. This procedure ensures also a ready selection of the *second* remedy, since the record will answer all the necessary questions and determine the right course to be pursued.

(*i*) The first and foremost rule is to *wait and watch* further development, as the selected homeopathic remedy simply stimulates the vital forces to reaction and we must await results.

(*ii*) No further interference is called for when any one of the following conditions presents itself:-

- *Short aggravation of the symptoms.* This is a curative effect of the remedy, and so should not be interfered with unless the aggravation continues and the general condition of the patient is worse, in which case an antidote, *i.e.*, a homeopathic remedy for the latest symptoms is indicated.

Usually one dose of such an antidote is all that is required to modify the condition and then the case can progress without further interruption.

- *General amelioration of the symptoms:* This condition should not be disturbed by further medication. If the disease gets better from within outward, or from above downward, from more vital to less vital parts, the improvement is permanent and radical.

- *Reappearance of old symptoms:* The return of some of the older symptoms, if not too severe, indicates a curative action of the remedy administered, *if they appear in the reverse order of their development* i.e., if the *latest* symptoms disappear *first*.

- *Appearance of new symptoms:* If such symptoms come on after the adminstration of a remedy, they may be clinical symptoms of the remedy, and if there is at the same time *general improvement,* they need not be considred, as they will disappear. If they persist, the homeopathic antidote will soon rectify the passing increase of the morbid phenomena. Under all these conditions, no further medication is required. So long as improvement is thus progressing, it is wrong to change the remedy, or even to repeat the dose.

(*iii*) If this progressive evolution of the symptoms towards health should cease, *a further review of the case is required, and a new remedy should be choosen* when–

- the mental state shows an embarrassed, helpless state instead of the tranquility of improvement
- When no change of any kind follows, the first prescription after waiting long enough for reaction, which is, however, a variable matter, according to

the chronicity of the case and character of the remedy chosen, the shortest period to be allowed in chronic disease being one week, and preferably a longer time.

- When *new* and *important symptoms and old modalities especially aggravations that persist,* characterise the case, proving that the remedy was not Homeopathic to the case, and acted only as a pathogenetic agent in producing new symptoms. This is the danger of selecting a remedy only remotely similar, instead of the similimum. The second remedy will often be found a complementary remedy of the first.

Three precautionary rules of Hahnemann

Hahnemann in "The Chronic Diseases," has established three precautionary rules, which he has impressed in the most urgent manner upon the minds of his disciples, and which no homeopahtic physician can violate without committing the greatest faults in practice. They are–

(i) To suppose that the doses which he had recommended for every anti-psoric remedy, and which experience had taught him to be the proper doses, are *too small*.

(ii) The improper selection of a drug.

(iii) The too great haste in administering a new dose.

Precautionary rule No.1 Smallness of dose

Hahnemann arrived at the necessity for the minute dose after considerable experience and very careful observation for a number of years. In connection with homeopathic aggravation after large doses, he says *"If the original symptoms of the disease continue with some intensity in the succeeding days as in the beginning, or if this intensity increases, this is a sure sign that, although the remedy may be homeopathic, yet the magnitude of the dose will make the cure impossible*. The remedial agent, by its powerful disproportionate action, not only neutralises its genuine homeopathic effects but established, moreover in the system, a medicinal disease by the side of the natural disturbance, which is even strengthened by the medicine."

Finally Hahnemann observes in this connection:

"Nothing is lost by giving even smaller doses than those which I have indicated. The doses can be scarcely too much reduced, provided the effects of the remedy are not disturbed by improper food. The remedial agent will act even in the smallest quantity, provided it corresponds perfectly to all the symptoms of the disease, and its action is not interfered with by improper diet. The advantage of giving the smallest dose is this, that it is an easy matter to neutralise their effects in case the medicine should not have been chosen with the necessary exactitude. This being done, a more suitable anti-psoric may be administered."

This advice ought to be carefully considered especially by beginners, together with the warning which Hahnemann has expressed in the preface to his work on 'Chronic Diseases.' "What would they have risked, if they had first followed my indications and then employed small doses? The worst which would have be fallen them was, that these doses would have been of no avail. It was impossible that they should do any harm. But instead of exhibiting small doses, they employed from a want of sense and of their own accord, large doses for homeopathic use, thus exposing the lives of their patients, and arriving at truth by that circuitous route, which I had travelled upon before them with trembling hesitation, but the end of which I had just reached with success. Nevertheless after having done much mischief and after having squandered the best period of their lives, they were obliged, when they were really desirous of curing a disease, to resort to the only true method which I had demonstrated to them a long while ago."

(e) General Hints on Health and Diet

Disease

"Disease is intrinsic to the body, created by the body itself, through manufacture of acid, end-products of digestion and metabolism, ashes of the body itself, and the oxidative processes by which it maintains its activities. When these ashes or end-products are manufactured in amounts greater than can be fully eliminated, we suffer from retention of these, and a state develops that is variously called autointoxication, acid intoxication, toxemia, self-poisoning, expressing this manufacture and retention of these irritating end products.

How to Maintain Perfect Health

If you eat those foods required by the body for replenishing, in their natural form, as far as possible, if you take those of unrefined character, that chiefly appeal to you sense of taste and enjoyment, if you combine these with the respect to their chemical requirements, then even if you do neglect exercise, sun, air, rest, play, you can keep normal health.

How we Depart from Health

By far the greatest share of these acids develop from the wrong type of foods, or the wrong combinations of even the right types, so acid accumulation is very largely a matter of what we eat, and how we combine them.

Protein foods, such as, meat, fish and cheese, when oxidized, leave behind the greatest amount of the most irritating debris, and we need to little of this class of foods that it is easy to overdo our needs. When we eat so much more than what we need, this excess protein does not reach the form of its final ash, urea, but stops as a sub-oxidation ash, a partially converted or imperfectly consumed ash represented by very acid and very irritating salts, such as, uric acid, acid urates, xanthin, hypo-xanthin, creatine, creatinin and a host of others.

Another cause for the departure from health is the very free use of the refined and thoroughly denatured things, such as, white flour preparations, *white sugar,* refined starches or sugars of any kind. These are acid-forming in high degree and do not leave behind, in the system, enough of the natural alkaline elements necessary for normal health.

The *third* source of acid formation is the wrong selection of foods, and their wrong combination.

When we eat natural foods in their natural form, we are not troubled with acid formation, as nature balances these foods nicely for our digestive ability. Anything that depletes our alkaline reserve depletes our functional activity.

All the vegetables, all the fruits, some of the nuts, all the raw vegetable salads, leave behind an alkaline ash or base, while all the starches and also the sugars, as well as the concentrated proteins, the meats, eggs, fish and cheese leave behind an acid ash. Therefore, the more we eat of the vegetables, salads and fruits, and the less we eat of the proteins and starches, the concentrated foods, the easier is it to maintain a competent alkaline reserve.

Balancing the Diet

"The proper proportion of acid-forming foods to base forming foods is two parts of the former, to eight parts of the latter. Four-fifths of the daily foods should therefore consist of the base-forming things, the vegetables, raw salads, fresh fruits. With this class can be combined either milk or butter milk."

(*Quoted from Dr. W.H. Hay in "A New Health Era"*)

Food Combinations

A correct food combination is essential, because unfavourable food combinations cause still graver disorders, such as hypertension, Bright's disease, Diabetes, Acidosis, and a host of other disorders. We may consider the reasons for observing a plan of food combination. It is a physiological certainty that foods like breads, chapaties, rice, oat-meal, cakes, potatoes, puddings, sweets, sugars– the carbohydrates require an alkaline environment at every step of their digestive process, acid encourages fermentation of these foods. It is equally a physiological fact that foods of the protein class, as fish, meat, eggs, and cheese require an acid solution to initiate their first separation into simpler units. For this purpose, the stomach produces a strongly hydrochloric acid fluid whenever concentrated proteins enter thats organ. When other non-concentrated protein foods form part of the meal, a much weaker hydrochloric acid fluid is secreted. For a carbohydrate meal, no free hydrochloric acid is produced.

Protein foods require a strongly acid stomach digestive fluid for their reduction, and these same protein foods leave a very acid ash in the blood, after they have been split up by the digestive process. Therefore, it is inadvisable combining at the same meal, such other highly acid-ash-forming foods, such as bread, rice, macaroni and puddings.

The best combination always with proteins is green vegetables, both cooked and raw, as salads. Tomatoes go well with proteins, as to citrus fruits but not the sweet fruits. Cereal foods may be comined at the same meal with cream, butter, butter-milk, or curds, sweet fruits, or green vegetables. They should not be taken at the same meal with acid fruits, nor with concentrated protein foods, as meat and eggs.

INTRODUCTORY

(f) Diet And Other Restrictions During Treatment

The following instructions should be followed in regard to the administration of medicines and the restrictions about diet during the treatment.

(*i*)   All medicines should be taken early in the morning on an empty stomach. In acute conditions, it may be taken half an hour before or two hours after any food or drink. In chronic cases, one hour's interval may be allowed before any food or drink is take. During this time the patient should have rest from any active physical or mental work, but should not sleep.

(*ii*) It is of the utmost importance that the food taken should be *light,* of *easy digestion and nutrition* and in quantities just sufficient to satisfy hunger. It is better always to wait until the patient has some desire for food and calls for it, for then its judicious administration will afford valuable assistance in his restoration from disease. Food should on no account be forced on the patient in a routine manner much against his will. It must be remembered that one important reason why certain articles are prohibited and the use of others are restricted is that the homeopathic remedies are given in such small doses and are so powerful in action, that nothing should be taken which by their chemical or medicinal action may disturb the normal action of these remedies and neutralise good effects which they may otherwise produce. In order to obtain quick relief and permanent results, it is absolutely necessary that the restrictions mentioned here should be rigidly observed.

(*iii*) The following are prohibited while the homeopathic medicines are being taken:

- *Coffee* in any form, *strong tea*, aerated water, camphor, flavouring essences, strongly smelling flowers, perfumes of all kinds, sandal, scented or medicated soaps, scented sticks or smokes, strongly scented hair oils, or pomades, tooth pastes and tooth powders containing chalk or any medicinal substances, chunam with betel leaves, spices, such as masalas, cardamoms, cloves, nutmeg, cinnamon bark, saffron and asafoetida.

- Onions and garlic, radish, pickles and all vegetables with bitter taste,
- All kinds of medicines, medicinal foods, tonics, disinfectants, such as phenyle in lavatories and naphthalene,
- All external medications, ointments, plasters, etc.
- Medicinal herbs or vegetables, castor oil, and all saline or mercurial purgatives or salts.

(*iv*)   The following are allowed:

- In place of coffee, cocoa, ovaltine, Bourne-Vita, oats porridge, Instant Postum cereal coffee, such as Ragi malt, wheat or whole-green gram, gently fried in an earthen pot to a brown color and converted into powder, or any form of conjee prepared out of broken wheat or rice may be used. Very light or weak tea may be used but even this should not be taken frequently and is *better* avoided in chronic troubles.
- For cleaning the teeth, powdered charcoal, or charred paddy husk, or finely powdered bark of babul or gum tree, mixed with table salt may be used. Plain table salt may also be used. Tooth brush may be used with water after cleaning the teeth as above.
- For the hair, *unscented or unmedicated,* plain coconuts, or other oil may be used. In place of

INTRODUCTORY

perfumed, or medicated soaps, (such as carbolic soap, cuticura soap, sandal soap, etc.) plain soaps such as glycerine soap, Godrej toilet soap No.2, Turkish Bath soap or Tata's Hamam Soap may be used.

- If one is accustomed to the use of tobacco in any form, it is better if it is used in moderation or avoided altogether, but none should be used within three hours of taking any medicine.

(g) General Instructions About Diet

The following general hints, as regards proper diet, are applicable for all persons who wish to maintain normal health. In the case of person who are suffering from particular diseases, foods or other articles which are objectionable and should be avoided are specifically indicated.

(*i*) All articles prepared with Bengal gram flour (Besan) should be taken to a limited extent by persons in normal health as they are indigestible in a high degree, but should be avoided completely by those having digestive troubles.

(*ii*) Milk and milk products such as cream, ghee, etc. should be reduced in quantity by all after a certain age, and avoided when their digestion is poor.

(*iii*) White sugar should be avoided generally as it causes irritation in the stomach and is not easily assimilated. Jaggery or brown sugar has better food value and should always be preferred. Honey which is nature's sugar has a tonic effect on the system generally and may always be taken with great advantage by every one and especially by those in weak health.

(*iv*) *Coffee* and *tea* should be avoided by every one as they are *merely stimulants and have no food value,* and if used continuously and without limit of quantity during youth, will bring about nervous depression, and various other disorders in the system, such as diabetes, dyspepsia, nervous debility, kidney and bladder troubles, and high blood pressure in later age, and a general decline in health will naturally follow which it will be hard to retrieve.

(v) *White bread* prepared out of flour from which bran has been removed, and all strong spices and condiments which stimulate the system and cause constipation, should be avoided.

(vi) The hours for meals should be regular in order to help the movement of the bowels regularly.

(vii) You should take plenty of time to eat, and *chew you food slowly as chewing stimulates the salivary glands* and helps the free flow of saliva which promotes digestion and *stimulates the action of the colon in pushing the residues along more feely.* Milk should also be taken in *small quantities* and swallowed *slowly* to enable it to be digested properly–that is, to put it more vividly, *milk should be eaten but not drunk.*

(viii) Foods prepared out of *whole* grain should be eaten, i.e., milled rice from which the outer bran is removed in the process of polishing should not be eaten because this has no nourishing elements to give strength, but *hand pounded rice (preferably parboiled rice)* which is merely pounded but not polished further, should be used instead. Cereals should also be used with their outer skin on, of all purposes, as the essential salts which they contain make them easily digestible and give the necessary nutriment to the constitution.

(ix) Plenty of tomatoes, greens and fresh vegetables which are cooked or boiled and without the essential liquid in which

INTRODUCTORY

they were cooked being removed, should be eaten as these contain the natural salts, not only for giving strength to the body but also to supply the necessary roughage for the free movement of the bowels. Potatoes and other root vegetables should be boiled along with the skin as in this process the essential salts are absorbed by them, and the potatoes should be eaten with the skin in order to make them easily digestible and to avoid gas trouble.

(x) Articles *fried* in ghee or other oils should be avoided by those who suffer from chronic digestive troubles.

(xi) Butter-milk may be taken freely by all who can do so without any discomfort.

(xii) Plenty of open air exercise of some kind is essential for good health.

For dyspeptics. *Foods to be wholly avoided:* All articles *fried* in ghee, or oils, all articles prepared with Bengal gram flour or dehusked wheat without bran, milk or milk products, roots growing underground, coffee or tea, white sugar or sweets prepared out of it. *Foods which may be taken*: All articles boiled or cooked in water or steam, butter-milk and its products in place of milk, greens, tomatoes (raw or boiled) and all other tender vegetable which are easily disgestible, parboiled rice in preference to raw rice.

Diabetics. *Foods to be wholly avoided:* Coffee, tea cocoa, sugar, sweet fruits, honey, saccharine, potatoes, plantain and other vegetables containing starch, pickles, condiments, alcoholic drinks, meats. The common use of saccharine tablets by Diabetic patients is a dangerous practice. It is a laboratory product of coal-tar and contains sugar in a concentrated form. It is highly irritating to the digestive system and is much more harmful in the long run then even ordinary sugar and should, therefore, be strictly avoided. *Foods* *which may be taken:* Milk and milk products in limited quantities, butter-milk in plenty, nuts, peas, beans and lentils, tomatoes (raw or boiled), greens and fresh vegetables.

Chronic constipation. The following instructions will be useful for those suffering from chronic constipation:

(*i*) The meals must be regular to make the movement of the bowels regular. Don't miss a meal. If nothing else is available at the time, drink a cup of butter-milk and eat also, if possible, one or two oranges or plantains (bananas).

(*ii*) Eat fresh sprouted green gram raw (not boiled) on empty stomach in the morning or with each meal.

(*iii*) Eat plenty of tomatoes (raw or boiled), green, fresh vegetables, plantains (bananas), dates, figs and prunes.

(*iv*) Drink a glass of cold water at bed time, on rising in the morning and every time the bladder is emptied.

(*v*) Never neglect a 'call'. Visit the latrine at least once a day even at some inconvenience. It may be better to attempt this after taking some food or drink, or after meals. Deep pressure just above the left groin often aids the free movement of the bowels.

(*vi*) Every morning and evening lie on the back and raise the extended legs as high as you can up to forty times, or take a long morning walk after drinking a glass of cold water.

(*vii*) Take a bath in cold water every morning.

(*viii*) Avoid all laxative or purgative medicines or salts, herbs and mineral waters, as they merely irritate the bowels and force an evacuation and so make the constipation worse therefore and create the necessity for a continuous use of the same medicines by force of regular habit.

Skin diseases. *Articles to be avoided*: Chillies in any form, mustard, much of sugar or articles prepared out of sugar, too much of salt in food, and vegetables like brinjals which produce heat in the system. For external application, gingelly or Sessamum oil should be avoided as it causes much irritation to the skin, coconut oil should be applied for washing as they irritate the skin and keep it dry. Green-gram powder being preferable may be used instead. *Articles which may be used:* Pepper may be substituted for chillies and jeera (cumin seed) for mustard. Green gram dhal is preferable to the common dhal (Thuvarai dhal) when it can be had. Butter-milk may be used liberally and so also tomatoes, greens and other vegetables.

Diarrhea and Dysentery. Milk should be used sparingly unless there is fever also at the same time. Light conjee prepared out of broken parboiled rice or sago with butter-milk is alway preferable. In the case of children either light conjee without milk or with whey may be used.

Headaches. As the coffee and tea habit is largely responsible for this trouble, they should be omitted. Acid fruit juice such as lemon juice may be taken in a little hot water for relief.

High blood-pressure. To be avoided. Tea, coffee, tobacco, condiments and fresh foods and eggs should be avoided. Salt should be reduced as far as possible and is better avoided when the pressure is high. *Foods which may be taken:* Low but nourishing diet may be taken with plenty of fruit juices. Potatoes and other root vegetables may be substituted for cereals. Fruits and greens should be taken in large quantities.

Epilepsy and Hysteria: Tea, coffee, mustard, pepper, chillies and condiments of all sorts, pickles, and meat foods should be avoided. It is best to avoid salt altogether and reduce the sugar. Over-eating should also be guarded against.

Fevers: Light diet such as conjee, prepared out of broken rice or sago with a little milk, butter-milk, or whey and fruit juices may be taken. *Foods to be avoided:* Solid foods of rice or wheat, pickles, condiments, much salt.

Chronic rheumatism: It is better to reduce the intake of the normal quantity of food temporarily and also substitute more of potatoes and other root vegetables in place of rice, wheat and other cereals, eat more greens and other vegetables and use acid fruits. Meat should be rigidly excluded.

Disorders of the Liver and Gall Bladder.

To be avoided: Tea, coffee, tobacco habit, the use of alcohol, use of purgatives of salts of any kind, high protein diet of any kind, much of cream, butter and fats generally. *Foods which may be taken*: Greens, and fresh vegetables, fruits and fruit juices, plenty of butter-milk, simple digesting food.

Diseases of the Kidneys, Bladder and Albuminuria.

To be avoided: Excess of proteins in foods, salt, mustard, pepper and other condiments, tea and coffee, smoking of cigars, and cigarettes, raw or insufficiently cooked eggs and meats of all kinds. *Foods which may be taken:* In general, *low protein diet,* greens and fresh vegetables, fruits and fruit juices, nuts, cereals such as parboiled rice, barely and puffed rice, butter, honey, butter-milk in plenty, ragi and green gram in limited quantity.

Appendicitis.

To be avoided: Meats and fresh foods of all sorts. This applies also to those who have had their appendix removed.*Foods which may be taken*: Greens and fresh vegetables, fruits and fruit juices, plenty of butter-milk, simple digesting food.

Asthma.

To be avoided: Tea, coffee, alcohol, vegetables which contain much of fluid content such as cucumbers and gourds, strawberries and other fruits to which they are sensitized, inhalation of various substances to which the body is sensitized, over-eating and especially eating after sunset, and particular kinds of foods which give rise to the attack. *Foods which may be taken:* Greens and all fresh vegetables which generally agree, all fresh and cooked fruits and fruit juices, tomatoes, specially useful, butter, butter-milk, all cereals especially those with unhusked bran which don't cause much flatulence.

During pregnancy.

To be avoided: Tea, coffee, condiments of all sorts, and all kinds of irritating foods and cravings for particular articles which have a bad effect on the constitution. *Foods which may be taken:* Simple, purely nutritious foods but not excessive so as to upset the system, plenty of milk, greens, fresh vegetables, fruits and fruit juices, and generally foods rich in lime, iron, vitamins and roughage. *For lying-in-women:* The food should generally be of easy digestion, moderate in quantity, and not stimulating. During the first two days, the diet should consist of conjee with milk of butter-milk (either of parboiled rice or quaker oats) bread, simple fruits, or fruit juices. After the third day, the quantity and kind of nourishment may be increased. Coffee and tea should be avoided absolutely.

The Study of the Materia Medica

Some hints on the study of the *Materia Medica* will be useful to the beginners.

The artist who has to paint his picture or has to carve in stone, studies his model until he feels the lines and shadows, and sees in his mind the image on canvas or carving in stone, before he commences his work. Similarly, the student of the *Materia Medica* must study a proving until the feels the image of the totality of sick feelings of all the provers, as if he himself and proved the remedy and felt all the morbid feelings of the provers. The doctor that prescribes for symptoms as they look on paper, fails to feel the weight of responsibility of the true healer. The physician that first places all the morbid feelings of his patient on paper and then ponders over that complexity of symptoms until he feels and sees what the patient suffers from, and next searches the *Materia Medica* till he finds the same image, will be able to cure the sick as Hahnemann did. This gives him the sphere of stickness either produced by disease or by drugs. This sphere is an important feature of the study of sick-making causes and cure. Through this study we discover the sphere of action of *Aconite Nap.* as it differs from *Sulphur,* of *Belladonna* as it differs from *Calcarea Carb.* of the natural successors, complements and inimicals. The careful study of each picture of sensations may reveal to the student the sphere of medicinal powers and curative possibilities, while even a wide study of Pathology may not reveal what we need in art of healing the sick. The allopathic doctor has to assign a name to every case of sickness expressive of the hypothetical and pathological condition, and sick physiology of the patient, which amounts purely to a generalisation, while the homeopathic physician has to individualise each case and record all the symptoms of the patient in detail. The sick patient has symptoms belonging to him as an individual, and so has every remedy in the *Materia Medica,* symptoms belonging to it exclusively. If we read the *Materia Medica* rightly, we perceive at once the characteristic symptoms of each remedy i.e., symptoms which are peculiar to it. They may be mental symptoms, or a peculiar kind of pain, the direction in which these pains appear, or the conditions under which they are aggravated or ameliorated, or peculiar concomitant symptoms, or the periodicity of them, or the

INTRODUCTORY

time of the day at which all or any of them generally appear and these symptoms all, or many, or some of them, show the reader of the *Materia Medica* in what particulars it differs from those having in common with it similar symptoms.

A few illustrations will serve to elucidate our position.

(*i*) We find a case of black vomit with putrid involuntary stools, with much thirst and restlessness, black tongue and great debility. The symptoms–coverer will at once read in this case *Arsenicum Alb.*, but the observing physician also finds that the patient is averse to being covered, and while in this case-taken from clinical experience-all and every symptom observable on the sick is to be found under *Arsenicum alb.*, the very fact that he objects to being covered, excludes *Arsenicum alb.* as the similar curative remedy. A truly similar homeopathic remedy which covers this important characteristic symptom has to be found. While *Arsenic Alb.* finds an amelioration from heat, and therefore seeks it, and desires to be warmly covered, *Secale cor.* finds a very decided aggravation from heat, therefore, dose not seek heat, but desires to be uncovered and seeks a cold room.

A further study of *Materia Medica* discloses that *Secale Cor.* is a true similimum and covers all the characteristic symptoms of the case.

(*ii*) A case of pneumonia presents itself, the characteristic pains and fever are present, the patient is afraid to move, because it aggravates the pain. The symptoms at the outset appear to refer to *Bryonia* as the suitable remedy, but on a further examination of the symptoms, it is found that the patient cannot lie on the painful side at all, and if he tries it, the pains become much worse, and this symptom is not necessarily present in pneumonia, but the physician has to find a similar remedy to cover this symptom also. From a further study of the *Materia Medica, Belladonna* is found to cover all the symptoms, especially aggravation from motion, and when lying on the painful side, and hence has to be selected though it is not indicated as a remedy for pneumonia, it works on Pharmacodynamics. And pathologists cannot explain why one patient suffering from pneumonia can lie best on the painful side, and another patient suffering from precisely the same disease cannot lie on the painful side.

Dr. Hering's advice on the study of *Materia Medica* is very valuable and may be quoted. This is what he says:

"The student should first memorize a few of the most characteristic symptoms of a dozen remedies. He should carefully go over an abstract of the *Materia Medica* and should find, say, of twelve remedies, the prevailing mental symptoms, the prevailing pains, the action on one or more ameliorated or aggravated, and finally the concomitant symptoms, he should now compare one of them with the other eleven, and finally, after having compared them all, he may become conscious of many strong characteristic differences in the effect of all these drugs. He now proceeds to make more comparisons between them and all their known sympoms. If a much easier task to acquire the knowledge of every next similar, and when, years after, he reads a new remedy, he will master it quickly, finding at once its characteristic similarities with other remedies, as well as the characteristic differences."

As regards the book on *Materia Medica*, which may be got by beginners, the most useful one of study and for obtaining a clear symptom-picture of each remedy, is Kent's *Lectures on Materia Medica'*. The best book to get the characteristic symptoms of each remedy at a glance, for purposes of memorizing and studying selected remedies of the *Materia Medica* as advised by Dr. Hering, is H. C. Allen's *'Keynotes and Characteristics'*. Nash's *'Leaders'* is a very interesting book giving essentials of each remedy in delightful language. Boger's *'Synoptic Key'* contains the characteristics of a large number of remedies set forth clearly for ready reference and has also a small repertory for ordinary use.

Boericke's *Pocket Book of Materia Medica* is a very useful book for quick reference, and contains also a comprehensive repertory, which will serve for ordinary purposes where a larger repertory is not available.

The latest publication is Dr. Margaret Tyler's *Drug pictures*. It is a very good book giving clear symptom-pictures of a wide range of remedies, with the leading characteristic symptoms of each remedy indicated clearly in clear type and includes also important notes from Kent, Nash and Farrington.

PART – II
TREATMENT OF DISEASES

CHAPTER – I

AFFECTIONS OF THE HEAD

1. GIDDINESS, VERTIGO

Giddiness sometimes arises out of disordered stomach, profuse evacuations, narcotic medicines, and falls or blows on the head, and at other times due to a general decline of health.

Nux Vomica and *Pulsatilla*, when due to disordered stomach.

Bryonia Alba, for vertigo with nausea and disposition to faint, worse on rising from a lying position and on motion, with constipation.

China, for vertigo associated with weakness or bloodlessness, also vertigo from debility, losses of fluids, etc.

Phosphorus, especially in nervous vertigo when caused by nervous debility, sexual abuse, occurring in the morning with an empty stomach, with fainting and trembling.

Rhus Tox., vertigo especially in old people which comes on as soon as the patient rises from a sitting position, associated with heavy limbs, and is probably caused by senile changes in the brain.

2. HEADACHE

Principal Remedies : *Bell., Nux Vom., Bryonia Alba, Ipecac., Mercurius Sol., Pulsatilla.*

Leading Indications :

Kinds of Headache:
- Congestive–Bell., Pul., Rhus Tox, Glonoine.
- Catarrhal–Nux Vom., Mercurius Sol., Arsenicum.

- *Rheumatic–Cham., Puls., Nux Vom., Mercurius Sulph.*
- *Bilious (Sick)–Sang., Bell., Ipec., Spigelia.*
- *Neuralgic (Nervous)–Coffea, Nux Vom., China, Cham.,*
- *Ignatia, Puls., Bry., Silicea, Sulphur, Calc carb., Sepia.*
- *One-sided–Bry., Nux Vom., Puls., Sulph., Sang., Spig.*

Caused by :
- Chill–*Aconitum, Nux Vom., Mercurius Sol.*
- Joy–*Coffea.*
- Coffee or want of coffee–*Nux Vom.*
- Fright–*Opium, Aconitum.*
- Grief–*Ignatia.*
- Mental exertion–*Nux Vom., Bell.*
- Sedentary occupation–*Nux Vom., Sulphur.*
- Spritis–*Nux Vom.*
- Suppressed eruptions–*Antimonium Crud.*, Sulphur.
- Overloaded stomach or Constipation–*Nux Vom.*
- Exposure to Sun–*Aconit Nap., Bell., Glonoine.*
- Suppressed menstruation–*Bell., Puls., Bryonia Alba.*
- Headache from constipation–*Nux Vomica, Bryonia Alba,*
- Pulsatilla, Opium, Ipecac. and Lycopodium.

Made worse by :
- Strong light–*Bell.*
- Mental effort–*Nux Vom.*
- Movement–*Bryonia Alba.*
- Noise–*Bell.*

Time of increase :
- Morning–*Nux Vom., Bryonia Alba., Ignatia, Spigelia.*
- Evening–*Puls., Bryonia Alba*

- Night–*Mercurius Sol., China, Sulphur, Silicea.*

Improved by :
- Closing the eyes–*Sepia, Calcarea Carb.*
- Bandaging the head–*Pulsatilla, Sepia, Calcarea Carb.*
- During rest–*China, Sepia, Spigelia.*
- During sleep–*Sepia.*

In the treatment of this common complaint, it is very necessary to enquire into the *cause* of the pain, as also the *complaints which accompany it,* and the *kind of pain* from which the patient suffers. As headache appears in many forms and arises from several causes, it has been divided under several heads.

(*a*) **Congestive Headache** : Frequently presents symptoms of an inflammatory nature, *a high excitement of the circulatory system*, face flushed, pulse full and quick, eyes bright and glassy or suffused and heavy, pain pulsative or throbbing, occasionally with beating noises in the ears, *great sensitiveness to light and noise, pain aggravated by moving, sitting up or talking.* There are also, at times, nausea and vomiting with coldness of the extremities.

Aconitum Nap., when there is violent throbbing, heaviness, fullness in the forehead and temples, with a sensation as if the head would burst, burning sensation in the whole body, congestion of blood to the head, with redness of the face and eyes, also when the pain is accompanied with *incoherent talking and raving, worse on moving, talking, drinking or rising up.*

Belladonna, especially when the pain is deep seated, is *oppressive* and heavy, and the face pale and haggard, *with unconsciousness, incoherent talking, murmuring drowsiness.*

Pulsatilla, when the pain is dull, oppressive, and affects *only one side of the head,* pain extending from the back part of the head to the root of the nose, *relieved by pressure, worse* towards evening, when sitting or looking upward, *better* by walking in open air, if the head is heavy, the face pale, with dizziness, inclination to weep, great agitation.

Rhus Tox., burning, throbbing pain, with fullness of the head, pain as if the brain were torn, tingling in the head, stitching headache, day and night, extending to the ears, root of the nose and cheek bones, when there is a *sensation as though everything in the head were loose and particularly when it comes on after meals.*

Glonoine, when the attack *comes suddenly* or *by exposure to the sun,* when the blood is felt rising up to the head with severe beating pain, almost causing delirium, and the throbbing headache is increased by the slightest movement, pain temporarily *relieved* by the application of cold water.

In this form of headache, the application of cold water in the form of wet packs is especially useful.

(*b*) **Catarrhal Headache** : Usually consists of a *severe, dull pain, and sense of weight* in the forehead and pain in the eyes, and is usually accompanied by a *sense of chilliness and lassitude.* In its severe form, the symptoms correspond to those under "congestive headache".

Aconitum Nap., pressing, dull feeling in the forehead, *better in the open air,* fever intermixed with chills, running in the eyes and nose.

Nux Vomica and Mercurius Sol., often useful for headaches which *accompany epidemic catarrh or influenza,* and when there is pressing pain in the forehead and over the roots of the nose, with constant sneezing and running of the nose, heaviness of the head, especially in the forehead.

Arsenicum Alb., throbbing pain in the forehead, *with excessive discharge of an acrid, burning water from the nose,*

AFFECTIONS OF THE HEAD

also with hoarseness and restlessness, buzzing in the ears, with hardness of hearing, as though the ears were stopped, pains are *aggravated by other people's talking*, and *relieved by external warmth*.

Most of the cases can be cured with *Arsenicum Alb.* or *Nux Vomica* and with the 200th potency.

(c) **Rheumatic Headache** : It is usually complicated with similar pains in other parts of the body down the neck, for instance, and into the shoulders. The pain in the head is heavy, distracting or aching and attended with a sense of coldness, sometimes accompanied by congestive symptoms.

Chamomilla is the best remedy when the rheumatic pains in the head which change their seat frequently have been excited by suppressed perspiration, tearing pains in one side of the head which extend down into the jaw, tearing and stinging ear-ache.

When *Chamomilla* fails, give *Pulsatilla* or *Nux Vomica,* the latter especially when there are shooting pains in the side of the head, head painful externally, worse in the open air or when stooping.

Mercurius Sol., burning or shooting pains which extend into the face, teeth and ears, *worse in bed and at night*.

Ipecac., will be useful when the pains are gnawing and tearing and are *relieved by heat and vomiting*.

Sulphur, when there is tearing, piercing, beating *on one side of the head, particularly if it reccurs every week, with vomiting and desire to lie down.*

(d) **Bilious Headache** : It is attended with a dull aching or racking pain which moves from one place to another, there is, also, often tenderness of the scalp, the digestive systems is deranged, the tongue is coated, breath foul, and bowels are constipated, there are sometimes nausea and vomiting, flatulency, coldness of the extremities, pain in the eyes, the mental faculties are weakened, and exertion of the mind is irksome.

Sanguinaria, severe pain affecting right *half of the head* and attended with bitter vomiting, coming on early in the morning and lasting till night, with fullness of the head as if it would burst, pain *worse upon the right side and aggravated by motion, or by stooping forward,* pressing pain in the eyes from within outward, shooting, beating pain throughout the head, *headache attended with chills,* tongue coated, nausea, with empty eructations, inclination to lie down.

Belladonna, is the next best remedy when the pains are *worse on the right side,* when the external part of the head is very sensitive, the veins of the head and hands being swollen– *painful sensation as of waves in the head,* buzzing in the ears and dimness of vision. It is also helpful for the worst pains extending to the eyes and nose, in one side of the head, with a pressing, bursting, waving, splashing sensation, *increased by every motion, by turning the eyes, by a bright light, by every noise, the sound of steps, in fact by every concussion,* when there is a *jolting sensation* in the had and forehead *at every step,* or *on going upstairs,* also *when the pain returns every afternoon, and continues till after midnight, aggravated* by the warmth of the bed, or on lying down, *worse when in a draught.*

Also in pains which commence very gradually, changing into an acute pain, affecting half the head, sometimes piercing momentarily, but so penetrating and severe as to deprive the sufferer of his senses.

In the case of women, headache connected with uterine complaint, especially falling of womb, accompanied with severe pressing down.

Ipecacuanha, stitching headache with great heaviness, giddiness when walking, pressure in the head, especially the forehead, pains affecting all the bones of the skull, through even to the root of the tongue, coldness of the hands and feet, aversion to

AFFECTIONS OF THE HEAD

every kind of food, tongue coated white or yellow, nausea and vomiting.

In all cases of headache which commence with nausea and vomiting, and are accompanied with a bruised sensation about the head.

It may be followed by *Nux Vomica* when there are shooting pains in the side of the head, which are *worse in the open air and when stooping.*

Spigelia, pain in the *left side of the head,* with beating in the temple, which is *aggravated* by the least exercise, or noise, or even opening the mouth, pain in the *whole left side* of the head, in the face and teeth, also deep in the orbits of the eyes, headache appearing at a regular time each morning, increasing in severity as the day advances, shocks in the head when walking, pain in the eyes, especially when moving them.

It may be given after *Belladonna.*

In obstinate cases, when the pain is particularly violent over the *right eye,* piercing and boring, so that the patient screams, with nausea and vomiting, *worse* when shaking or moving the head, even when stooping, give *Sepia.* For the same pain on the *Left side,* give *Aconitume Nap.* and if no better after several hours, give *Sulphur* or *Silicea.*

In selecting a remedy, the following special indications may be taken as guiding :

Belladonna, if the pain is accompanied with great sensitiveness to light.

Spigelia, if there is great sensitiveness to noise.

Sulphur or *Aconitum Nap.,* if there is great sensitiveness to *all kinds of odours.*

Sanguinaria, if the pain is accompanied with great sensitiveness to the walking of others in the room.

Sepia, if the patient dislikes to be touched, complains of his bed, is very sensitive and made worse by thunderstorms, cold air, vexations, etc.

Note– As a general rule, the remedy which best corresponds to all the symptoms in a given case, and especially to its *characteristic* or *distinguishing features,* should be administered, no matter whether such remedy be found under the 'Bilious', 'Nervous', 'Rheumatic' or any other form or division of the disease.

(*e*) **Nervous Headache or Neuralgic Headache** : It is characterized by acute, excruciating, lancinating, or darting pains, at times, the pains are constrictive, or attended with a sensation, as though the temples were being pressed together. It is sometimes attended with dizziness, or a feeling of sinking down, also with great nervous agitation of restlessness, exertion, either physical or mental, is almost impossible, vision is more or less affected, the patient frequently seeing small dark spots flickering before the eyes. The neuralgic headache comes quite suddenly without any warning, unlike other forms of headache. The pain is usually *confined to a single spot, or a single nerve,* and is at times, so severe as to drive the sufferer mad.

This kind of headache is more common among those accustomed to coffee drinking, who use strong coffee and use it more frequently. As the headache is due more to this habit, it is advisable to stop the use of coffee while the attack is on and use the medicines prescribed below.

Coffea, pain as though a nail was driven into the brain, or headache, as if the brain would be torn, shattered or crushed, pain which seems to be intolerable, almost driving the patient mad, the pain is excited or aggravated by the slightest noise, a footstep or even music. For headache arising from cold, vexation, mental exertion or excitement.

AFFECTIONS OF THE HEAD

Coffea, may be repeated every half hour, or hour, and if there is no relief, may be followed by *Nux Vomica* or *China off.*

Nux Vomica, headache in the *morning* after breakfast, *worse after every meal,* increased by motion, or stooping forward, with nausea and sour vomiting, when there are shooting, drawing, tearing or stitching jerks in the head, *worse upon one side, especially after the excessive use of coffee, or wine, fits of anger or constipation.* Pain as though a nail were driven into the brain, or as through the head would fly to pieces, from a pressive pain from within outwards, heaviness of the head, with a buzzing noise and giddiness when walking, especially early in the morning, or when moving the eyes, shaking of the brain at every step, headache when reflecting, as though the brain would be crushed, face pale and dejected, when the pain beginning in the morning, grows worse and worse as the day advances. Headache from loss of sleep or long night watching.

China off is most suitable for sensitive persons, and when the pain is oppressive, and prevents them from sleeping at night, or when there is tearing in the temples, as if the head was bursting, boring in the top of the head, while the brain feels as if bruised, jerking, tearing, rolling and bursting.

Worse when stepping, at every motion, and on opening the eyes, *relieved* by lying down and remaining quiet, the skin is tender to the touch. For discontented persons, stubborn, disobedient children who are fond of sweets and have a pale complexion.

Chamomilla, relieves pains in the head which are *caused by* a cold, or by drinking coffee, when there is a rending or drawing pain on one side, extending to the jaw, acute, shooting pains in the temples, heaviness over the nose, or very troublesome throbbing, when the eyes are painful, attended by a sore throat or cold on the lungs, or a bitter, offensive taste.

It is useful for children, and also for persons unable to bear the least pain and are quite unmanageable.

Ignatia, aching or pressing pain above the nose with nausea, pain lessened by bending the head forward, pressing in the head from within outwards, boring, stitching, throbbing, tearing or shooting pain deep into the brain, sensation *as though a nail had been driven into the head*, with nausea, dizziness of sight, and pale face. The pains *relieved,* for a moment, by change of position, but frequently returning after eating or on waking in the morning, the patient is full of fear, inclined to start, despairs of his health, is irresolute, impatient and wants to be alone. For headaches caused by grief, fear or exciting news.

Pulsatilla, pain of a jerking, stitching or tearing character, especially when confined to one side of the head, and accompanied by giddiness, sickness at the stomach, dimness of sight, humming in the ears, or jerking, tearing pain in the ears, countenance pale or yellowish, and haggard, loss of appetite, no thirst, chilliness, palpitation of the heart, and great nervous agitation, pain as if the brain would be torn, or as if the head were in a vice, or as if the skull would fly to pieces, especially when moving the eyes, cracking or snapping in the head when walking.

Headache *worse* in the evening, or early in the morning in bed, *worse* in the evening, and continuing all night, *increased* by rest, or sitting still, but *relieved by being out in the open air,* and by pressure of a tight bandage.

It is most suitable for *mild* good natured persons, also, for headache *caused by suppression of the menses.*

Bryonia, great fullness and heaviness of the head, with pressive or burning pain in the forehead, worse when walking, with a sensation, when tooping, as though everything would be forced out through the forehead, pressing in the brain, either from within outward, or from without inward, external, tearing pains, which

AFFECTIONS OF THE HEAD

extend to the face and temples, jerking, throbbing headache or rending in particular spots, heat in the head and face, with red cheeks and thirst, dizziness and headache, tongue coated yellow, insipid or foul taste in the mouth, everything tastes bitter, nausea and vomiting.

The headache is worse when moving about, or walking about, or when first opening the eyes, *especially indicated in warm and damp weather, also for persons suffering from rheumatism. Rhus Tox.* will be useful after *Bryonia Alba.*

Silicea, headache ascending from the nape of the neck to the crown of the head, headache from getting heated, stitches in the head, especially in the temples, throbbing headache, pain extends to the nose and face, rush of blood to the head, scalp painful to contact, hair falls out, perspiration of the head in the evening. Useful in stubborn and chronic cases.

Sulphur, headache with nausea, nightly headache, feeling of fullness and weight in the head, especially in the crown, pain as from a hoop around the head, pressing in the temples from within outward, throbbing, tearing pains, with heat principally in the morning, with *nausea worse* in the open air, *better* within doors, it *returns* weekly, loss of hair after suppressed skin eruptions, ulcers, or perspiration.

Arsenicum Album for the same kind of pains, if *worse within doors* and *better in the open air.*

Sulphur may follow any of the other remedies, and especially applicable to chronic cases.

Calcarea Carb., for children and young people who have vertigo, which is *worse* when stooping, and it becomes dark before the eyes, particularly if *Belladonna* has been insufficient.

Sepia, for piercing, boring or throbbing headache, chiefly about the temples, or under one frontal protuberance, which pains at the slightest touch, compelling the patient to scream, nausea and vomiting, *worse f*rom the slightest motion, better when keeping very still, in the dark, with closed eyes, desire to sleep, which soon follows, and after sleeping for some time the headache ceases.

When water affords relief, it may be applied either hot or cold accordingly as required.

CHAPTER – II

DISEASES OF THE EYES

1. GENERAL REMARKS

The eye is the most perfect and beautiful optical instrument in the world, but, like all other organs and parts of the body, this organ, upon the perfect working of which so much of our comfort and happiness depends, is subject to disease and decay. Its delicate structure renders it extremely liable to accidents of various kinds, and diseases of various forms. For all these, Homeopathy furnishes numerous effective *internal* remedies which do not fail to give relief in every case, if correct remedies are administered and in time. The allopathic treatment prescribes in every case external washes, lotions, ointments, etc., prepared out of caustics or nitrate of silver, and it may be confidently asserted that these external applications have done more damage and permanent injury to the eyes in several cases than could have happened if they had been left alone with mere application of nature's best gift, viz., pure cold water which is an excellent remedy for all affections. As the allopaths do not realise that the affections of the eyes are really *external* manifestations of *internal* troubles and that internal medicines are required to cure them, it is difficult for them to believe that such remedies could exist and that Homeopathy furnishes them.

2. SORE EYES OF YOUNG INFANTS

This affection is very common among young infants, setting in frequently when the child is but a few days old. It is caused either by some irritating substance getting into the eye-soap for instance, when the child is being washed, or by cold. In such cases, the eyes may be bathed in lukewarm water and a few doses (one drop in solution) of *Aconitum Nap.*, or if this fails, *Belladonna* may be given three times a day for two days, and these should ordinarily be enough.

If the eyes are swollen and glued together in the morning with yellowish matter, *Cham.* may be given in the same way.

Mercurius Sol. and *Puls.*, when there are small yellowish ulcers along the margin of the lids and a profuse discharge of yellow matter from the eyes, with redness of the whole interior of the eye.

Sulph. and *Calcarea Carb.* in chronic tendencies.

3. INFLAMMATION OF THE EYES-OPHTHALMIA

Aconitum Nap. in acute inflammation of the eyes of any kind due to exposure to cold, especially after falling of any foreign matter, such as coal or other dust, or sand, wounds, or burns or operations.

Arnica Mont., for inflammation from external injuries.

Belladonna, suitable for much inflammation, dry, injected eyes, total absence of tears, the *intensity and violence* of symptoms are characteristic of this remedy, great intolerance of light.

When the eyelids are inflamed inside, red and painful, burning violently and the eyes can scarcely be opened, give *Arsenicum Alb.* But if they seem to be forcibly closed, or swollen, difficult to open, and the pain is more cutting, with the edges ulcerated and scabs on the outside, give *Mercurius sol.,* and if this does not produce a favourable change, give *Hepar Sulph.*

Rhus Tox., useful for inflammations with great intolerance of light, so much so that the *eyes cannot be opened at night, gush of tears on separating the lids is an important symptom.* The secretion is scanty. There is much pain in the eyes and spasmodic closure of the lids.

DISEASES OF THE EYES

Gelsemium, soreness of the eye-balls, giddiness and pain in the eye-balls, double vision.

Sulphur, should be given after *Aconitum Nap.* or *Arnica Mont.* in cases in which the sensation of smarting still continues.

4. CHRONIC INFLAMMATION OF THE EYELIDS– CHRONIC OPTHALMIA

Arsenicum Alb. of main importance in chronic inflammation of the eyelids from whatever cause, especially in ulceration of the internal surface of the eyelids with a sensation of burning, and the discharge also pungent and corrosive.

Sulphur and then Calcarea carb., should be administered after *Arsenicum Alb.* when the immediate symptoms have yielded, but a susceptibility to irritation upon the least exposure remains, or when the irritation of the eyelids continues without active inflammatory symptoms.

5. STYE ON THE EYELIDS

A stye is simply a little boil upon the margin of the eyelid. Styes usually appear near the great angle of the eye. They are quite painful, suppurate slowly and have no tendency to heal.

Cold water is injurious, a warm poultice of boiled rice flour and milk left on during the night is better.

Pulsatilla, is the chief remedy and the first to be used unless there is local irritation, pain and heat and there is some fever, when it is preceded by one or two doses of *Aconitum Nap.*

Hepar Sulph., increased swelling, heat and throbbing, to expedite the ripening and bursting.

Sulphur, to remove the tendency to *re-occur.*

Silicea, scrofulous patients predisposed to styes should be given at long intervals this remedy in the 200th potency.

6. AFTER OPERATIONS ON THE EYE

Aconitum Nap.–Principal remedy.
Ignatia–Violent pain in temples.
Rhus Tox.–Pains shooting into head.
Bryonia Alba–Pains in head accompanied by vomiting.
Thuja–Stinging pains in temples.

CHAPTER – III

AFFECTIONS OF THE EARS

1. MUMPS

Definition : The salivary glands are six in number, three on either side of the throat, and are named, respectively, the *parotid*, so called or being situated below and in front of the ear, the *sub-maxillary*, because situated beneath the sub-maxillary or under jaw bone, and the *sublingual*, that is under the tongue.

The function of these glands is to furnish saliva or spittle, with which the food, during mastication, is moistened, so that when carried into the throat, it passes with ease through the esophagus into the stomach.

MUMPS is an inflammation of the largest and most important gland in this group, the *parotid*, hence the name parotitis. It often prevails as an epidemic. When it attacks one child in a family, or a school, several others are pretty sure to be affected also, either simultaneously or in succession. It is undoubtedly contagious. It chiefly attacks children and young persons, and rather curiously it seldom attacks them the second time.

Symptoms . At the commencement of the disease, there are no marked symptoms, except the swelling just below the ear. The swelling generally extends from the parotid, where it commences, to the sub-maxillary, and even to the sub-lingual glands. Sometimes only one side is affected and sometimes both, one after the other. The swelling is hot, dry and painful, and very tender to the touch. There is usually some fever and the motion of the lower jaw is interfered with from the swelling in the vicinity of the joint. The inflammation reaches its height in about four days, and then begins to decline, its whole duration being from eight to ten days.

Mumps is not considered dangerous unless from imprudent exposure, the patient catches cold, or from any other cause the disease is thrown into the system involving some of the vital organs. In many cases, under these circumstances, the swelling above the neck and throat subsides quickly on the fifth or seventh day, and shows itself upon the testicles in the male sex, and upon the breast in the female, and these parts become hot, swollen and painful. Another dangerous transfer of this disease, but particularly rare, is from the testicles to the brain.

Treatment

Mercurius Sol. is the principal remedy, as it has a specific action on the salivary glands. The special symptoms are tenderness, salivation, offensive breath and threatening suppuration. It is always best to commence the treatment with two globules dissolved in one ounce of water, and teaspoon doses given every three hours till there is a change. A few doses will very often be enough to prevent further development of the trouble.

Belladonna, will be better, if, in the beginning, the glands are swollen, hot and red and sensitive to pressure, worse on the right side. The pains are flying and lancinating and extend to the ear. It is also useful when the swelling suddenly subsides, and is followed by throbbing headache and delirium. If the testicles are affected, or the breasts are swollen, *Pulsatilla* may be given, and followed after several days by *Mercurius Sol.* or *Sulphur.*

Bryonia Alba, sometimes useful when the swelling suddenly disappears, and brain symptoms develop.

Rhus Tox., when the swelling is dark red and the left side is affected.

AFFECTIONS OF THE EARS

Carbo Vegetablis, when the patient has a slow fever the *swelling becomes harder* and does not go away, or when striking in, it affects the stomach, also when *Merccurius Sol.* does not give relief in the commencement, also if the patient had taken much calomel. *If Carbo Vegetablis* is not sufficient, it may be followed by *Cocculus.*

Lycopodium Clav., also useful when the stomach is affected.

Hyoscyamus Nig., useful for the symptoms indicated under *Belladonna,* when it does not produce a favourable change in thirty-six hours.

Arsenicum Alb., when the swelling appears after malarial fever, or after suppression of scald head.

Pilocorpine (Jaborandi), considered as a specific and prophylactic for mumps. It has specific action for the metastasis to testes or mammae.

2. INFLAMMATION OF THE EAR–EARACHE

Aconitum Nap. for recent inflammation *from cold.*

Belladonna, rush of blood to the head, redness of the face, shooting pains extending to the throat with tendency to delirium.

Pulsatilla, is almost a specific remedy for this complaint, especially when there are sticking or tearing pains in and behind the ear, swelling, and a feeling as if the ears were closed. It is especially suited to the earache of children, and after the inflammatory symptoms have been controlled by the former remedies.

Chamomilla, earache from cold or *suppressed perspiration,* stabbing, tearing pains in the ears, *extreme* sensitiveness and irritability.

Nux Vomica may follow *Chamomilla,* if the pains extend to the forehead and temples.

Hepar Sulph., may follow *Belladonna* when it is insufficient, and there is throbbing and buzzing in the ears.

Mercurius Sol., after *Pulsatilla* or *Chamomilla,* if these are insufficient, and also when there is tearing pain extending to the cheeks, chilly sensation in the ear, *worse from the warmth of the bed.* When *Mercurius Sol.* affords partial relief, a dose or two of *Hepar Sulph.* will subdue the remaining symptoms.

Sulphur, if the pain returns frequently, is on the left side, or is aggravated in the evening or before midnight.

Rhus Tox., is very useful if the earache is caused by getting wet in rain, or by bathing in river, or by suppressed perspiration.

3. RUNNING OF THE EARS

This is a troublesome complaint which should be carefully attended to. Local application of all kinds should be avoided as they produce serious consequences. Even oil should not be dropped into the ear. The ear should be *gently* syringed out several times daily with warm water, and then a little fine cotton should be put into the ear to protect it from the cold air, to hinder insects from crawling into it, and to prevent the discharge flowing out on to the cheek. When the syringe is used, the ear should be pulled up and backward to straighten the canal and the nozzle of the small syringe inserted a short distance into the canal.

This disorder generally follows other causes and should be treated accordingly.

When it follows after inflammation of the ear, or measles, give *Pulsatilla* and then *Sulphur.* When it follows small pox, *Mercurius Sol., Sulphur* or *Calcarea Carb.*

When the matter discharged contains pus, give *Mercurius, Hepar Sulph., Pulsatilla* or *Calcarea Carb.*

AFFECTIONS OF THE EARS

When the matter is very offensive, *Mercurius Sol., Hepar Sulph., Lycopodium Clav., Pulsatilla, Sulphur.*

If upon a sudden suppression of this discharge, after local applications or other causes, the glands of the neck should become hard and swollen, give *Pulsatilla* followed by *Mercurius Sol.* or *Belladonna.*

If severe headache and fever are present, give *Belladonna* and *Bryonia Alba.*

If after such a suppression, the testicles begin to swell, give *Nux Vomica* and *Pulsatilla.*

4. HARDNESS OF HEARING

If due to great dryness of the canal of the ear or want of wax, *Carbo Veg.* or *Lachesis.* The passage may be moistened by glycerine applied on a little cotton wool.

If connected with running of the ear, give *Pulsatilla, Mercurius Sol., Sulphur, Calcarea Carb.*

If it is after measles, *Pulsatilla* or *Carbo Veg.*

If it is after small pox, *Mercurius Sol.* or *Sulphur.*

If connected with cold in the head, followed by sore throat, *Chamomilla, Arsenicum Album* or *Mercurius Sol.*

If after Rheumatism, *Bryonia* Alba or *Sulphur.*

If after Typhoid fever, *Phosphorus.*

If caused by suppressed eruptions or ulcers by external ointments, *Sulphur* or *Antimonium Crudum.*

If after piles, *Nux Vomica.*

If with nervous fever, *Arnica mont.* or *Phosphoric acid.*

If tonsils are enlarged or swollen and cause hardness of hearing, *Mercurius Sol.* and *Staphysagria.*

CHAPTER – IV

AFFECTIONS OF THE NOSE

BLEEDING FROM THE NOSE–EPISTAXIS

CAUSES: A slight blow, a fit of sneezing, or the heat of summer is sufficient to make the nose bleed. In young girls it sometimes comes on periodically, with or at the time the menses should appear, and frequently in fevers and many other diseases. A moderate hemorrhage from the nose is generally succeeded by a sense of relief. Bleeding from the nose in young children is generally harmless and may be ignored and left to work its own cure.

Very often severe hemorrhage may be stopped by getting the patient to hold his hands high above the head.

When the bleeding is caused by a fall, give *Arnica mont.*

When it is due to a rush of blood to the head, *Aconitum Nap., Belladonna* or *Bryonia Alba.*

If in the morning, *Nux Vomica* and *Bryonia Alba.*

If it occurs principally at night, give *Bryonia Alba* and *Belladonna.*

When it arises from over-heating, give *Aconitum Nap.* and *Bryonia Alba.*

In the case of children with worms, *Cina* and *Mercurius Sol.*

In females periodically, or with scanty flow during the periods, give *Pulsatilla.*

AFFECTION OF THE NOSE

For those subject to frequent attacks, give *Sulphur, Carbo Veg., Lycopodium Clav.*

In acute severe attacks, the medicines may be given in watery solution in teaspoon doses every ten or fifteen minutes. If the attack is not so severe, the doses may be given once in an hour or two hours.

CHAPTER – V

DISEASES OF THE ORGANS OF RESPIRATION

1. CATARRH OR COMMON COLD

This disorder which consists of an inflammation and consequent thickening up of the mucous membrane lining the nasal passages, occurs as a distinct disease, but it is also connected with the inflammation of the lungs, with measles, but more particularly with scarlet fever. As a general rule, exposure to cold is the exciting cause. It usually commences with shivering, some little fever, sneezing, obstruction and dryness of the nose. This dryness is soon followed by a discharge, more or less profuse, with watering of the eyes, pain through forehead and temples, as well as about the root of the nose.

Leading Indications

Early Stage–Icy cold : Cold subjectively and objectively. *Camphor* 6 frequently effective in arresting the progress of symptoms.

Feverishness, due to exposure to dry cold air: *Aconitum Nap.* Through the day, with frontal headache: *Nux Vom.*

Nose remains dry and obstructed, headache over the root of the nose persists and is aggravated by motion, lips are dry and there is much thirst, even after above remedies have been given: *Bryonia Alba.*

Second State–Running of the nose: *Mercurius Sol., Allium Cepa, Arsenicum Alb.*

Third Stage–Thick yellow discharge : *Pulsatilla, Sulphur.*

DISEASES OF THE ORGANS OF RESIRATION

Loss of taste and smell–Pulsatilla.
Chronic Cases : Sulphur.

Detailed Treatment

Camphor 6: It is useful only in the very first stage of a cold when there is icy coldness, subjectively and objectively, nose stopped, dry and pointed, the head aches in front, even throat. The medicines should be given in watery solution every two hours. If given promptly, a few doses will be enough. If this stage is passed and fever sets in, then *Aconitum Nap.* is called for.

Aconitum Nap.: There is feverishness due to exposure to *dry cold air*, chill or coldness followed by fever, heat and restlessness, headache at the root of the nose, not much running of the nose as yet, burning and pricking in the throat.

Nux Vomica: Another splendid remedy for the first stage of a cold. The nose is blocked, or *stops at night and runs through the day,* there is *frontal headache,* throat sore and very sensitive to *inhaled cold air.* The most characteristic indications is that the patient is *chilly on the least motion or uncovering* and even during the fever must be covered and keep quiet.

These three remedies are ordinarily enough for the first state. If, after these remedies, the nose remains dry and obstructed and the headache over the *root of the nose* persists and is *worse* on motion, the lips are parched and dry, and there is much thirst, *Bryonia* Alba follows well.

If the first stage is passed and watery discharge from the nose sets in, i.e., in the *second stage,* following remedies can be used.

Mercurius Sol.: Creeping chills, worse in the evening and night, even in bed, the nose discharges thin water with sneezing, watering of eyes, and sore throat, which *stings* and pricks, with constant inclination to swallow saliva which accumulates in plenty with a bad smell from the mouth, slight fever with *profuse sweat which does not relieve.*

Allium Cepa: There is profuse discharge from the eyes and nose, with burning, biting and smarting in the eyes, and *corroding the nose and upper lip* and is *worse* in the evening and indoors and *better* in *open* air. This remedy is particularly useful in children, when the profuse coryza or cold extends downward to the bronchi, with a *profuse secretion in the tubes, with cough and much rattling of mucus.*

Arsenicum Album : If the discharge becomes more burning in character, throat also burns, but is relieved by *hot drinks,* general relief from *heat* of room or hot local applications, great weakness and prostration, and all troubles worse at night, *especially at midnight.*

In the third stage, when the discharge becomes thick.

Pulsatilla: Bland, thick, yellow discharge from nose or some discharge from the throat, loss of smell and taste, or bitter taste, no thirst and generally poor appetite.

Sulphur: Cases becoming chronic with thick yellow discharge, or running into the chronic form with thick discharge of offensive smell.

2. COUGH

Cough is not a disease in itself, but rather a symptom denoting an abnormal condition of the throat or lungs. In fact, it is but an effort on the part of nature to remove some obstruction, or to throw off some accumulation which disease has created. During the course of an inflammation of the lungs, there is always more or less mucus secreted, and were it not for these forcible and violent expirations, the air passages would become clogged up and respiration materially interfered with. Cough is often combined with cold in the head, both originating from the same cause, viz., exposure to cold. In the

DISEASES OF THE ORGANS OF RESIRATION

majority of cases, cough is but a slight inflammation or irritation of the throat, or upper part of the windpipe, accompanied with more or less fever. In such cases, a few doses of *Bryonia Alba* 30 or *Nux Vomica* 30, will be sufficient to remove the trouble in a few days. But there are a great many *indirect* causes which produce coughs, such as elongated palate, enlarged tonsils, or they may be nervous cough, worm cough or stomach cough. In these cases, it is necessary to ascertain the cause of the trouble, and select a remedy which will cover the most important and largest number of symptoms present.

Aconitum Nap., generally *dry*, short cough with constant irritation, *worse* in the evening or at night *during expiration*, excited by dry cold winds, deep inspiration, smoking or drinking, accompanied by short breath, stitching pains, fever and restlessness, indicated in the first stage of all acute inflammatory diseases of the respiratory organs.

Nux Vom., dry fatiguing cough, seldom loose, in the first stage, *worse* after eating or drinking, mental or physical exertion, when lying on the back, when breathing cold air, and *early in the morning, better* by covering up or when quiet, hoarseness, with roughness or sense of rawness in the nose and throat, pain in head and stomach on coughing, accumulation of sticky mucus in the throat, is often the best remedy in the acute stage of common colds, especially if *Aconitum Nap.* has only half cured the case.

Belladonna, short, dry, hoarse, with little or no expectoration, excited by *dryness, scraping* or *burning* in the throat, *worse* in the evening and at night and *on lying down, better by sitting up*, eating or drinking warm things. Red, injected sore throat, cough connected with inflamed tonsils.

Bryonia Alba, predominantly *dry, worse on motion, eating or drinking, coming from cold air into warm room* and *on breathing deeply, better* by perfect quiet, pressing hand upon chest, intense thirst, dry mouth and lips.

Ipecac., sometimes dry, at others loose, worse on motion and in open air, better by warmth and quiet, fine rattling or wheezing in throat with large accumulation of mucus, loses breath with cough, nauses and vomiting with cough, whooping cough with nose bleed.

Hepar Sulph., dry and hoarse, at other times *loose and rattling,* wheezing, caused by exposure to dry, cold air, worse on slightest portion of body becoming uncovered, eating or drinking anything cold, *towards early morning, better* by covering or keeping warm, very sensitive to pain and touch, mentally irritable.

Antimonium Tart., predominantly loose, *coarse rattling of mucus, chest seems loaded with it,* accompanied by yawning, dozing and sleepiness, *worse* as the accumulation increases and when lying down, *better* on throwing out and on sitting up.

Phosphorus, dry, tickling cough, hollow, harsh, irritating cough, loose cough with expectoration, *worse* when entering a room, or going from warm into *cold air,* and *lying on left side, better* after sleeping, lying on right side, from cold drink and pressure on chest, accompanied by tightness across chest, aching pain in throat, and burning in back between shoulders.

Mercurius Sol., racking cough in the evening or *at night, worse* by dampness, accompanied by sore throat with salivation, bad breath, flabby tongue with indented edges, heat and *profuse sweat which does not relieve, can't lie on right side.*

Pulsatilla, dry cough at night or evening, after lying down, *loose* cough with plenty of expectoration of *bitter* or tasteless mucus, *worse* on lying down, and *better* by sitting up, and in *cool air.*

Sulphur, dry, short, violent, worse at nights, at other times, loose cough with *rattling and gagging,* expectoration greenish lumps, or sometimes blood mixed *with pus,* sputa offensive, *worse* by eating, talking, breathing in cold air, lying, and *better* sitting up, soreness in upper portion of left chest, weakness in chest, flushes of heat all over, burning in feet, wants windows and doors open.

3. CROUP

(catarrhal or diphtheritic)

It is divided into two separate and distinct forms, viz., Spasmodic or Catarrhal and Membranous or Diphtheritic.

SPASMODIC CROUP: It is almost peculiar to children and occurs during the period of first denition, i.e. about the second year. However, children from one to ten or twelve years of age are liable to it. Spasmodic croup from whatever cause it originates, consists in a simple, ordinary inflammation of the upper part of the windpipe, the larynx, with a violent spasmodic action of that organ. It is more common in cold, damp climates than in warm dry ones, and rapid and frequent changes of season, weather and temperature also cause it. The symptoms appear suddenly without warning. The child going to bed suffering from a slight cold and husky voice, is aroused from sleep before midnight with a spasmodic fit of coughing which is rough, barking and accompanied by a shrill, sharp sound. During the paroxysms of cough, the breathing is spasmodically oppressed, at times almost to suffocation. The face and neck are at first highly flushed, but when the paroxysms become more violent they become dark. The veins swell and there is perspiration on the face or the whole head. The voice, during the attack, becomes almost extinct. The attack may last from fifteen to twenty minutes, or from half an hour to an hour in the first instance, but is apt to reappear toward morning. If suitable remedies are given at the very commencement, the attack need not recur.

MEMBRANOUS COUGH: It is closely allied to and is often connected with the spasmodic form and consists of inflammation, generally of a highly acute character, of the larynx (upper part of the windpipe), or the trachea (windpipe proper), or of both, which terminates in the majority of cases in the exudation of false membranes more or less abundantly upon the affected surface. In this severe form, the child has croupy cough and hoarseness of voice for two or three days, and then the voice becomes weak and the child speaks or cries in a whisper.

Detailed Treatment

Aconitum Nap. is always the remedy in the beginning of croup. It generally occurs as the result of exposure to *dry cold air, attacking* the child in the evening or the first part of the night, with great excitement, high fever, tossing and gasping for breath, and with cough of the *driest* kind, loud and barking, and no expectoration. Two globules of *Aconitum Nap.* 30 in one ounce of water in *teaspoon* doses, once in 10 or 15 minutes, until the child becomes more quiet, and then at longer intervals until the fever subsides, will be all that is necessary in the beginning. If, however, the cough persists with a rough, croupy sound as of a *"saw driven through a wooden board"*, and there is hard breathing between the paroxysms, *Spongia Tosta* 30 is the remedy to follow, and may be given in watery solution in teaspoon doses every three hours till there is relief. If the cough becomes more rattling but still croupy, as if the mucus would come up but does not, and the cough is worse in the latter part of the night, or early in the morning, and all symptoms are made worse by cold air striking the patient, *Hepar Sulph.* is indicated and *Hepar Sulph.* 6 may be given in watery solution every three hours till there is relief.

In the first or inflammatory or spasmodic stage, if *Aconitum Nap.* failed and if the restlessness and fearful agony was displaced by a condition of great heat, but there was more of a semistupor, twitching and jerking, and delirium, *Belladonna* will be more useful. *Kalium* is useful in cases where *ropy mucus* is discharged from the mouth and sometimes from the nose.

When the violence of the attack has been broken by the foregoing remedies but there remains a tendency for relapse, the child grows worse again every evening, or the cough goes down in the tubes and lungs, *Phosphorus* is especially useful. It will often clear up the case, in desperate cases where other remedies have failed in both forms of croup.

4. BRONCHITIS

It is simply an inflammation of the mucous membrane lining the bronchial tubes. The bronchial tubes are formed by the division of the windpipe–trachea–and they lead directly to the lungs. Upon entering the lungs, they divide into two branches and each branch divides and sub-divides, and ultimately terminates in small sacks or cells of various sizes. The function of these tubes is to convey air into the lungs. In mild cases–ordinary bronchitis, or cold on the chest as we commonly call it, the inflammation which is only slight is confined to the larger tubes, there is little or no difficulty of breathing, moderate cough and slight fever, while in the severer forms, the inflammation extends down into the most minute cells, and all the symptoms from the beginning are of a severe nature.

The most frequent and perhaps the only exciting cause of the disease is sudden changes from a warm to a cold atmosphere.

First (Inflammatory) Stage

Aconitum Nap., chill with high temperature, quick pulse, dry heat and dry skin, great restlessness, *fear* and tossing about, short dry cough, after exposure to *dry cold air*, suitable for sanguine, full blooded subjects.

Ferrum Phos., suitable in delicate, pale or weakly subjects, not so much of the nervous excitability as with *Aconitum Nap.*, but the fever is very great and congestion to the lungs more liable.

Belladonna, follows when *Aconitum Nap.* has quieted the great excitement so far as the *anxious* restlessness is concerned, but the heat still continues, though there is a disposition to sweat on the covered parts. There are more brain symptoms, such as red eyes, flushed face, *throbbing carotids and delirium,* and especially if the child starts and jumps in sleep. One of these three remedies will either check the disease in the first stage, or modify its character as to call for one of the following remedies.

Bryonia Alba., still high temperature, great thirst, mouth dry and lips parched, short respiration, dry, hard cough, which hurts the head and chest, splitting headache, and all symptoms greatly aggravated on the least motion, wants to lie perfectly still. It is especially indicated if the trouble extends downwards, threatening the lungs and pleura.

Mercurius Sol., the whole mucous membrane catarrhal, but, unlike *Bryonia,* high fever, *moist mouth,* with great thirst, salivation, tongue flabby, showing prints of the teeth upon it, and offensive breath, profuse *sweat, which does not relieve.* The more the sweat, the more the suffering.

Chamomilla, especially useful in this stage, especially in children, if the heat is accompanied with profuse sweat on the head. The sweat is very hot while that of *Mercurius* may be cold or clammy. There is great pain and restlessness, child wants to be carried, one cheek *red and hot,* while the other is *pale and cold.* The disposition is ugly, nothing pleases.

If these remedies have broken the violence of the attack, but convalescence is slow.

Sulphur, may now come in. There is still some fever which comes and goes in *flashes of heat,* which passes off with a little sweat and debility and there are *faint, weak spells,* which may be generally due to a psoric or constitutional taint. A dose of *Sulphur* 30 will clear the case and effect prompt recovery. If, however, the

DISEASES OF THE ORGANS OF RESIRATION

case seems to settle down into a persistent form, it becomes the *second stage* and calls for the following remedies.

Second Stage

Hepar Sulph., loose rattling cough with choking or wheezing breathing, worse even on slight exposure to cold air, even if a hand becomes uncovered, cough worse in the early morning hours.

Phosphorus, throat painful with inability to talk, *especially worse* in the evening and *lying on the left side*, cough hurts and the patient holds the breath and lets it out with a moan because it hurts him so.

Antimonium Tart., almost always loose cough with much *coarse rattling of mucus* which is abundant, but the patient feels choked and cannot raise, particularly indicated in children and old people.

If notwithstanding the use of this remedy, the rattling and weakness increases, the extremities and breath become cold, and the patient gasps and wants to be fanned as hard as possible, *Carbo Vegetablis* will help in this case.

If the patient improves until the inflammatory symptoms are mainly gone, but there is considerable cough with loose rattling of mucus which needs clearing up, then *Pulsatilla* comes in.

Third Stage

Pulsatilla, expectoration green and bitter, bad taste in the mouth, appetite poor, patient wants open air or cool room.

If this does not do all that is necessary, *Kalium Sulph.*, which is its chronic, will do the rest.

5. ASTHMA

It causes spasms of the glottis, or opening at the top of the windpipe, caused by an affection of the spinal system of nerves.

The entrance of air into the lungs is entirely prevented by the spasmodic contraction of the opening into the windpipe. Difficult breathing is the first symptom, the inspirations are prolonged and laboured, the air as it passes through the narrowed opening, produces a wheezing sound, or the breathing may be momentarily arrested. In severe cases, when the closure is complete, the patient gasps for breath, the body is thrown violently backward, the face turns pale, the forehead is bathed in sweat, the nostrils dilate and the eyes are fixed and staring. It may be due to several causes, such as atmospheric changes, odours of different kinds–agreeable and disagreeable–smoke, dust, gases, metallic and other particles floating in the air, vapour of sulphur, also irregularities of diet, especially taking food in too large a quantity, or of improper quality, abuse of alcoholic liquors, the suppression of any accustomed discharge or of skin eruptions by external medication, over-exertion and mental emotion.

Leading Indications

SPASMODIC–*Ipecac. Arsenicum Alb.*

DRY VARIETY–Arsenicum Alb.

AFTER HAY FEVER–*Natrium Sulph., Ipecac, Arsenicum Alb.*

WORSE IN WET WEATHER–*Natrium Sulph., Dulcamara.*

WORSE IN DRY COLD WEATHER–*Hepar Sulph.*

WORSE IN ALL SEASONS–*Ipecac., Arsenicum Alb.*

CHILDREN AND HERIDITARY CASES–*Natrium Sulph.*

AGED PERSONS–*Arsenicum Alb., Antimonium Tart., Kalium Carb., Carbo Veg.*

DUE TO GASTRIC DISTURBANCES–*Nux Vomica.*

FROM SUPPRESSED ERUPTIONS–*Arsenicum Alb., Hepar Sulph., Sulphur, Psorinum.*

DISEASES OF THE ORGANS OF RESIRATION

FOR ANTI–PSORICS, ANTI–SYPHILITICS AND ANTI-SYCOTICS–*Sulphur, Psorinum, Silicea, Kalium Bich., Tuberculimum, Drosera, Thuja, Medorrhinum.*

Detailed Treatment

Ipecac, spasmodic form, *violent contraction* with rattling or *wheezing* in the bronchial tubes, seems as if would suffocate from constriction, worse on motion, and often accompanied with nausea or vomiting, expiration is especially difficult. The cough is constant, the chest seems full of phlegm, yet none is thrown out and the extremities are covered with cold prespiration.

Arsenicum Alb., has oppression of breathing as severe as *Ipecac,* but much *worse at night,* especially from 1 to 3 A.M, also on lying down, must sit up for fear of suffocation. It is also *worse* on the least motion, particularly on ascending a height, and is *better* by warm applications, warm air or room, accompanied with great *anguish, restlessness* and thirst for small quantities of water at a time. The asthma of *Arsenicum Alb.* is accompanied by general sweat, great debility, and burning in the chest. It followed *Ipecac.* well in chronic cases, and when the difficult breathing is habitual and *dry* and the patient aged.

Natrium Sulph., the symptoms are moist asthma, generally worse during, or brought on by change to *damp weather which is often the case,* there is also great rattling and wheezing, and the patient sits up and *holds the chest with his hands, as it hurts him so to cough,* the attacks generally come on about 4 or 5 o'clock in the morning, oftenest useful in the chronic form and also in children and adults who have inherited from their parents.

Dulcamara, is useful when there is much accumulation of mucus, and like *Natrium Sulph.*, is *worse* or brought on by *damp cold weather.*

Kalium carbonicum, useful especially in elderly people, where the patient has *to sit bent forward* to breathe, and the cough is decidedly worse at 3 A.M. *Anemia with baglike swelling of upper eyelids is strongly characteristic.*

Antimonium, Tart., is beneficial in the cases in which cough become very *loose, coarse rattling* with inability to expectorate, especially suitable for the asthmatic attacks of the aged, and the dyspnea of young children when due to lung affections. The sensation that the patient cannot get air enough is characteristic of the remedy.

Kalium Bichronicum, the attacks come on about three or four o'clock in the morning compelling the patient to sit up to breathe, the expectoration of *stringy, yellow mucus* is characteristic of the remedy.

Hepar Sulph., asthma *worse* in dry cold weather, in cold air, *better* in damp, wet weather, breathing anxious, wheezing, rattling, short, deep breathing, threatens suffocation, must bend head back and sit up, after suppressed eruption (*Psorinum*).

Psorinum, asthma, dyspnea, *worse* in open air, sitting up, *better lying down* and keeping arms stretched far apart *(reverse of Arsenicum),* despondent, thinks he will die, after suppressed eruption.

Nux Vomica, useful for athmatic attacks brought on by gastric disturbances due to over-eating or eating wrong foods, drinking coffee in excess or liquor.

Carbo Vegetablis, asthma of the aged who are much debilitated and are greatly oppressed for breath, belching wind gives relief.

Sulphur, to complete the cure in chronic cases.

Silicea, "humid asthma, coarse rattling, chest seems filled with mucus, seems as if he would suffocate. Asthma of old 'sycotics', or of children of such, pale, waxy, anemic, with prostration and thirst." Asthma from suppressed gonorrhea

(Thuja). Worse cold, draught, thunderstorm. *From checked perspiration* or foot-sweat.

Tuberculinum, in prsons with a T.B. history or family history. Takes cold every time he gets a breath of fresh air, yet craves fresh air.

Dosera, asthma with T.B. history, or family history, or after whooping cough. Worse at night.

Thuja, cases that follow vaccination, many vaccinations, or bad vaccination.

After Gonorrhea, or offensive green discharges. PECULIAR SYMPTOMS, *sweat only* on *uncovered parts.* Worse, cold damp *(Natrium Sulph.),* 3 A.M. *(Kalium Carb.).* A left side remedy. "Often the chronic of *Ars. Alb.*"

Medorrhinum, asthma, choking from weakness or spasm of epiglottis. *Only better by lying on face and protruding tongue. Better seaside (Brom).* Where asthma is connected, even remotely with gonorrhea *(Thuja).*

In *acute* troubles which occur principally at nights, it is best to administer the indicated remedy in watery solution in *tea-spoon* doses every two to four hours according to the severity of the case, till the acute spasms subside and other times, in single doses morning and evening for a few days, till there is relief. For the better action of the remedy, the watery solution should be *stirred well each time* before the doses are taken. For chronic troubles, the indicated remedy may be given weekly, or at longer intervals.

It is always best to commence the treatment of this complaint in all cases, unless other remedies are specially indicated, with *Ipecac* 30 in repeated doses as explained above, and this will diminish the intensity and frequency of the attacks, after which, if there is continued oppression and tightness of breathing between the paroxysms, with expectoration of a tenacious mucus, a few doses of *Sulphur* 30 at intervals, will remove the remaining symptoms. In chronic cases of some years standing, if *Ipecac* 30 does not relieve the acute spasms, *Ipecac* 200 may be used instead, in the same way.

If, however, there are still dyspnea and attacks of anxiety at night, especially from 1 to 3 A.M. *Arsenicum Alb.* 30 may be given in *repeated doses*, as described above, for the relief of acute symptoms. For the chronic complaint, *Arsenicum Alb.* 30 may be given at weekly intervals, and then *Arsenicum Alb.* 200 fortnightly at first, and later at longer intervals.

In children and adults who have inherited the disease from their parents, or in patients when the attack is brought on, or is worse, during damp wet weather, *Natrium Sulph.* is better indicated. For recent attacks, it is better to commence the treatment with the 12 X *Trituration)*, and give it in repeated teaspoon doses for the acute spasms at nights (1/2 grain being dissolved in one ounce of water), and single doses, morning and evening, at other times, till the symptoms subside.

In chronic cases, the 30th potency may be used in the same way for the acute spasmodic attacks, at nights, and single doses morning and evening for 3 days at a time, allowing an interval of 2 or 3 days, and later at weekly intervals. If the remedy is given in the 200th potency fortnightly or at longer intervals, the chronic tendency may be cured.

These remedies will be enough to treat a majority of cases. Other indicated remedies will be necessary for other characteristic symptoms in particular cases.

6. WHOOPING COUGH

This is one of the peculiar class of diseases that seldom, if ever, attacks the same individual but once during a life time. It is essentially a disease of childhood. It usually prevails as an epidemic and is contagious. It is probably most easily communicated in the second stage after the disease has become fully established, and during the decline. Its duration is, according to general belief, from six weeks to six months.

It has been usually divided into three stages–the *first*, catarrhal stage, resembling ordinary symptoms of a common cold, with sneezing, watering from the eyes and nose, irritation and tickling of the throat, loss of appetite, restless, uneasiness, often chilliness, with flushes of heat, indisposition to do anything but worry and complain, sometimes fever with a hollow cough, which, at first, is quite dry, but afterwards with expectoration of thick, tough mucus. This stage may last from a few days to a fortnight.

The *second*, the spasmodic or convulsive stage. It consists of violent spasmodic paroxysms, or fits of coughing. These paroxysms occur at longer or shorter intervals, and last from a quarter to a half or three quarters of a minute. A rapid succession of them may occur so close together as to make almost one continual paroxysm, lasting from ten to fifteen minutes. These paroxysms are made up of a succession of quick forced *expirations*, without any intervening *inspiration*, until the child gets blue in the face and appears upon the very point of suffocation. This is followed by one long drawn act of inspiration, which produces the peculiar, shrill sound or whoop, as it is called, from which the disease derives its name. This alternation of several short coughs, expelling all the air from the lungs, followed by one long inspiration, again filling them, usually ends in the expulsion of a quantity of thick, ropy mucus, or else in vomiting.

The duration of this period varies from two or three weeks to some months, but it can be cut shot in most cases if suitable remedies are administered in time.

The *third,* the stage of decline consists of the paroxysms growing shorter and shorter and less violent and frequent, the whoop gradually disappears, and the cough does not differ from that of ordinary cough and gradually ceases.

First (Inflammatory) Stage

Belladonna, dry, hollow, harsh, barking cough, *worse at night.*

Nux Vomica, dry and hard, hurts the head and stomach or abdomen on coughing and *worse in the morning* or after eating.

Second (Whooping) Stage

After the whooping stage begins,

Ipecac., considerable wheezing and spasmodic coughing with blueness of the face during the cough, also gagging and vomiting.

Deep sounding hoarse cough.

Corallium Rub., violent spasmodic cough occurring in rapid succession so that the child *turns purple* or black in the face, i.e. when it is definitely known that the cough is whooping, and in whatever stage it may be, it is best to give *Corallium Rub.* 30 in watery solution every four hours for four or five days.

Drosera, hoarse cough with a metallic sound, dry spasmodic cough with retching, worse at night, or upon repose, pain in the side, just under the short ribs, when coughing, the child presses with its hand upon the pit of the stomach, severe fits of coughing following each other in quick succession, with bleeding from mouth and nose, expectoration of thick, cough phlegm, the cough is excited by talking or laughing. *Drosera* 200 acts very well in such cases, and should be given in watery solution every six hours.

These three remedies will be ordinarily sufficient for a majority of ordinary cases. For severe cases, the following will be useful.

DISEASES OF THE ORGANS OF RESIRATION

Cuprum Met., useful in one of the worst forms of the disease. Cough very violent and long continued, *completely prostrating* the patient, the child becomes rigid, turns blue or black in the face, lies as if dead, sometimes vomiting after the attack and rattling of mucus between. 200th potency is useful when the 30th does not help.

Veratrum Album, child coughs itself into regular collapse, falls *exhausted* wtih cold sweat, especially on the forehead. Follows well after *Cuprum Met.* in violent cases.

Arnica Mont., 'a wonderful whooping–cough remedy'. Violent tickling cough if child gets angry. *Begins to cry* before cough (*Bell.*), knows it is coming and dreads it.

Third (Loose or Rattling) Stage

Pulsatilla, expectoration thick, green and the patient craves fresh, cool air, and is better in a cool room.

Antimonium Tart., much coarse rattling of mucus difficult to raise, as if a cup full of mucus would come.

Sulphur, to finish the case, especially in *Psoric cases.*

Hepar Sulph., particularly useful during convalescence, and to prevent a recurrence of the trouble.

7. PLEURISY OR PLEURITIS

DEFINITION: The lungs are enclosed and their structure maintained by a serous membrane called the *Pleura*. This membrane forms a shut sack, and the lungs fit into it as does a boy's head into his cap, when it is inverted or folded partially within itself. Pleurisy or pleuritis consists of an inflammation of this membrane.

CAUSES: The exciting cause, as a general rule, is exposure to cold or damp. It may also arise from severe injuries to the chest, as from a blow or a fall.

SYMPTOMS: Pleurisy, from the beginning, is marked by a sharp, stabbing pain, on a level with or just beneath one or the other of the breasts, preceded or accompanied by chilliness or shivering, a dry ineffectual cough is usually present, with no expectoration, or, if any, very little, and of a frothy whitish look, some difficulty of respiration, hot dry skin, loss of appetite, headache and sometimes bilious vomiting.

The pain is always aggravated by deep inspiration, change of position, or by pressing upon the parts. The patient cannot lie upon the affected side, at least during the first stages of the disease, as that position increases the pain, however, as the pain subsides and serous fluid is formed, he is unable to lie on either side, on account of the pressure made upon the sound lungs by the effused serum, which produces great difficulty of breathing. The patient is, therefore, compelled to lie upon his back, or nearly so.

Treatment

Aconitum Nap. is the chief remedy, and if it is given in the 6th or 30th potency, in repeated doses, once an hour to three hours, according to violence of the symptoms, and continued until the pain, heat, thirst and cough have sensibly diminished, it will often check the disease in from 24 to 48 hours.

If, however, *Aconitum Nap.* does not remove all the trouble, or the stage of effusion had already begun when the treatment was started, when the sharp stitching pain continues, and the thirst and fever also, the pain and suffering is aggravated on the *least motion* and the patient feels better lying on the painful side, the tongue is coated white, then *Bryonia Alba* is the most appropriate remedy and will act more positively on the serous membrane, and promote the effusion, and complete the cure which *Aconitum Nap.* could not do. If the remedy acts favourably, it may be continued for some days, morning and evening, till a cure is effected. If the case seems to get a little better and relapses again and again, the fever comes and goes in fitful flashes, followed by spells of sweat and debility, there is burning, especially of the feet, diarrhea worse in the mornings, and the lips are very red, *Sulphur* is necessary to finish up the case and to absorb the large quantities of effusion.

These three remedies will, in a majority of cases, be enough to effect a cure.

In severe cases, or when the attack is sudden, the medicines may be given in repeated doses, every three or four hours, increasing the intervals between the doses as the severity of the symptoms diminishes. The following remedies may also be required :

Arnica Mont., where pleurisy is due to external violence of injuries, or when the fever has been subdued by *Aconitum Nap.* but there is still pain and difficulty of breathing remaining.

Mercurius Sol., when there are copious night sweats, more or less difficulty and shortness of breathing, *after* the fever has been subdued by other remedies.

Arsenicum Alb., if extensive effusion has taken place, and there is considerable prostration.

In chronic cases, when through neglect, bad management or constitutional pre-disposition, there is danger of consumption following, with purulent expectoration, protracted cough, dropsical swelling and other complications, *Lycopodium Clav., Arsenicum Alb.* and *Phosphorus* will be required.

8. PNEUMONIA

Definition : Pneumonia is an inflammation of the *substance* of the lungs, but the majority of the cases of pneumonia are attended with more or less inflammation of the serous membrane lining the interior of the chest, and inverting over the lungs, that is, there is some pleurisy also. Bronchitis is also a frequent accompaniment.

Pneumonia may be either single or double, one lung may be affected, or both. It is more common upon the right side than upon the left, and generally commences in the lower lobes.

Cause : As a general rule, Pneumonia or inflammation of the lungs does not occur as a primary affection, but follows as a complication of some other disease, such as measles, whooping cough, inflammation of the bowels, or bilious remittent fever. As cold is an active, exciting cause, pneumonia is more frequent during the winter than during the summer months. A severe blow or fall upon the chest, the inhalation of irritating or poisonous gases may also produce it.

Symptoms : Pneumonia commences with a chill or shivering, followed by heat, and an increased frequency of the pulse. Cough is always present, at first dry and deep, or quick and spontaneous. Pain or more properly speaking a stitch in the side, usually the right, on taking a long breath or deep inspiration. This is the *first* stage of the disease.

First stage

(Stage of congestion of blood in the lungs)

If there is chill followed by high fever, great heat, dry skin, intense thirst, restlessness, *fever* and anguish, and the patient tosses in bed, with dry cough, a few doses of *Aconitum Nap.6 or 30*, repeated every hour, will produce profuse perspiration, and relief of all symptoms. If there is no relief in 24 hours, *Sulphur* 30 given in small doses in watery solution, once in 2 hours, will give relief in the first stage. These two remedies will abort many cases. If, with the high fever there is delirium, eyes are red, the face is flushed, and there is sweat on *covered parts*, and the blood seems to mount to the brain as well as the chest, *Belladonna* 30 is suitable.

Second Stage

If the inflammation develops and mucus is forming, the fever still continues, being only partially continues, being only partially controlled, the breathing is short, expiration shorter, and the patient wants to *lie quiet on the painful side*, has much thirst *with dryness of mouth and lips* and complains of stitching pains in the chest, *Bryonia* Alba 30 or 200 may be given in watery solution every four hours. If this is followed by *Sulphur* 30, it will cure the case.

If, however, there is greater oppression in the chest and the patient feels as if there is a load pressing it down, the temperature is very high, and the expectoration is often very profuse, and there is pain on the lower and of the *right* lung, and the patient feels *worse* lying on the *left* side but better the right side, *Phosphorus* 30 or 200 will help, and may be followed by *Sulphur* 30, or *Lycopodium Clav.* 30 to cure. If the chest seems full of mucus, with coarse rattling and cough, which seems as though it must bring up large quantities but it does not, *Antimonium Tart.* 30 is indicated. It is oftenest found in children and very old people.

Ipecac., which has also great accumulation of mucus, is again useful in children, but the oppression of breathing is accompanied with *wheezing breathing* instead of the coarse rattling of *Antimonium Tart.*

Third Stage

(Resolution and Clearance)

Sulphur, will occupy the first place to clear the remnants of the case. Burning in chest, skin, or locally in many places, and especially of the feet which must be kept out of the bed to cool them, weakness, or weak, empty gone feeling in the stomach, especially *worse at* 11 A.M., white tongue with very red tip and borders, bright redness of the lips or any of the borders.

Calcarea Carb., suitable for fat or flabby persons, with coldness of the extremities instead of burnings, cough *worse* in the morning, the external chest becomes sensitive to touch and sore, sensation in feet and legs as if the patient had on cold, damp stockings, night sweats, general and especially local sweats which the patient was always subject to, such as sweaty head as a child.

Lycopodium Clav., one of the best remedies for the later stages of typhoid or neglected pneumonia, and especially when there is copious expectoration, circumscribed redness of the cheeks, especially from 4 to 8 P.M., often red sand in the urine and fan-like motion of the flaps of the nose, *especially indicated in cases with liver complications and windy condition of the stomach.*

Hepar Sulph., when there is wheezing sound in the throat, and the least cold air makes the cough worse.

Pulsatilla, when the expectoration becomes thick, profuse, green and with bitter or offensive taste, and the patient feels chilly, but yet cannot bear the atmosphere of a close warm room.

Tuberculinum Bovinum, will promptly clear pneumonia cases hanging fire in persons of a *tuberculous family history.*

Psorinum, patients convalesce very slowly, are chilly, offensive, with despair of recovery.

Psorinum is a chilly *Sulphur.*

CHAPTER – VI

DISEASES OF THE HEART

LEADING INDICATIONS

1. INFLAMMATIONS (Carditis, Pericarditis)–*Aconitum Nap., Bryonia Alba, Bell., Puls., Arsenicum Alb., Kalium Carb., Apis Mell.,a Sulph.*
2. ENDOCARDITIS, RHEUMATISM OF THE HEART–*Bell., Bryonia Alba, Puls., Spig., Phos., Kalmia, Aurum Met., Arsenicum Alb, Calcarea Carb.*
3. PALPITATION OF THE HEART–Caused by debilitating influences-*China off., Puls., Phos.*
   BY GOING UP AN EMINENCE–*Sulph.*
   IF AT NIGHT–*Arsenicum Alb., Puls., Phos.*
   IF AFTER EATING–*Phos., Lycopus Vir.*
   IF ACCOMPANIED BY GREAT ANXIETY–*Aconitum Nap., Arsenicum Alb., Spig., Puls., Aurum Met.*
   IF BY SYNCOPE, WEAKNESS–*Arsenicum Alb.*
   BY GREAT DYSPNEA–*Aconitum Nap., Phos., Spig.*
   CHRONIC PALPITATION–*Sulph., Arsenicum Alb., Aurum Met., Phos., Calcarea Carb., China off.*
4. NEURALGIA, PAIN OF THE HEART–*Angina Pectoris, Arsenicum Alb., Spongia, Arnica Mont., Aurum Mur., Latrod.*
5. HYPERTROPHY (Abnormal enlargement) of the heart–*Puls., Spig., Arsenicum Alb., Lycopodium Clav., Kalmia, Calcarea Carb.* For resulting dropsy–*Lycopus Vir.*
6. ANEURISM (Dilation of an artery) of the heart–*Arsenicum Alb., Spig.*

7. VALVULAR DISEASES–*Arsenicum Alb.*, *Spongia.* For thickening of the valves–*Spig., Kalmia.*
8. *Cyanosis* (Blue discolouration of the skin)-*Dig.* (especially for new-born infants)–*Sulph., Calcarea Carb., Lach.*

Some important remedies are :

Arnica Mont., pain in the region of heart, as if it were squeezed together (*Cact., Lil Tig.*) or had got a shock, or blow *(Angina Pectoris)*. Heart, first rapid, then extremely slow, stitches in cardiac region, stitches left to right, pulse feeble, hurried, irregular, horror of instant death, with cardiac–distress in the night, imagines he has heart, disease, one of our gretest remedies for tired heart dilated after strain or exertion–*our greatest pick me-up*, tired out from physical or mental strain, feels bruised, beaten, sore–bruises easily, restless, because bed feels too hard, does not wish to be touched, fears approach.

Aconitum Nap., great distress in heart and chest, dreadful oppression of the pericardial region, inward pressign in the region of heart, palpitation with great anxiety and difficulty of breathing, anguish with dyspnea, sensation of something rushing into head, with confusion and flying heat in face, sudden attacks of pain in heart with dyspnoea. *Aconitum Nap.* is *anxious*, restless with fears, fear of death, sudden acute conditions from chill, shock, fright, all ailments and fears, worse at night.

Spigelia, violent beating of heart, so that he frequently could hear the pulsation, or so that the beats could be seen through the clothes, palpitation aggravated by sitting down and bending forward (rev. of *Kalium carb.*), heart seemed to be in tremulous motion, worse for deep inspiration, or holding breath, heart sounds may be heard several inches away, must lie on right side, or with head very high. *Spigelia's* pain are *stitching,* sharp neuralgic pains, (chest, head, heart, eyes etc.) *worse* from slightest motion.

DISEASE OF THE HEART

Lycopus Vir., protrusion of eyes, with tumultuous action of heart (*Spig.*), eyes feel full and heavy, pressing outwards, cardiac irritability, pulse frequent, small, compressible or quick, hard, wiry, not comprersssible, trembling hands. (*Lycopus* is useful in exophthalmic goitre.)

Kalium Carb., stitching pains in heart, chest, extort cries, stitches about heart and through to scapula, heart's action intermittent, irregular, tumultuous, weak, mitral insufficiency, leans forward, resting on arms to take weight off chest (rev. of *Spig.*), *Kali Carb.* has stitching pains (like *Bry.*), but also independently of motion and respiration (unlike *Bry.*), its worst hours are 2 A.M. to 4 A.M., has profuse sweat, puffiness about the eyes. Complementary to *Carb Veg.*

Lilium Tig., dull pressive pain in heart, sharp quick pain, with fluttering, roused from sleep by pain as if heart were violently grasped, the grasp gradually relaxed, interrupting heart beat and breathing, sensation as if heart was grasped or squeezed in a vice *(Cactus),* as if blood had all gone to heart, must bend double (rev. of *Spig.*), heart alternately grasped and released, heart feels over-loaded with blood, violent palpitation with throbbing of carotids, depression of spirits, weeps.

Characteristic, hurried feeling, as of imperative duties and inability to perform them, pressure on rectum and bladder, terrible urging to stool, to urinate, all the time, bearing down with heavy weight, as if whole contents of pelvis would issue through vagina, but for upward pressure of hand.

Cactus Grand., palpitation of the heart, heart squeezed, sense of constriction in the heart, as if an iron band prevented its normal movement, several violent irregular beats of the heart, with sensation of pressure and heaviness, small irregular heart beats, with necessity for deep inspiration, congestion in chest. It is the nature of *Cactus* to constrict. Tightness and constriction about head, chest, diaphragm, heart, uterus clutchings. Cactus has a profound curative action upon the heart. Fear and distress, such violent suffering, screaming with pain, determination of blood to an organ–chest, heart, strong pulsation felt in strange places–stomach, bowels and even extremities, 11 O'clock remedy, 11 A.M. and 11 P.M.

Sepia, violent palpitation of the heart, and beating of all the arteries, in bed, stitches in heart, violent palpitations in heart, as if, it would force its way through chest wall, *relieved by walking a long distance and walking very fast.* The *Sepia* patient is very indifferent, hates fuss, tendency to ptosis (abnormal depression of organs) and dragging down, especially, in pelvic organs *(Lil Tig.),* profuse perspirations, especially axillae, general relief from motion, food, sleep.

Digitalis, sensation as through heart stood still, with great anxiety, must hold breath, *pulse, very slow,* thready, slow, intermittent, heart had lost its force, beats more frequent, and sometimes irregular, sensation as if heart would stop beating if he moved *(Gels. must move, or it will stop),* respiration difficult, sighing, stops when she drops off to sleep, *Digitalis* affects heart and liver, jaundice–white stools, *with very slow pulse (Kalm.),* diarrhea and nausea with heart disease.

Kalmia, violent palpitations of the heart with faint feelings and oppressed breathing, wandering rheumatic pains in region of heart, extend down to the left arm *(Lat., Mact, Med.),* heart disease after frequent attacks of rheumatism, or alternating with it, hypertrophy and valvular insufficiency, or thickening after rheumatism, paroxysms of anguish about heart, dyspnea and febrile excitement, remarkable slowness of pulse *(Dig.),* pulse very feeble, or heart's action very tumultuous, rapid and visible *(Spig.), when rheumatism has been treated externally and cardiac symptoms ensure.*

Naja, heart weak. Post-diphteritic heart. For a heart damaged by acute rheumatism.

DISEASE OF THE HEART

Aurum Met., frequent attacks of anguish about heart, and tremulous fearfulness, violent palpitation of the heart, congestion of heart, notably with the *Aurum Met.* mental symptoms, rheumatism that has gone to the heart, *(Kalmia)*. Acute rheumatism with desperate heart conditions, extreme dyspnea, impossible to lie down. A queer symptom–*heart seems to shake, as if loose, when walking.* The *Arum Met.* mental state is profound despondency and melancholy, disgust for life, tendency to suicide, great anguish, increasing into self–destruction, absolute loss of enjoyment in everything, terrible melancholy, after the abuse of mercury, pains wander from joint to joint and finally settle in the heart.

Aurum Mur. angina Pectoris (next to *Arnica* Mont., indispensable), heaviness, aching, sensation of rigidity in heart, cardiac anguish, sticking in heart.

Lactrodectus Mac., violent peri-cardial pains extending to axilla and down left arm and forearm to fingers with numbness and apnea, violent peri-cardial pains and pained left arm which was almost paralyzed, pulse uncountable, quick and thready, (*A great medicine for Angina Pectoris*).

Spongia, constricting pain (*Cardiac*) with anxiety, attacks of oppression and cardiac pain worse lying with head low, anxious sweat, palpitation are strviolent, with pain, gasping respiration, suddenly awakened after midnight, with suffocating *(Lach.)*, lips blue *(Lach.)*, Angina Pectoris, contracting pain in chest, heat, suffocation, faintness, anxious sweat (Exophthalmic Goitre).

Lachesis, cramp-like pain in peri-cardial region, causing palpitation with anxiety, heart feels too large for containing cavity, bluish lips–cyanosis *(Spongia),* intolerance of touch or pressure on throat–larynx, stomach, abdomen, as if something swollen in pit of throat would suffocate him. *Worse after sleep (Spongia).* Lacheis is one of our most useful remedies in troubles of heart, acute or chronic, the peculiar suffocation, cough, and aggravation from constriction, being the guiding symptoms.

Arsenicum Alb. useful in advanced and desperate cases. Palpitation with anguish, cannot lie on back, worse going upstairs, heart beats irritable, palpitation, and tremulous weakness, after stool, *Angina Pectoris*–sudden tightness above the heart, agonising pericardial pain, pain extends into neck and occiput. *(Lacto dect. and Kalm.)* to left arm and hand, breathing difficult, fainting spells, least motion makes him lose his breath, sits bent forward, or with head thrown back. *Worse at night especially from* 1 A.M. to 5 A.M. Rheumatism affecting heart, with great prostration, cold, sticky sweat, great anxiety and oppression, burning about the heart. Pulse small, rapid, feeble, intermittent, valvular disease, with dyspnea, anasarca. *Hydropericardium* with great irritability, anguish and restlessness.

N.B.– *The cardinal symptoms of Arsenicum Alb.* are *generally present-extreme restlessness, driving out of bed, or from bed to bed, thirst for small quantities, often, aggravation from cold, relief from heat* (rev. of *APIS*).

Apis, sudden edema, dyspnea, and sudden lancinating or *stinging* pains, restlessness and anxiety. Think of *Apis Mell.* for burning and stinging pains anywhere. *Apis Mell. is generally* thirstless, is *worse,* after sleep, from warm room and heat, *better,* cold air and cold room, cold application (rev. of *Ars.)* Skin alternately dry and hot or perspiring.

Sulphur, anxious palpitation, violent palpitation, rush of blood to heart, heart feels enlarged, great orgasm of blood, with burning hands, stitches heart and chest, worse deep breathing, *Sulphur* is hungry, untidy, argumentative. Worse heat, intolerant of clothing, fond of fat. Complaints relapse, suppressed eruptions.

Pulsatilla, rheumatic irritation of heart, where pains shift rapidly about the body, heart symptoms reflex from indigestion, heaviness, pressure, fullness (heart), violent palpitation with anguish, sight obscured, patient nervous, weepy, intolerant of heat, craves air and fuss.

DISEASE OF THE HEART

Phosphorus, palpitation, violent, on slightest motion, violent, lying on left side, pericardial anguish from emotion, heaviness, chest as if a weight lying on it, constriction, pressing sensation about heart, burning pain between scapula *(Lyc.).* The *Phos.* type–tall, fine, fear being alone, dark, slender, thirst for cold drinks.

In case which do not respond to treatment and have a history of tubercle, sycosis or syphilis, the following remedies will be necessary :

Tuberculinum Bacillinum, heart cases, where there is a familial past history of tubercular manifestations, palpitation, heaviness, pressure over heart, irritable, irritable on waking, nothing pleases, nothing satisfies, wants to travel, cosmopolitan condition of mind, suffocates in a warm room *(Puls.).*

Medorrhinum, useful in sycotic cases. Heart felt very hot, beat very fast, with burning sensation, or feeling of a cavity where heart ought to be, sharp pain at apex, worse motion. Great pain, heart, extending to left arm *(Latro mac.)* and throat. Intense pain in heart, radiates to all parts of left chest, worse least movement. The troubles of *Medo.* are worse by day, sunrise to sunset. Those of *Luet.*, by night, sunset to sunrise, *Medo.* is rich in mental symptoms, *everything seems unreal* like a dream. Time moves so slowly–things done an hour ago, as if done a week ago *(Cann ind.)* anguish, introspection, always anticipating evil happenings. Cannot concentrate, forgets what she is reading, cannot spell simple words. News coming seems to touch her heart before she hears it.

Lueticum, pain and pressure behind the sternum. Lancinating pains in heart *at night*, base to apex *(Medo.* is worse by day).

Diphtherium, with history of diphtheria, feeble, irregular or intermittent pulse, quick or slow, with vomiting and cyanosis.

Crataegus, acts on *weak heart–muscles,* and is said to be a heart tonic, chronic heart, disease, with extreme weakness, very feeble and irregular heart action, general anasarca, very nervous with pain in back of head and neck, pulse irregular, feeble, intermittent. High arterial tension, is a sedative in cross, irritable patients with cardiac symptoms.

Dose– Tincture, one to fifteen drops, must be used for some time to obtain good results.

CHAPTER VII

BLOOD PRESSURE

1. HYPERTENSION–HIGH BLOOD PRESSURE

High Blood pressure is not a disease– it is a symptom like fever. Blood pressure essential for life, and every living man or woman carries some degree of blood pressure. In certain pathological states, the blood pressure rises above normal figure– sometimes reaching such heights as to become a source of imminent danger to life. This raised blood pressure is not a disease by itself, but a sign or manifestation of a pathological process–just as fever is not a disease but a measurable external index of an internal malady. It might be said in consonance, both with reason and science, that the rise of blood pressure is a *conservative* or *compensatory process*, by which adequate circulation of blood is maintained in the tissues in spite of increased resistance or obstruction to the flow of blood. If the blood pressure would fail to rise, while the obstruction to the flow of blood is increasing, the inevitable result would be death from failure of circulation. To bring the analogy closer between fever and increased blood pressure, it may be explained that a rise of blood pressure is a necessary evil to support life in adverse circumstances of blood flow as much as fever is an unpleasant reaction but, nevertheless conducive to the body to fight out the invading disease.

But both fever and blood pressure should remain within safe limits, and every effort should be made to reduce them when they assume alarming proportions. It must be borne in mind, however, that a drastic reduction of fever or blood pressure by drugs is brought with grave consequences, and should, by no means be attempted.

Removal of the cause to which the body reacts by fever or increased blood pressure is, therefore, the ideal method of treatment.

Causes of Hypertension

(a) HEREDITY: Herdity plays an important role in its causation. If both the parents have high blood pressure the children rarely escape. If one of the parents is hypertensive, the chance of hypertension in the children is less present, but less so than in the former case.

(b) AGE: Hypertension is mostly found in people after the age of forty. But younger people even below the age of twenty and also children of about 10 years of age are found to suffer from hypertension. The cause of hypertension may not be the same in all these cases. Hypertension in children is mostly due to a chronic inflammation of the kidneys.

(c) SEX: More cases are found amongst men than women. In the case of women, the period of "menopause" is about the time when they suffer from hypertension.

(d) OVERWEIGHT AND OBESITY: More cases of hypertension are found in over weight and obese people than in thin and under-weight ones. They are often of low stature, with stumpy limbs and short neck.

(e) THOSE WHO PRESENT DEFINITE SYMPTOMS OF DISEASE OF THE KIDNEYS: In these persons, the cause of the kidney trouble may be the use of alcohol, tobacco, tea or coffee, a heavy meat diet, or constipation.

(f) CASES IN WHICH THE ARTERIES ARE HARDENED: The hardened and sometimes tortuous arteries may be felt at the wrist, in the arm, at the temples, and elsewhere in the body. In some cases, the changes in the arteries may be seen in the funds of the eye by the ophthalmoscope or in the large vessels near the heart by the aid of the X-ray. The most common causes of these blood-vessel changes are syphilis and auto-intoxication.

(g) In cases in which both the conditions referred to in clauses (e) and (f) are present, the kidneys being diseased as shown by examination of the urine, and the arteries also hardened.

(h) In case in which although the blood pressure is high, no other evidence is present of either disease of the kidneys, or of the arteries, the cause of high pressure is generally to be found in erroneous habits of life, especially the excessive use of tea, coffee, tobacco, beer and other alcoholics. It is also probable that poisons absorbed from the colon are about the most common of all causes.

(i) MENTAL STATES: People who are unfortunately placed in life, and suffer from continual anxiety or worry for many years, are liable to become hypertensive. A continued and sustained rise of blood pressure over a long period, may become a permanent disease.

(j) PERSONALITY: A type of high blood pressure known as "Essential Hypertension" is often associated with a distinctive personality type. They are usually hyperactive individuals, with great exuberance of mental and physical energy. They are always restless, usually sensitive and short tempered. They may, otherwise, appear to be in normal health.

Symptoms: Ordinarily, the nervous symptoms appear first, which are noticed either by the patient himself, or by his friends and relations.

Irritability of temper, nervousness, change of disposition, inability to concentrate the mind, throbbing headache, insomnia and giddiness, are some of the common initial symptoms. Rapid failure of vision, or even sudden blindness due to retinal hemorrhage, may be the first symptom to attract attention to the blood pressure.

With deterioration of the function of the kidneys, the urinary symptoms appear, and puffiness, more or less, under the eyes is noticed in the morning. When the heart is embarrassed by the increased load of peripheral resistance, breathlessness on slight exertion, and cough make their appearance. Soon after, edema of the ankles starts, which is particularly marked in the evening after the day's work, but may disappear in the morning after a good night's rest. Peri-cardial distress and even anginal pain, may be experienced. When heart failure becomes very marked, there are great dyspnea, even at rest, cough with bloody expectoration, anasarca, and scanty high coloured urine.

Hemorrhage in and from different parts of the body is met with cases of hypertension. Bleeding from nose and gums is common, and is deemed beneficial-since such bleeding may be considered as safety-valve action. Bleeding in the lungs is also met with, which reveals itself as hemoptysis of different intensity. Hemorrhage in the brain, known as 'apoplexy', is a very serious condition, which kills the patient outright, or leaves him to the miserable existence of a paralytic, only occasionally, a complete or almost complete recovery is seen.

Treatment

There are many drugs which will reduce blood pressure temporarily, or as long as the drug is used. Nitro-glycerine and nitrate of soda are especially active, but the effect is disastrous, and death is hastened. Blood pressure should be reduced by removal of the cause. Pressure is never any higher than it needs to be. The injury is not from the high blood pressure, but from the poisons which produce the high pressure and cause degenerations in the heart, kidneys and other organs. Pressure-lowering drugs are not indicated, and should not be used.

The best and the safest means of reducing blood pressure are the avoidance of meats, tea, coffee, alcohol, tobacco,

BLOOD PRESSURE

condiments. Much benefit may be derived from the systematic use of warm baths, rest and moderate exercise, and steps taken for the free and regular movement of the bowels daily. The use of suitable Homeopathic remedies stirs up the natural curative agencies of the body and helps towards a general restoration of normal health as far as possible.

The best diet for high blood pressure

AVOID OR ELIMINATE: Tea, coffee, cocoa, chocolate, cold beverages, pepper, mustard, spices, horse-radish, and "hot" sauces of all sorts, as they rapidly wear out the liver and kidneys, vinegar and pickles, foods and beverages in which appreciable amounts of oxalic acid are present, such as rhubarb, sorrel, cocoa powder, and black tea.

USE VERY SPARINGLY: Salt, breakfast cereals, as well as other acid-free foods (on account of the excess of Phosphoric acid which they contain, which tends to induce acidosis).

DISCARD ALTOGETHER: Meats, white bread.

USE VERY SELDOM, if at all : Eggs, which are high up in acid-ash class of foods and encourage intestinal putrefaction. The diet should consist chiefly of fresh vegetables, greens, fruits, nuts and dairy products.

The Bill of Fare should be–Potatoes in place of cereals, spinach, lettuce, string beans, apples, citrus fruits and melons. Papaya, foods rich in vitamins and food minerals are most important, whole wheat, and par–boiled unpolished rice.

Therapeutic Hints

Aconitum Nap., dry heat and red face. Thirsty and restless. Chilliness and formication down back. Formication and numbness. Sleeplessness with tossing about. Bursting headache, as if the brain were moved by boiling water. Vertigo, worse on rising

(Nux Vom. Opium).Pulse full and bounding, almost incompressible. Fears death, but believes that he will soon die. Pains are intolerable, they drive him crazy. Bitter taste of everything except water. Burning from stomach to esophagus. High tension is reduced by this remedy.

Alumen, great weakness of chest. Asthma of old people. Copious, ropy expectoration in the morning. *Hemoptysis Palpitation from lying down on the right hand side. Obstiante constipation, no desire for stool for days together. Marble like masses pass, still the rectum feels loaded.* Vertigo, mental paresis, dysphagia, especially to liquids. Every cold settles in throat.

Amyl Nitrate, palpitation of the heart and similar conditions are readily cured by it, especially the flushing and other discomforts at climacteric. *Hiccough and yawning. Surging of blood to head and face. Sense of constriction in the throat. Collar seems too tight. Dyspnea and asthmatic feelings. Great oppression and fullness of chest.*

Pericardial anxiety, tumultuous action of the heart. Much flushing of heat, sometimes followed by cold and clammy skin and profuse sweat. Throbbing throughout the whole body. Constant stretching for hours.

Apis Mell., lids swollen, red, edematous, pale, waxy, or oedematous countenance. Thirstlessness, vomiting of food. Craving for milk. *Urine suppressed, albuminous, loaded with casts, scanty and high colored urine.* Constipation. Feels as if something would break on straining. Hemorrhoids with stinging pains. Feels as if he could not draw another breath. Sudden puffing up of the whole body.

Arnica Mont., this remedy is valuable in cerebral arteriosclerosis, vertigo of the aged, heaviness and cerebral affections, plethoric people who have a tendency to hemorrhages.

Arsenicum Album, great thirst, drinks much, but little, at a time. Nausea, retching and vomiting, after eating or drinking, craves acids, coffee and pungent things. Heartburn. Long-lasting eructations. *Is unable to lie down, fears suffocation. Asthma, worse at midnight. Wheezing respiration. Palpitation.* Albuminous urine, scanty and burning urine. Great prostration, Gradual loss of weight from impaired nutrition. *Great anguish restlessness. Despair derives him from place to place.* Arsenicum Iodatum is very useful in senile hearts with aortitis, myocarditis, and fatty degeneration.

Aurum Metallicum, hopeless, despondent, and great desire to commit suicide. *Palpitation and congestion. Is particularly useful as an anti-venereal and anti-scrofulous constitution. Arterio-sclerosis,* high blood pressure, nightly paroxysms of pain behind sternum. Weakness of memory. Roaring in head. *Violent headache, congestion to head, double vision, upper half of objects invisible, sees fine objects.* Horrible odour from the nose and mouth. *Obstinate constipation,* stools hard and painful, urine turbid, like butter milk, dyspnea worse at night. *Sleeplessness. Pulse rapid and irregular. Cardiac hypertrophy.*

Aurum Muriaticum, is indicated by hypertrophy of the heart, congestion to the chest and head, strong palpitation. Paraesthesias about the heart, stitches and heaviness. It corresponds with the old age if the characteristic mental symptoms of *Aurum* are present. It has special affinity to the arteries of the head.

Baryta Carb. affects glandular structures, and useful in general degenerative changes, especially in coats of arteries, *aneurism* and senility. Blood vessels soften and degenerate, become distended, and aneurisms ruptures and apoplexia result. Loss of memory. Irresolute.

Baryta Mur., is the most useful in arterio-sclerosis of the large blood vessels and aorta similar to senile atheroma. It has headache which is more or less severe, but which is rather heaviness of old people. Apoplexy or threatened apoplexy with buzzing in the ears. It also corresponds well to pulmonary arterio-sclerosis. The potencies recommended are 3, 6 and 30. It should be continued for a long time.

Belladonna, has a marked action on vascular system, skin kand glands. *Hence, its complaints are always associated with hot, red skin, flushed face, glaring eyes, throbbing carotids, excited mental states, etc.* Vertigo with falling to the left side or backwards. Intense headache, worse from light, noise, jar, lying down and in afternoon, better by semi-erect position. Constant moaning, great thirst for cold water. Palpitation from least exertion.

Bryonia Alba, excessive dryness of mucous membranes of the entire body. Lips and tongue dry, parched, cracked, stool dry, as if burnt, cough dry, hard, racking, with scanty expectoration, urine dark and scanty. *Great thirst for large quantities at long intervals. Pressure as from stone at pit of stomack,* relieved by eructation *(Nux V., Puls.),* Nausea and faintness when rising up. Mind exceedingly irritable and faintness when rising up.Everything puts him out of humour. Bursting or splitting headache, as if everything would be pressed out.

Calcarea Arsenicum, violent rush of blood to head with vertigo. *Headache better from lying on the painful side. Weekly headache. Albuminuria, passes urine every hour. Slightest emotion causes palpitation.* Great mental depression. Craving for alcohol. Fleshy women at climacteric. *Slightest emotion causing palpitation.*

Calcarea Carbonicum, headache with cold hands and feet. Vertigo, worse from ascending and when turning head. *Much perspiration over the head, wetting the pillow far around. Palpitation. Extreme dyspnea. Longing for dry climate and weather.* Incarcerated flatulence.

Conium Mal., very useful for the treatment of high blood pressure, when accompanied by great dizziness onl changing position, such as turning over in bed, or rising or lying down, or turning the head from side to side, especially of old people. Difficult gait, trembling, sudden loss of strength while walking, painful stiffness of legs, as ususally found in old people. Sexual nervousness, with feeble erection. Testicles hard and enlarged. *Much difficulty in voiding urine, it flows and stops again, frequent urging for stool. Tremulous weakness after every stool.*

Crataegus, it acts on the muscles of the heart and is a heart tonic. Myocarditis. Failing compensation. *Irregularity of heart. General anasarca. Arterio-sclerosis. Said to have a solvent power upon crustaceous and calcareous deposits in arteries.* Apprehensive and despondent. Air hunger. Dyspepsia. Irregular pulse and breathing. Painful sensation of pressure in left side of chest below the clavicle.

Fluoric acid, especially adapted to chronic diseases with syphilitic and mercurial history. Acts especially upon lower tissues, and indicated in deep destructive processes, ulcerations, varicose veins and ulcers. Patient is compelled to move about energetically. Complaints of old age, or the prematurely aged, with weak, distended blood vessels. Hob-nailed liver of alcoholics. Easy decay of teeth.

Glonoine, a great remedy for congestive headache, hyperemia of the brain, etc. Violent convulsions, associated with cerebral congestion. *Surging of blood to head and heart. Confusion with dizziness. Bad effects of sunheat, sun stroke. Cannot recognise localities. Head feels enormously large, as if the skull were too small for the brain.* Laborious action of the heart. Fluttering or palpitation along with dyspnea. Cannot go up hill. Any exertion brings on rush of blood to heart and fainting spells. Throbbing in the whole body up to finger tips.

Iodum, rapid metabolism, *loss of flesh* with great appetite. *Great debility, the slightest effort induces* prespiration. Abnormal vaso-constriction, capillary congestion followed by edema, ecchymosis, hemorrhages and nutritive disturbances are the pathological conditions at the basis of its symptomatology. Acute catarrh of all mucous membranes, rapid emaciation notwithstanding good appetite and glandular atrophy call for this remedy, in numerous wasting diseases and in scrofulous patients. *Iodine* is warm, and wants cool surroundings.

Lachesis, gums swollen, spongy, bleeding easily, tongue trembles, on attempting to protrude it, or catches on the teeth. Trigeminal neuralgia, worse on the left side. *Palpitation, with fainting spells, especially during climacteric. Constricted feeling in the chest. Irregular beating of the heart. Feels he must take a deep breath.* Cramp-like distress in the pericardial region. Breathing almost stops, on falling asleep. Hemorrhage from the bowls, like charred straw. Cannot bear anything tight anywhere. General burning.

Nux Vom., is the greatest of all polychrests, because the bulk of its symptoms correspond with those of the commonest diseases. Frontal headache. Congestion in the brain. Head feels distended. Photophobia, much worse in the morning. *Oppressed breathing, especially* after eating. *Shallow respiration. Cough brings on bursting headache, bruised pain in the epigastrium. Nervous palpitation. Bad effects of coffee and sexual excesses. Spermatorrhea, with* weakness, backache and irritability. Liver engorged, with stitches and soreness. Difficult belching. Wants to vomit, but often fails. Frequent, ineffectual urging for stool. Incomplete and unsatisfactory stools.

Phos. Acid., heavy and confused feeling in the head. Crushing headache. Cannot collect his thoughts, or find the right word. Memory impaired. *Frequent flow of urine. Polyurea, worse at night. Sexual power deficient. Scrotal eczema. Difficult* respiration. *Weak feeling in the chest, worse from talking. Pressure behind the sternum, rendering obstruction in breathing. Palpitation.* Pulse irregular or intermittent. Carves juicy or pungent things. Shows dislike for sour or acid substances. Distension and fermentation in the bowels.

Phosphorus, vertigo, worse after rising. Heat comes from the spine. Is restless and fidgety. Loss of memory. Oversensitive to external impressions. Vexed easily. Cough from tickling in the throat. *Feels tightness across chest* or great weight on chest. *Repeated hemoptysis. Violent palpitation, worse lying on left side. Heart dilated, especially the right chambers. Feeling of warmth in the heart.* Lack of sexual power, although there is irresistible desire. Involuntary emissions, with lascivious dreams. Constipation, stools narrow and long, like a dog's, difficult to expel. Burning sensation in the palms and soles.

Plumbum., Hyper-tension and arterio-sclerosis. Excessive and rapid emaciation. Loss of memory. Slow perception. Amnesic aphasis. Paretic dementia. Face looks pale and cachetic, and cheeks sunken. Cardiac weakness. Palpitation. Wiry pulse, or soft and small pulse. Paralysis of the lower extremities as a result of apoplexy. Albuminous urine. Chronic interstitial nephritis, with scanty urine. Excessive colic, readiating to all parts of the body. Obstructed evacuation, from impaction of faeces. It suits the anemic, pale, emaciated patients with extreme weakness.

Pulsatilla, averse to fat and warm food and drink. Heart-burns. Thirstlessness. Vomiting of food substances eaten long before. Pressure as from a stone in the abdomen, must loosen clothing. Cough with thick, bland and easy expectoration. Short breath, anxiety and palpitation when lying on the left side. Smothering sensation on lying down. Wakes languid and unrefreshed. Intolerable burning heat at night with distended veins. Heat in parts of body with coldness in other. One-side sweat. Longing for open air.

Strophanthus, it acts on the heart increasing the systole and diminishing the rapidity. May be used with advantage to tone the heart, and run off dropsical accumulations. Anemia, with palpitation and breathlessness. Arterio-sclerosis, rigid arteries of the aged. Irritable heart of tobacco-smokers. Scanty and albuminous urine. Temporal headache, with double vision. Extremities swollen, dropsical. Edema of lungs. "*Strophanthus* occasions no gastric distress, has no cumulative effects, is a greater diuretic, and is safer for the aged, as it does not affect the vaso-motors."

Sulphur, constant heat on the top of the head. Beating headache with vertigo, worse from stooping. Heat and burning in the eyes. Bitter taste, especially in the morning. White coated tongue, with red tip and borders. Great acidity, sour eructation. Drinks much, eats little. Difficult respiration. Wants windows open. Heat throughout chest. Flushes of heat in chest, rising to head. Palpitation. Frequent micturition, especially at night. Must hurry-sudden call to urinate. Hard, knotty, insufficient stools, cat-naps, slightest noise awakens. Unhealthy skin, every little injury suppurates. Itching of the genitals, when going to bed.

2. HYPOTENSION-LOW BLOOD PRESSURE

The reason why hypotension has not received so much attention from the Medical Profession as hyper-tension, is that the latter is more often associated with grave danger and consequence, while the former is not so dangerous to life, provided there is no serious associated conditions.

Primary and Secondary Hypotension

Primary hypotension is a condition for which no specific cause could be ascertained. Probably the factors responsible for this condition may be traced to family heredity, but even this is not quite so common.

Secondary hypotension is, however, more common. The cases are numerous, and are always the result of some primary malady.

The causes of secondary hypotension may be classified as follows:

(a) *Acute infections*: Excepting cerebro-spinal meningits, all acute infective diseases cause a fall in the blood pressure.

(b) *Chronic wasting diseases*: Diabetes, turberculosis and malnutrition, from whatever cause.

(c) *Endocrine disease*: Addison's disease.

(d) *Fluid loss from the body*: Hemorrhage, profuse diarrhea, cholera, etc.

(e) *Cardio-vascular diseases:* Dilation of the heart, myocarditis, mitral stenosis, arterio-sclerosis (in some cases), and failing heart before death.

(f) *Nervous Diseases*: Neurasthenia, after epileptic fits, and after lumbar puncture, exhaustion, anaphylactic and surgical shock.

(g) *Blood dyscrasias*: Anemia–primary or secondary, leukemia, and poly polycythemia with splenomegaly.

(h) *Intoxication:* Chloroform and tobacco (Chronic).

Symptoms : Those who suffer from hypotension are unable to carry on with their normal pursuits in life with normal vigour and, in bad cases, may bot be able to live comfortably even while at rest. Any change of posture-particularly when assuming the upright position from recumbent position-causes a fall in the pulse pressure, due to the low vascular tone, specially in the splanchnic vessels. The fall causes giddiness, and may even cause fainting, due to a temporary poverty of blood in the brain.

Hypotension is also a contributory cause in the production of cerebral, as well as coronary thrombosis. In diseased arteries, (arterio-sclerosis) a slow blood stream, which is inevitable with hypotension is an important cause for extra vascular clotting. In fact, most cases of coronary and cerebral thrombosis are met with in people who have been suffering from arterio-sclerosis with hypotension.

Also, a hypotensive has a poor resistance to infection, which, when contracted, would worsen his condition by a further reduction of pressure.

General Management and Treatment

In the treatment of secondary hypotension, the primary cause of the trouble should be taken into account, and treated in accordance with the characteristic symptoms presented by the patient. If the primary cause is amenable to treatment, the associated hypotension will disappear in the ordinary course. Thus, a course of constitutional treatment as explain in chapter XXII is called for to start with, and is important in dealing with such cases.

General Management

(a) The hygiene of the mouth, teeth and throat should be attended to. Constipation should be corrected by suitable diet, and enemas when necessary. Strong purgatives should be avoided in any case.

(b) Mal-nutrition should be corrected by suitable appetising, wholesome foods and foods rich in vitamins, and easily digested should be used, avoiding over-loading which may lead to indigestion or diarrhea. The articles of food suitable for hypertension, as detailed in clause 1, may be used in these cases also. All irritating articles of food should be avoided.

(c) Rest is an important factor. It is desirable to retire early to bed and rise early, if possible. Rest for an hour in bed after each meal is also necessary.

(d) Massage and exercise are also necessary. General massage has a stimulating effect. A gentle oil massage before bath is helpful. Suitable and gentle bodily exercise, in the open air or in bed, in accordance with the capacity of the patient, and so as not to cause even the least sense of fatigue to the patient, will also be helpful.

(e) Hydrotherapy:

 (i) Hot and cold shower bath is the best when available. The patient should stand under a shower of warm water, which should be gradually and slowly changed to hot, and then the hot shower turned off, and when the shower of cold water is started, it should be gradually and slowly changed into as cold as could be comfortably borne.

 (i) Hot and cold sponge bath : A hot sponging may be given to the whole body, except the head. Then a sponge, with cold fresh or salt water may be given. After this, cold water may be poured over the whole body including the head.

 (iii) After the bath, the whole body may be dried with a dry towel. The patient may rest in recumbent position for half an hour, covered with blankets or sheets.

(f) Intoxicants: Excessive indulgence in tobacco, alcohol, tea and coffee, should be avoided.

Therapeutic Hints

Calcarea, Phos., effects of chronic wasting diseases: Chlorosis and phthisis. Forgetfullness of what had been done a short time ago. Writes wrong words, or same words twice. Wishes to be at home, and when at home, to go out, goes from place to place. Staggering when rising from a seat. Vertigo, on motion, when walking in open air. Weakness, with other symptoms. Drowsiness all day. Disturbed sleep, worse before midnight.

Carbo Animalis, scrofulous constitutions after debilitating diseases, with feeble circulation and lowered vitality. Confused, does not know whether he had been asleep or awake. Desires to be alone, sad and reflective, avoids conversation. Alternate cheerfulness and melancholy. Low spirited. Vertigo and confusion on sitting up, better, when reclining, nausea. Weak, want of energy, head confused, prostration. Sleeps all forenoon, yawning, sleep full of wild fancies, talks, groans, sheds tears.

Carbo Veg., disintegration and *imperfect oxidation* is the keynote of this remedy. The typical *Carbo Veg.* patient is sluggish, fat and lazy, and has a tendency to chronicity in his complaints. Blood seems to stagnate in the capillaries, causing blueness, coldness and ecchymosis. Body becomes blue, icy-cold. A lowered vital power from loss of fluids, after drugging, with quinine and coal tar products, such as saccharine tablet, etc., after other diseases, in old people with venous congestions. The patient faints easily, is worn-out, and must have fresh air. Very debilitated. The patient seems to be too weak to hold out. *Persons who have never fully recovered from the effects of some previous illness.* Weakness of memory and slowness of thought.

Causticum, disturbed functional activity of brain and spinal cord, from exhausting diseases or severe mental shock, resulting in paralysis. Ailments, from long-lasting grief and sorrow, from loss of sleep, night-watching, from sudden emotions, fear, fright, joy, from anger or vexation. Broken down seniles. Vertigo, bending forwards and sideways, at night in bed, on rising and on lying down again, on looking fixedly at an object. Weakness and trembling. Faint-like sinking of strength.

China off., debility from exhausting discharges, from loss of vital fluids, together with a *nervous erethism.* Vertigo, after loss of animal fluids, from anemia, head feels weak, can hardly hold it erect. Constant sopor or unrefreshing sleep. Paralysis from loss of fluids. Dislike to all mental or physical exertion. Low-spirited, gloomy, has no desire to live.

Gelsemium, centres its action upon the nervous system, causing vaurious degress of *motor paralysis.* General prostration. Dizziness, drowsiness, dullness, and trembling. Mental exertions cause a sense of helplessness from brain weakness, inability to attend to anything requiring thought, Vertigo, confusion of the head, spreading from occiput over whole head. Excessive irritability of mind and body, vascular excitement.

Kalium Phos., prostration: weak and tired. Conditions arising from *want of nerve power*, neurasthenia, mental and physical depression. Marked disturbance of the sympathetic nervous system. Cerebral anemia. Very nervous, starts easily, irritable, loss of memory. *Slightest labour seems a heavy task.* The causes are usually excitement, overwork and worry.

Lycopodium Clav., suitable for older persons in whom the skin shows yellowish spots, earthy complexion, uric acid disthesis, in kidney-affections, *red sand in urine,* backache, in renal region, worse before urination. *Pre-senility,* Weak memory, confused thoughts, mixes up letters and syllables, or omits parts of words in writing. Impending cerebral paralysis. *Lycopodium* patient is thin, withered, full of gas and dry. Lacks vital heat, has poor circulation, cold extremities.

Natrium Mur., "The prolonged taking of excessive salt causes profound nutritive changes to take place in the system and there arise not only the symptoms of salt retention as evidenced by dropsies and edema, but also an alteration in the blood causing a condition of anemia and leucocytosis. There seems also to be a retention in the tissues of effete materials giving rise to symptoms loosely descibed as gouty or rheumatic gout" (Dr. Stonham). Great debility,most weakness felt in the morning bed. Coldness, emaciation most noticeable in neck. Great liability to take cold. *Great weakness and weariness.* After-effects of certain forms of intermittent fever, anemia, chlorosis, many disturbances of the alimentary tract and skin.

Picric Acid, degeneration of the spinal cord, with paralysis. Neurasthenia. Muscular debility. Heavy tired feeling. Progressive, persistent anemia. Writer's palsy. Inflammation of kidneys with profound weakness, dark bloody scanty urine, urine contains much indican, granular cylinders and fatty degenerated epithelium.

Silicea, in imperfect assimilation and consequent defective nutrition, neurasthenic states and increased susceptibility to nervous stimuli and exaggerated reflexes. Lack of vital heat. Prostration of mind and body. Great sensitiveness to taking cold. Want of grit, moral or physical.

Stannum Met., chief action is centred upon the nervous system and respiratory organs. Debility very marked, especially of chronic bronchial and pulmonary conditions, characterised by profuse muco-purulent discharges upon tubercular basis. Talking causes a very weak feeling in the throat and chest.

Sepia, tubercular patients with chronic hepatic troubles and uterine reflexes. Weakness, yellow complexion, bearing down sensation, especially in women, upon whose organism it has most pronounced effect. General dragged-down feeling, pulsation throughout the body, desire for sours, relief from violent exercise to their own surprise, empty, all-gone feeling in the epigastrium before lunch, liver spots, indifference to life and to family, and also those loved best.

Psorinum, very useful in all psoric manifestations, *extreme sensitiveness to cold, wants to keep head warm, wants warm clothing, even in summer,* lack of reaction i. e., when well-chosen remedies fail to act, cardiac weakness, skin symptoms very prominent. Scrofulous patients. Profuse sweating. Easy walking. Offensive discharges.

Tuberculinum, especially adapted to the light-complexioned, narrow-chested subjects. Lax fibre, low recuperative powers, and very susceptible to changes in the weather. Patient always tired, motion causes intense fatigue, aversion to work, wants constant changes. Rapid emaciation, general exhaustion. Nervous weakness. Trembling. Very sensitive mentally and physically

CHAPTER – VIII

AFFECTIONS OF THE THROAT

1. SORE THROAT

This is specially brought on by exposure to cold in the cold months of the year, and during cold, damp weather.

An excellent remedy for sore throat when it first comes on, is to put two or three thicknesses of cloth, which has been dipped in cold water, around the neck and over his flannel folded double may be tied. The patient should at once go to bed covering himself up warmly. By the next morning the sore throat will have gone and the patient will feel better.

If, however, the sore throat develops, the following remedies will be useful.

Aconitum Nap., in the beginning when the patient has difficulty and pain in swallowing or speaking, when the throat is much more red than usual with a burning, pricking or contracting sensation, accompanied by fever, anxiety and uneasiness, to be followed by *Belladonna,* when the fever is very high, pulse full and bounding, great dryness and brightness of the throat, tonsils are swollen and enlarged, constant desire to swallow, swallowing produces spasms of the throat, which forces the liquids partaken of out through the nose, pains shooting into the tonsils and up into the ears, swelling of the outside of the throat, red and swollen face, pain in the forehead. *A great aversion to drink with the sore throat is characteristic.* These two are the most appropriate remedies to commence the treatment with, and in the majority of cases will suffice to effect a cure if the above symptoms are present. If, however, there are other symptoms, the following remedies will be necessary.

AFFECTIONS OF THE THROAT

Bryonia Alba, especially after taking cold, or after getting over-heated, or after eating ice or drinking ice water in the summer, hoarseness, oppressed respiration, pricking and painful sensibility of the throat, *pain on turning the head, dryness of the throat with* difficulty of speech, swallowing painful, pain in the limbs, back and head. These symptoms are frequently accompanied by fever, dry mouth, either with or without thirst, and great irritability.

Rhus Tox., for symptoms similar to those under Bryonia, except that the pain extend further down. The glands under the ears are much swollen, and the patient is extremely restless, a bloody saliva runs out of the mouth during sleep.

Chamomilla, especially useful for children, when the sore throat was induced by taking cold from exposure to a draught of air, or while in a state of perspiration, swelling of the tonsils, tingling in the throat, hacking cough, hoarseness, *child cross and irritable and wishes to be carried in the arms.*

Mercurius Sol., useful in the beginning of an attack, especially when sore throat arises from taking cold, *accompanied with rheumatic pains in the head and nape of the neck,* violent throbbing in the throat and tonsils, extending to the ears and glands of the neck, especially when swallowing, *disagreeable taste in the mouth, profuse discharge of saliva,* chills in the evening, or heat followed by perspiration, swelling and inflammation of the parts affected, ulcers and tendency to suppuration in the throat. When the ulcers *are not painful, and appear gradually, Belladonna is of no use, but Mercurius Sol. should* be given. After *Belladonna or Mercurius Sol.* is given, the patient should avoid catching cold. If, however, the patient catches cold, and there is the tendency to the formation of pus, *Mercurius Sol.* should be continued to hasten the formation of pus, and if pus is formed it should be followed by *Hepar Sulph.* to help the discharge of pus.

Hepar Sulph., in the beginning, if the pricking pains are very violent when swallowing, extending to the ears or to the glands of the throat, and to the lower jaw, *if the patient feels as if a splinter or fish-bone were in the throat,* when the burning in the throat scarcely allows the patient to swallow, with stitches in the swollen tonsils, and a very disagreeable taste in the mouth, the gums and back part of the tongue swollen, with abundant discharge of saliva, in the evening, chills or heat, followed by perspiration, which does not relieve, uneasiness or aggravation of all the symptoms during the right, also worse in the cold air or early in the morning, accompanied by violent headache, and drawing in the nape of the neck. It may also be given when there are several small ulcers, which appear slowly and are not painful. When the suppurated tonsils begin to discharge, this remedy should be given to hasten the discharge. After *Hepar Sulp., Mercurius Sol.* may again be given if there is no improvement.

Lachesis, will be found useful when *Belladonna* or *Mercurius Sol.* has been used without effect, also *when there is a constant* disposition to swallow, dryness of the throat, extensive swelling of the tonsils with threatened suffocation, if the uvula is swollen, *the throat is very sensitive to the touch, even to that of the bed clothes,* it is especially indicated when there are white or gray patches on the tonsils or throat, *particularly when the disease began on the left side, the symptoms are worse* in the evening, sometimes in the morning, *but always after* sleeping.

Nux Vomica, in cases similar to those mentioned under Chamomilla, especially for a sensation as if there were a swelling like a plug or lump in the throat, particularly when swallowing, with pains rather pressing than shooting, *worse on swallowing the saliva.* The throat feels raw and excoriated, or as if scraped and rough, the cold air affects the throat painfully, sometimes the uvula is swollen and red.

Pulsatilla, for the same sensation on swallowing as described under *Nux Vomica,* or the throat appears too narrow, as if obstructed by swelling, redness and sensation of scraping, *dryness of the throat without thirst,* shooting pains in the throat when swallowing, but *worse when not* swallowing, a feeling of tension in the throat, the glands of the neck are painful when touched, the *interior of the throat is more of a bluish red,* the fever is *unaccompanied by thirst,* chilliness in the evening followed by heat.

Sulphur, for frequent or continued sore throat, especially in weak constitutions. *Sulphur* is a valuable remedy to hurry forward the suppuration process when an abscess seems certain to burst,, also, after the discharge of an abscess, when the cavity is slow in headling, or when many abscesses form in succession. In order to hasten the healing, *Silicea* may be given.

In persons pre-disposed to sore throat, *Sulphur, Graphites,* and *Silicea* have been found useful in over coming this constitutional tendency. In such cases, a dose of the remedy suitable for the constitution of the patient may be taken in the 30th potency every fourth day untill six doses are taken, if it has to be repeated after some time, it may be given in the 200th potency, 3 or 4 doses at fortnightly intervals.

2. TONSILITIS OR INFLAMMATION OF THE TONSILS

(a) *Definition–Causes*

Acute tonsilitis has already been considered under 'Sore throat'. Chronic enlargement will now be dealt with.

The tonsils are two oblong, somewhat rounded bodies, placed between the arches of the palate. In some they can scarcely be said to exist, as they are not clearly visible, while in others they fill up the throat to such an extent as to impede swallowing, or even respiration. The use of these glands is to secrete a fluid which makes passage to the stomach smooth and slippery, for the easy transmission of the food we swallow.

Enlargement of these glands from chronic inflammation, or enlargement either congenital, or arising from excessive nutrition which is not assimilated by the system, constitutes the disease under consideration.

Symptoms : The first symptom that attracts attention, is the habitually loud breathing of the patient during sleep, or in other words, his snoring. This caused by the enlarged tonsils pressing upon the palate, which partially closed that passage through the nose, the air being forcibly drawn through this narrowed opening produces that horrid noise. The voice becomes thick and inarticulate. These symptoms and that of snoring become aggravated upon the slightest attack of cold or catarrh.

Deafness is also another symptom and originates from a similar cause–the enlarged tonsil pressing upon the Eustachian tube, which is a small canal leading from the throat to the internal ear. But the most serious consequence of long-continued enlarged tonsils is the effect it produces upon the chest, enlargement of the tonsils, and the "pigeon chest", usually go together. The obstruction preventing the free entrance of air into the lungs, these organs are but imperfectly developed, how this imperfect expansion of the lungs produces the prominence of the breast bone, it is unnecessary to explain in this place, but this is a fact which may be impressed on all.

It will, therefore, be seen that the enlargement of the tonsils, though it may appear to be of slight importance, may lead to serious results.

A weakly child, with slight enlargement of the tonsils, will often get rid of the ailment as he gains strength, and at the age of fourteen or fifteen have entirely outgrown it.

Treatment : The application of Nitrate of silver (Caustic), Iodine, Alum, or to cut the tonsils out, as allopathic physicians generally do, is worse than useless, as in the majority of such cases,

AFFECTIONS OF THE THROAT

after such barbarous operations, the lungs become affected, and sooner or later, as the result, the patient dies of consumption. If there is a patient with a hereditary taint of, or a pre-disposition towards consumption, these external applications or operations are certain to bring about this result.

As the tonsils have a natural function to perform, and are not, therefore, redundant in the man body, it is irrational to torture them by external medications or to have them removed as if they were unnecessary or useless. The only rational way of *curing* these enlarged tonsils is to put the patients under a strict course of homeopathic treatment which will bring them to a normal condition and enable them to function normally. This may take a long time, but it is certainly better and safer in the interest of the patient.

(b) *Acute Tonsilitis*

Baryta Carbonica, in mild cases in the beginning, for those who have an attack from any exposure. If it is given in repeated doses in the 6th potency in the early stages, it removes the predisposition to the attack. *Aconitum Nap.,* if it starts with fever, to be given in teaspoon doses, should be given every three hours, after which, if the tonsils are very much swollen.

Belladonna should be given if the right side is affected and the patient complains of a good deal of headache, and rush of blood to the head. If this does not help, *Hepar Sulph.,* should be given if the pains during swallowing are very severe and reach up to the ear and cervical glands with severe drawing pains in the nape of the neck, also if the affection was the result of mercurial medicines, like calomel.

Lachesis, if the *left side is* affected, and if the neck is very sensitive to the tonsils continue even after *Belladonna and Hep. Sulph.*

If an abscess begins to form after *Belladonna, Mercurius Sol.* should be given which causes the abscess to discharge. This should not be given prematurely, for if it is given before the abscess is ripe for discharge, it will increase the inflammation and render it more obstinate. In obstinate cases, especially on *the left side*, if they don't break, *Silicea* should be followed.

Ignatia, if the tonsils become hard, and have also flat open ulcers. If the ulcers break out rapidly and spread *extensively*, *Belladonna* is required, but if they arise slowly and are rather painless, *Mercurius Sol.* is the chief remedy.

Sulphur, when, after the bursting of the abscess, the parts still remain irritated, and the patient does not recover as fast as he should.

Lachesis, if the uvula is the most swollen part.

(c) *Chronic Enlargement of the Tonsils*

In all cases, it is better to commence the treatment with a dose of *Hepar Sulph.* 200, in water (three doses at two hour intervals on the first day), and after a week or later, the indicated remedy may be given according to symptoms.

Baryta Carbonica, is a very important remedy for children who have a chronic enlargement of the tonsils, and also enlarged glands in other parts of the body, tonsils worse on the right side, backward children, slow to learn and generally shy, slow development of the mind and body as a whole.

Baryta muriatica, mentally weak children with recurrent tonsilitis from taking cold, enlarged tonsils, elongation of the uvula with sore throat, suppuration of the tonsils, swallowing very difficult, worse on the *right* side.

Calcarea Phosphorica, chronic enlargement of the tonsils in delicate children and also adenoid growths, the tonsils are flabby pale, with inflammation and *impaired* hearing.

Lycopodium Clav., chronic enlargement of the tonsils, which are covered with small ulcers.

AFFECTIONS OF THE THROAT

Sulphur and *Psorinum,* in chronic cases.

Tuberculinum Bacillinum, adenoids are greatly benefited and are often permanently cured by a weekly dose of *Bacillinum 30,* and fortnightly doses of *Tuberculinum Bov 200.*

3. ENLARGEMENT OF THE UVULA OR FALLING OF THE PALATE

This is merely an inflammation or swelling of the uvula. It may be remedied right in the beginning by repeated doses of *Nux Vomica* every two hours till the unpleasant feeling subsides. If this does not help, *Mercurius Sol., Belladonna,* or *Sulphur* may be tried in the same way.

4. DIPHTHERIA

Symptoms : It generally commences with slight chills and flashes of heat, some little irritation of the throat, but no great amount of pain or difficulty in swallowing, stoppage of the nose or fluent discharge, aching in the bones, general prostration and weariness, occasionally with high fever and severe pain in the head, disordered stomach and loss of appetite, followed in the course of twenty-four on forty-eight hours by a more or less decided aggravation of the throat trouble, the glands about the neck becoming sensitive and swollen, with an increased flow of saliva or water in the mouth. In more severe cases, the patient early complains of soreness of the throat and stiffness of the neck, externally, the tonsils are found enlarged and tender, internally, the inflammation is plainly visible, sometimes appearing bright and glassy, at others almost purplish, and dotted over with spots of false membrane. These spots may vary in size from a split pea to a half inch in diameter. When the membrane becomes detached, it leaves the surface beneath looking like a piece of raw meat in many cases, there is fever, with headache almost unbearable, the breath is extremely offensive. A *characteristic symptom* is the *extreme prostration* with which all these cases are attended.

A rash on the skin, resembling sometimes measles, at other times scarlet fever, often accompanies this disease, it breaks out sometimes at the beginning, sometimes at a later period, in a large number of cases it does not appear at all, it may last only a few hours, or remain a longer time, or reappear after having been absent for several days.

Treatment

Bryonia Alba, the patient is *quickly prostrated, avoids all motion* and complains on the slightest movement of pain everywhere, white tongue, dryness of the mouth without thirst, or else desire for large quantities of water.

Belladonna, the patient is restless, complains of sore throat, the faces look highly inflamed, the pupils are enlarged, he feels drowsy but yet unable to fall asleep, starts suddenly out of sleep.

Lachesis, when after *Belladonna,* by next evening there is no marked change for the better, or when he is even worse in the morning after some sleep, with a distinct development of the skinny patches on the tonsils, *worse on the left side,* or when cough symptoms appear, and the patient cannot bear anything touching his neck and throat.

Lycopodium Clav., when the appearance of the throat is rather *brownish red,* worse on the right side, and worse from swallowing *warm* drinks, when the nose is stopped up, and the patient cannot breathe with his mouth shut, he keeps his mouth constantly open, slightly projecting his tongue, which gives him a silly expression, the nostrils are widely dilated with every inspiration, on awakening out of a short nap, he is very cross, or he jumps up in bed, stares about and does not recognise anybody, frequent jerkings of the lower limbs, mostly with a groan, awake, or slumbering, great fear of being left alone.

AFFECTIONS OF THE THROAT

Rhus Tox., when the child is restless, wants to be carried about, wakes up every now and then complaining of pain in the throat, bloody saliva runs out of the mouth during sleep, the parotid glands are very much swollen, there are transparent jelly-like discharges from the bowels as stool, or afterwards.

Apis Mell., great debility from the beginning, the membrane assumes at once a *dirty-greyish* colour, or there is a great edema of the soft palate and uvula, puffiness around the eyes, pain in the ears, when swallowing, an *itchy, stinging eruption on the skin,* a sensation of weakness in the larynx, numbness of the feet and hands and even paralysis.

It *acts almost as a specific when edema stands first among the indications.* When all other remedies fail, this should be tried in every case. It *should not, however, be given either before or after Rhus Toxicodendron.*

Antimonium Tart, difficult breathing, gasping for air, *rattling in the chest, retching, vomiting of tenacious mucus,* small circular patches, like small-pox pustules, in and upon the mouth and tongue, edema of the lungs.

Ignatia, in many cases this remedy is alone required. There is more or less membrane in the throat, usually in greater abundance *on the right side. Much prostration.*

Mercurius cyanatus, tongue coated thickly white or yellowish. *Much salivation, glands swollen.* Much membrane on tonsils. It is *especially a remedy in the malignant type of diphtheria and when the disease invades the nostrils. Extreme debility even from the beginning.*

Kalium Bichromicum, yellow coated or dry, red tongue, thick, tenacious exudation, pain extending to neck and shoulders.

It is most useful in the later stage of the disease, when the line of demarcation has formed and the slough has commenced to separate.

Diphtherinim, when the attack from the onset tends to malignancy, painless diphtheria. Symptoms almost or entirely objective. Patient weak, apathetic, stupor. Dark-red swelling of tonsils and throat. Breath and discharges very ofensive *(Merc Cy.)* Membrane thick, dark-grey or brownish black. Temperature low, or sub-normal. Pulse weak and rapid. Vital reaction very low. Epistaxis or profound prostration from the onset. Collapse almost at the very beginning. Swallows without pain, but fluids are vomited or returned through nose. Laryngeal diphtheria, post-diphtheritic paralysis *(Caust., Gels.)*

When the patient from the first seems doomed, and the most carefully selected remedies fail to relieve. To remove persistent diphtheria–organisms in 'carriers'. As a prophylactic, *Diphtherinim* 30 may be given *weekly.* Dose–Diphtherinum 30 and 200. *Must not be repeated too frequently.*

Post–Diphtheric Paralysis

Gelsemium, with regurgitations through nose *(Lycopodium Clav. Caust., Coculus Ind.).*

CHAPTER – IX

AFFECTIONS OF THE TEETH

CAUSES: This troublesome affection may arise from many causes— Some are hereditarily predisposed to it, while others suffer from every exposure, again, it may arise from disturbances going on elsewhere in the system, or it may be purely nervous. It is often rheumatic, often arises from carious teeth, also from abuse of coffee or calomel. Many are its causes, and as numerous as its forms. It may be confined to one tooth, or it may extend to many, one side of the face, both, or even the whole face may be affected. The pain may be of any and of all forms imaginable, from a dull, heavy ache to a sharp, shooting pain.

The principal remedies for toothache are: *Aconitum Nap., Arnica Mont., Antimonium Crud., Arsenicum Alb., Belladonna, Bryonia Alba, Chamomilla, Kreosote, Mercurius Sol., Nux Vomica, Pulsatilla and Sulphur.*

Leading Indications

TOOTHACHE IN CHILDREN–*Aconitum Nap., Bell., Cham., Mercurius Sol., Puls., Coffea.*

IN FEMALES–*Aconitum Nap., Bell., Cham., China off., Coffea, Hyosyamus Nig, Puls.*

DURING NURSING– *Aconitum Nap., Bell., China, Nux V.*

DURING MENSTRUATION–*Calcarea, Carb Alba, Cham., Puls., Bryorina Alba, Lach.*

DURING PREGNANCY–*Bell., Bryonia Alba, Nux V., Puls., Staph., Rhus Tox.*

FROM CALOMEL– *Carbo Veg., Hepar Sulp., Puls., Sulph.,*

Lach.

FROM TAKING COLD–*Aconitum Nap., Bell., Bryonia Alba, Dulc., Hyosyamus Nig., Mercurius Sol., Nux V., Rhus Tox., Phos., Puls.*

WITH SWELLED FACE– *Cham., Mercurius Sol., Nux V., Puls., Bryonia Alba.*

WITH SWELLED`GUMS–*Aconitum Nap., Bell., Mercurius Sol.,Nux V., Sulph.*

WITH SWELLED GLANDS– *Mercurius Sol.,Bell., Nux V.*

WITH FACEACHE– *Mercurius Sol., Acon Nap., Bell., Bryonia Alba, Cham.*

WITH EARACHE– *Cham., Mercurius Sol., Puls., Calcarea Carb, Sulph.*

WITH HEADACHE–*Bell., Glon., Nux V., Lach., Puls.*

OF A NERVOUS NATURE– *Aconitum Nap., Bell., Coff., Ign., Hyosyamus Nig., Cham., Nux Vom., Spig.*

OF A RHEUMATIC NATURE– *Cham., Mercurius Sol., Bryonia Alba, Bell., Sulph., Puls., Rhus Tox.*

OF A CONGESTIVE NATURE– *Aconitum Nap., Bell., Cham., Puls., China.*

OF A HYSTERICAL NATURE– *Ign., Cham., Hyosyamus Nig., Sep., Bell.*

ON THE LEFT SIDE– *Aconitum Nap., Cham., Phos., Sulph.*

ON THE RIGHT SIDE– *Bell., Bryonia Alba, Staph.*

IN THE UPPER JAW– *Bell., Calc Carb, Bryonia Alba.*

IN THE LOWER JAW– *Caust., Nux V., Staph., Sulph.*

Aconitum Nap., feverishness, with great anxiety and restlessness, violent throubbing or beating pain, rheumatic pain in the face and teeth, congestion of the head, heat, redness and swelling of the face, *toothache occasioned by cold*. If it does not give relief, follow with *Belladonna or Chamomilla.*

AFFECTIONS OF THE TEETH

Arnica Mont., when the pain is the *result of mechanical injuries*, as from extraction or plugging. If children fall and injure the teeth, at the same time bruise and cut the lips or cheeks, *Arnica tincture* may be used as a lotion by mixing one part of the tincture with six parts of water, and a linen cloth dipped in the lotion may be laid on the injured part, and renewed every three or four hours. When the injury is in the interior of the lips, or the teeth alone are affected, the mouth may be rinsed or gargled with this solution.

At the same time *Arnica Mont.* 30 may be given internally at intervals of three or four hours.

Antimonium Crud., for pain in hollow and decayed teeth.

Arsenicum Alb. is useful when *everything cold aggravates, the pain*.

Belladonna, when there is a sensation of ulceration at the roots of the teeth, drawing pain in the face and teeth, extending to the ears, *aggravated in the evening on getting warm in the bed, or on applying anything hot, heat and throbbing in the gums*.

Bryonia Alba. drawing, jerking toothache, with a sensation as though the teeth were loose and elongated, *especially during and after eating*, pain in decayed teeth, *toothache caused by wet weather*, or accompanying *rheumatic affections, pains relieved momentarily by cold water held in the mouth.* Bryonia is serviceable for *pains through the face generally*, and for pains which *shoot from one tooth* into another.

Chamomilla, violent, boring and throbbing pain, extending through the jaws to the ears, also into the temples and eyes, the child is cross and feverish, complains of pain in all the teeth, cannot tell which aches the most, *worse at night, when the patient is warm in bed, also after eating anything warm*, swelling and redness of the cheeks. *Chamomilla* is useful for *toothache before menstruation*.

Kreosote, for pain in decayed teeth, with swelling and congestion of the gums.

Mercurius Sol., for pains in hollow teeth, tearing pain through the root of the teeth, shooting pain, passing over through the sides of the face, extending to the ears, especially at night, *aggravated by cold food or drink,* swelling and inflammation of the gums.

Nux Moschata, especially for pregnant women, also sometimes for children, when it arises from taking cold.

Nux Vomica, toothache *arising from cold,* with throbbing, boring, or gnawing pain, throughout the teeth and gums, *aggravated by eating, or exposure to the open air,* tearing pain on one side, rheumatic pains deep down in the nerve of the tooth, with *pain as though the tooth were being wrenched out.* This may be followed by *Mercurius Sol.* if there is no relief.

Pulsatilla, is most suitable for young girls, or children of a mild or timid disposition, shooting pain that extends to the ear of the affected side, *jerking pain as though the nerve was tightened, and then suddenly relaxed, particularly on the left side, the pain increased by warmth and rest, better walking about, especially in the open air,* toothache accompanied by earache and headache.

Sulphur, tearing and pulsative pain, particularly *carious or decayed* teeth, extending of the upper jaw and into the ear, *pain worse at night, when warm in bed,* swelling of the gums attended with shooting pain, suits well after *Mercurius Sol.*

CHAPTER X

AFFECTIONS OF THE MOUTH

1. GUMBOIL, SORE MOUTH

Mercurius Sol., is indicated in almost every case for extensive, bright, inflammatory redness and swelling in the gums and root of the mouth.

If the swelling was brought about by the use of calomel or other mercurial preparations, *Carbo Veg.* should be given, and followed, if necessary, by *Hepar Sulph.* or *Nitricum Acidum.*

If the disorder is the result of excessive use of salt food, *Carbo Veg.* will be useful when the gums bleed much and the smell is very offensive, or *Arsenicum Alb.* if the ulcers burn violently and the patient is much debilitated.

Natrium Mur., when the ulcers spread slowly and the above remedies give no relief, the gums are swollen, bleed and very sensitive, everything cold or warm, or eating or drinking, affects them, when white blisters and small ulcers appear on the tongue, which bite and burn, and render talking painful.

Sulphur, at the end of the cure, or when other remedies fail, also when there is swelling of the gums, with pulsative pains.

Gargling of the mouth with lemon juice will be beneficial.

2. INFLAMMATION AND SWELLING OF THE TONGUE

Aconitum Nap. for inflammation and swelling of the tongue.

Mercurius Sol. after *Aconitum Nap.* or in the beginning when there is violent pain, swelling, hardness and salivation, also in ulceration of the tongue.

For inflammation of the tongue

(a)   Caused by wounds, *Aconitum Nap.* and *Arnica Mont.*

(b)   Caused by stings of bees, or the like, *Natrium Mur.*

(c)   Produced by biting the tongue during sleep, *Phos Acid.*

If children are slow in learning to talk, *Natrium Mur.* will be useful and may be given in the 30th potency at weekly intervals, and in the 200th potency at fortnightly intervals for some time.

CHAPTER – XI

AFFECTIONS OF THE STOMACH AND ABDOMEN

1. CATARRH OF THE STOMACH, HEARTBURN, WATERBRASH, SOUR STOMACH

DEFINITION–SYMPTOMS: Under these names are usually arranged the following symptoms; gnawing or a burning sensation at the pit of the stomach, accompanied with or followed by sour, acid eructations, or belchings, attended with nausea, coldness of the extremities, and often with faintings. These disagreeable symptoms are always aggravated when anything is taken into the stomach which does not exactly agree with it.

When these symptoms appears by themselves, unconnected with any other trouble, the following remedies will be useful:

Ipecac., should first be given, and then, if necessary, one of the following remedies :

Nux Vomica, if the symptoms come especially after eating. If this does not held and there is much flatulence or frequent rising of wind, *China* and then *Carbo Veg.*

For flatulence after eating fat food, *Pulsatilla,* if attended with colic, *Nux Vomica.*

For sour stomach in nursing infants, *Chamomilla, Ipecac.,* or *Nux Vomica.*

2. BILIOUSNESS

SYMPTOMS: The patient at first appears dull and languid, complains of headache, or rather, a giddy sensation in the head, great oppression, and a fullness at the pit of the stomach, with nausea, sometimes vomiting, eructations of offensive gas, the tongue is covered with a thick, slimy, yellowish coating, there is a disagreeable, bitter, putrid, or slimy taste in the mouth, especially in the morning. Bowels are either constipated or quite loose, the evacuations are dark, very offensive, and accompanied with a great deal of stinking wind.

Bryonia Alba, is useful when in addition to the above symptoms there is chilliness, followed by fever, rapid pulse, and headache.

Pulsatilla, when they are due to eating fatty foods.

Ipecac and Mercurius Sol., will be sufficient in a majority of cases.

3. NAUSEA AND VOMITING

Ipecac, the stomach is irritated by the least drink. Simple copious vomiting with an extremely sick sensation. Persistent nausea and vomiting is its chief indication.

Antimonium Crud., nausea, *thickly coated white tongue,* eructations, loss of appetite.

Arsenicum Alb., burning in the stomach and throat, excessive weakness, purging, coldness of the hands and feet.

Nux Vom., or Bryonia Alba, vomiting with dryness of the mouth, disturbed sleep and constipation, especially indicated if vomiting is due to strong drink, heavy food, or keeping late or irregular hours. Chronic or long standing cases require *Sulphur,* to be followed by *Calcarea Carb.*

AFFECTIONS OF THE STOMACH AND ABDOMEN

4. SEA–SICKNESS OR VOMITING FROM TRAVELLING IN A CARRIAGE, MOTOR CAR OR BY AIR

Nux Vom., and *Petroleum,* are good preventives if taken a day or some hours before the journey.

Cocculus and *Veratrum Alb.*, useful during the journey.

Arsenicum Alb., after severe and prolonged sea–sickness with great weakness.

Opium, has also given quick relief in some cases, and may be tried when the symptoms increase.

Belladonna, in air–sickness of aviators, give as *preventive*.

5. COLIC OR GRIPING PAIN IN THE BOWELS

Colocynth, violent pains cutting as if from knives, compelling the patient to *bend double and press something hard into the abdomen* which relieves the pain, with bilious colic, with bilious diarrhea and vomiting.

Nux Vom., from indigestible food, in brandy or coffee drinkers, suppressed monthly periods, or during pregnancy, with severe contracting pains low in the abdomen and relieved by pressure, from bowels not moving freely, or alternate constipation and diarrhea.

Chamomilla, particularly suitable for women and children.

Colic from anger, worse from warmth, flatulent colic.

Cina, Sulphur or *Mercurius Sol.* colic due to worms.

Opium, lead colic or colic of compositors who work in printing presses, or painters who use paints containing lead.

FOR COLIC IN PREGNANT WOMEN– *Chamomilla, Nux Vom., Pulsatilla.*

MENSTRUAL COLIC– Pulsatilla, Coffea, Belladonna, Cocculus Ind.

6. DYSPEPSIA OR INDIGESTION

Definition : The terms 'Dyspepsia' means difficult digestion or indigestion. It is a condition or state of the stomach, in which its function of digestion is disturbed or suspended giving rise to a train of numerous symptoms, such as want of appetite, sudden and transient distension of the stomach, eructations of various kinds, heart burn, water-brash, pain in the region of the stomach, uneasiness after eating, rumbling noise in the bowels, sometimes vomiting, and frequently constipation or diarrhea, with an endless string of nervous symptoms.

Causes : Sedentary occupations, especially when carried on in close rooms and factories, indolent habits, either of body or mind, long and intense study, insufficient exercise in the open air, excesses in eating, wrong modes of living, such as excessive use of coffee or tea, or indulgence in liquors, intoxicating drugs, or tobacco in any form, or the habitual use of purgatives.

Treatment : The treatment of this complicated disease may be divided under the following head.

FOR DYSPEPSIA OF ADULTS : *Antimonium Crud., Arnica, Bell., Bryonia Alba, Calcarea Carb., Carb., Veg., Allium Cepa, Chamomilla, China, Hepar Sulph., Ipecac., Lachesis, Mercurius Sol., Nux Vom., Pulsatilla, Sulphur.*

FOR DYSPEPSIA OF CHILDREN : *Bryonia Alba, Calcarea, Carb., Chamomilla, Ipecac, Puls., Sulphur.*

TRANSIENT OR ACUTE DYSPEPSIA : Arnica, Ant. Crud., Bell., Bryonia, Ipecac., Mercurius, Nux *Vom., Puls.*

HABITUAL OR CHRONIC DYSPEPSIA : *Arsenicum, Bell., Calcarea Carb., China, Hep. Sulph., Lachesis, Mercurius., Nux Vom., Puls., Sulph.*

AFFECTIONS OF THE STOMACH AND ABDOMEN 195

Arnica Mont., when the disorder is *caused by a fall, blow upon the stomach,* or by *lifting heavy weights,* with pain and a sensation as if the small of the back is broken, also with great sensitiveness and nervous excitement, frequent eructations with a putrid or bitter taste, tongue with thick, yellowish coat, some nausea with inclination to vomit, head full and giddy, also heaviness of the limbs. If *Arnica* is not sufficient, give *Nux Vomica,* or this failing, *Chamomilla.*

Antimonium Crud., particularly useful for disorders arising *from overloading* of stomach, with frequent eructations tasting of food last partaken of, mouth feels dry, or saliva flows from it, much thirst particularly during the night, great desire for sour things, accumulation of mucus in the throat, or vomiting of mucus and bile, *tongue coated with white or yellowish mucus,* stomach distended and tender to touch, also flatulency with griping pains or diarrhea. The *patient is drowsy and could sleep all the time.* If *Antimonium Crud.* does not help, try *Bryonia Alba.*

Belladonna, painful distension of the abdomen, with griping pains as if the bowels were grasped with the fingers, flatulent colic, hiccough, bitter erucations, nausea with loathing of food, vomiting of water, or bile, also dullness of the head or congestion of blood to the head.

Arsenicum Alb., in serious chronic cases, with great prostration of vital powers, sunken cheeks, extremities cold, face pale, dark circle around the eyes, nose pointed, tongue white, or of a brownish colour, dry and trembling, pulse irregular, small, frequent and weak. Also with severe cramps in the stomach, with sensation of coldness or much heat, when vomiting becomes excfessive, everything taken being thrown out from the stomach, the skin hot and dry, the patient becomes emaciated and the face pale. If *Arsenicm Alb.* does not prove favourable, give *Lachesis.*

Bryonia Alba, an important remedy for dyspepsia *occurring in summer, or in warm and damp weather, also when* accompanied with chilliness, headache, pain in the limbs, small of the back, etc. *Tongue dry and red, or coated* white or yellow, loss of appetite or perverted appetite, *bowels constipated, excessive thirst,* both night and day, and more *dryness in the throat and stomach.* If *Bryonia Alba* does not help, try *Antimonium Crud.*

Allium Cepa, no hunger but considerable thirst, particularly in the evening, greatest nausea, many eructations which relieved a little, sometimes frothy mucus is raised, weakness in the stomach, as if empty, pressure in stomach, more when bending forward, fullness in the head, much yawning, much flatulence, with pain in the stomach, tongue always coated, particularly towards the base, and early in the morning.

Carbo veg., loss of appetite, *digestion slow and imperject,* with distension of the stomach after eating, *empty eructations or belching up of air tasting of the fat and food eaten, flatulence fetid and offensive,* wind-colic, rumbling in the abdomen, water brash, hiccough, contractive or burning pain in the stomach, nausea in the morning, *tendency to diarrhea,* suitable for chronic dyspepsias of *old people,* follows well after *Nux Vom.*

Calcarea Carb., particularly for *fat children* who are *slow and sluggish, or weak children slow in learning to walk, with bloated abdomen, with sour eructations and sour vomitings, sour smelling diarrhea. Chronic dyspepsias of adults, with heart-burn after any kind of food,* sour vomiting of food, sour eructations, morning nausea, loss of appetite, at other times, canine hunger, distension of abdomen, pain in the stomach after eating, followed by nausea and vomiting, desire for wine, salt or sweet things.

Chamomilla, especially for gastric derangements brought on by a fit of a passion, bitter or sour eructations, regurgitation of food, nausea, vomiting of food, green phlegm or bile, cramps in the

AFFECTIONS OF THE STOMACH AND ABDOMEN 197

stomach, distension of the stomach, sometimes constipation, but generally diarrheal, especially in children, while the evacations are green or watery. Headache, fullness, giddiness, and staggering in the morning when getting up, sleep disturbed, tossing about, frequent awaking, face red and hot, eyes red and burning, disposition very sensitive. If this does not relieve, give *Pulsatilla* and it this also is insufficient, give *Nux Vomica*.

China off., especially applicable for that form of dyspepsia which is *caused by an impure atmosphere,* which is overloaded with exhalations of decayed vegetable matter, also for indigestion which precedes of accompanies chills and malarial fever.

Pressure in stomach as from a load, constant feeling of having eaten too much, constant eructations, aversion to food and drink, with feeling of fullness, flat or bitter taste in the mouth, morbid craving for all sorts of things, after eating, drowsiness, oppressive fullness in the stomach and abdomen, weakness and tired feeling, disposition to lie down, without being able to remain quiet, patient obliged to bend and stretch his limbs which are quite stiff in the morning, the patient melancholy and morose.

Hepar Sulph., important remedy for correcting chronic derangement of the stomach, caused by taking blue-pills or other preparations of mercury, or where the stomach appears to be very sensitive and easily deranged, though the patient may be healthy and very regular in his general habits. Nausea in the morning, with eructations, or vomiting of sour, bilious, or mucous substances, *appetite only for something sour or pungent, aversion to fat.* Distension in the pit of the stomach, as from wind, cannot bear tight clothes. Bowels constipated, stools hard and dry, or in children, a sour, whitish diarrhea. If *Hepar Sulph.* is not sufficient, try *Lachesis.*

Ipecac., the principal remedy for indigestion of children, due to imperfect mastication or taking improper food. It should be given in the beginning, when the tongue is coated white or yellowish, nausea with empty eructations, vomiting of undigested food, or of bile or bitter fluid, vomiting with diarrhea, and coldness of the face and extremities, *diarrhea with nausea, colic and vomiting.*

For adults, when the tongue is not coated, although the patient is sick at the stomach and vomits, aversion to food, especially rich fat food, headache with nausea and vomiting, for easy or violent vomiting when the vomit contains mucus, especially when accompanied by diarrhea, *also when the complaint returns every day, or every other day, at the same hour.*

Lachesis, in severe cases where *Hepar Sulph.* or *Arsenicum Alb.* is found insufficient, and *when the complaint is worse immediately* after meals, or *early in the morning,* when several days pass without any evacuation.

Mercurius Sol., acrid, bitter eructations, putrid, sweetish, or bitter taste in the morning, bilious vomiting, aversion to solid food, pressure at the pit of the stomach after eating, weak digestion, with constant hunger. Suits well before or after *Lachesis.*

Nux Vom., if caused by dissipation and late hours, by *drinking wine or coffee,* particularly if the patient has caught cold besides, mouth dry without thirst, tongue coated white, accumulation of mucus in the mouth and heartburn, no taste, water collects in the mouth, vomiting, pressure and weight in the stomach, the abdomen is distended, scanty and hard evacuations, or none at all, reeling, giddiness or dullness in the head, heaviness in the back part of the head, ringing in the ears, drawing in the limbs, want of energy and aversion to thinking, patient restless, quarrelsome, sullen, at times there is heat in the face, red pimples on the face.

If this remedy is not sufficient, give *Chamomilla.*

For chronic dyspepsia of old people, follow with *Carbo Veg.*

Pulsatilla, caused by over-eating, or *by the use of too much fat, meat, oily articles or articles fried in oil or rancid butter,* when the taste is bitter, saltish, or resembles that of putrid meat or fat, *aversion to food, especially to meat, bread, butter, milk* and any thing warm, *no thirst for water,* pressure in the pit of the stomach, especially after eating, wind colic at night, rolling and rumbling in the abdomen, slow, small evacuations of diarrhea, frequent urging to stool, waterbrash. The patient feels chilly, is weak, cross, sad, melancholy, annoyed at every trifle, not inclined to talk.

Sulphur, acts well after *Nux Vomica and Mercurius Sol.* in cases of long standing, or when there is loss of appetite, aversion to meat, difficulty of breathing, nausea after eating, belching or vomiting of food, colic immediately after eating, water-brash, sour stomach, flatulence and constipation. Mental depression, morose irascibility, dissatisfied with everything and everybody. Should be taken at *long* intervals in the *200th potency.* If it fails to effect a cure after a considerable time, give *Calcarea Carb. or Mercurius Sol.* and after these, *Sulphur* may act more favourably again.

7. CONSTIPATION

Causes

CONSTIPATION OF INFANTS: Generally appears in children who are wholly or practically fed upon artificial diet, and in those whose mothers take improper foods.

CONSTIPATION OF ADULTS AND OLDER CHILDREN: Is caused by improper diet, stimulating foods and drinks, such as coffee, strong tea, alcohol, etc., heavy sleep. Inattention to normal desire for evacuation of the bowels, and the habitual use of purgative medicines.

The fundamental difference in the method of treatment of constipation in the Homeopathic and all other systems of medicine is that, while the former aims at correcting the system and removing the cause of the disorder, the others consider this abnormal condition as a simple obstruction of the intestinal canal, and if the bowls are once opened by means of purgative, the trouble is over. The result is that while the Homeopathic medicines improve the general condition of the patient and make him healthy, the purgatives produce violent evacuations at first as a first effect, but habitual constipation, always requiring purgatives, is the final result.

The principal remedies are : *Nux Vomica, Bryonia Alba, Opium, Lycopodium Clav., Sulphur, Alumina, Plumbum, Platina, Graphites and Naturium Muriaticum.*

Nux Vomica, antidotes purgative medicines, constant ineffective urging to stool, that is, a *sensation as if a part remained behind,* irregular action of the bowels, constipation with nausea and sickness in the morning, distension and heaviness in the stomach, ill-humour, fullness of pain in the head, uneasy sleep. It is suited to constipation following intoxicating drinks, absence of coffee for those accustomed to its regular use, eating too much or different kinds of food at one time, over study, sedentary habits. Also when constipation is preceded by diahrrea, or accompanied by a feeling of general depression.

If *Nux Vomica* proves inefficient, give *Bryonia Alba,* if the disorder occurs in warm weather or is accompanied by disordered stomach.

Bryonia Alba, for those who are *regularly constipated* and have *dry mouth* generally and pass *large, hard, dry stools with great difficulty,* owing to weakness of the rectum, constipation with headache and irritability, in *bilious and rheumatic patients, and during warm weather* when accompanied with disordered stomachs.

AFFECTIONS OF THE STOMACH AND ABDOMEN

Opium, constipation from a general paralytic condition of the intestines with stools in the form of *hard, dry, black balls,* like sheep's dung, *obstinate constipation* with a feeling as if the anus were closed, headache, dizziness, dry mouth and thirst, *in chronic cases* from want to outdoor exercise, especially useful for the constipation of aged persons when the patient is drowsy and dizzy, in 200th potency is more useful in such cases.

Lycopodium Clav., Like *Nux Vom.,* sensation after stool as if something remained behind, but with tightness of the anus, useful for the *constipation of children and pregnant women,* mental depression, melancholy and apprehension.

Sulphur, ineffectual urging to stool with a sensation of heat and discomfort in the rectum and a general uneasy feeling all through the intestinal tract, habitual constipation with tendency to piles, either blind or bleeding, constipation, alternating with diarrhea, follows *Nux Vom.* very well, *Sulphur* 200 should be used at long intervals for *chronic cases.*

Alumina, chief remedy for *chronic* troubles due to dryness of the intestinal tract and want of action of the rectum, so that even soft stool is expelled with difficulty, no *urging to stool, stools hard and knotty like sheep's dung,* or soft, differs from *Bryonia Alba in inactivity of the rectum but* not in its weakness. One of the most useful in constipation of children, where the rectum is dry, inflamed and bleeding about the opening.

Plumbum Met., for obstinate constipation, tenacious, hard difficult stools, sometimes in hard lumps or balls, along with the urging there is a *colic with a marked retraction of the abdominal walls,* the anus feels as if drawn upward.

Platina, when, after much straining, the faces are evacuated in but small quantities, straining and itching at the anus, *shuddering over the whole body after every evacuation,* accompanied by feeling of weakness in the abdomen, with contraction, bearing down, oppression of the stomach, and ineffectual efforts to belch wind, suitable also for *constipation after or while travelling.*

Graphites, is very useful when there in no urging and the patient sometimes passes several days without a stool, and when it does come it is composed of little round balls, knotted together with shreds of mucus, and accompanied with great pain when passing, owing to the fissure in the anus. Excessive pain and soreness of the anus after stool.

Natrium Muriaticum, in tedious cases, where the above remedies have failed, and there is no *inclination whatever to evacuate,* also when the stools are scanty, hard and insufficient, and there is a *constant feeling as if something were being pressed down in the large intestine, without regular urging to stool.*

Conium Mac., ineffectual urging, hard stool. Inability to strain at stool, inability to expel contents because of the paralytic weakness of all the muscles that take part in expulsion. Strains so much at stool that uterus protrudes. At every stool, tremendous weakness and palpitation has dizziness, numbness, paralytic weakness, mental and physical.

A peculiar symptom, sweats copiously during sleep, on merely closing eyes.

FOR CONSTIPATION OF PREGNANT WOMEN–*Nux Vom., Opium, Sepia.*

FOR CONSTIPATION OF LYING–IN–WOMEN– *Bryonia Alba, Nux Vom.*

FOR CONSTIPATION OF NURSING INFANTS– *Bryonia Alba, Nux Vom., Opium, Sulphur.*

8. PILES OR HEMORRHOIDS

Nux Vomica and Sulphur are the principal remedies for piles.

Nux Vomica, in every form of piles, with a burning and

AFFECTIONS OF THE STOMACH AND ABDOMEN

constipated feeling in the rectum, and a bruised pain in the small of the back, due to sedentary habits, or due to intoxicating drinks, strong coffee etc., also when there is a discharge of light blood after each evacuation of the bowels, and a constant disposition to evacuate.

Sulphur is adapted for all forms of piles, and like *Nux Vomica* is especially called for, when there is constant, ineffectual inclination to stool. It is also useful when there is considerable protrusion of the tumours, so much so that it is difficult to replace them, also when there are violent, shooting pains in the back.

Nux Vomica, may be given at night and may be followed by *Sulphur* on the following morning.

When these two remedies, after two or three day's trial, fail to afford relief, then *Ignatia* may be given, especially if the pains, like violent stitches, shoot upward, or where, after the evacuation, there is painful contraction and soreness, or the rectum protrudes after each evacuation.

Pulsatilla, when blood and mucus are discharged with the faeces, with painful pressure on the tumors, pains in the back, pale countenance, disposition to faint. It acts better in the 200th potency. If it is insufficient, *Mercurius Sol.,* and afterwards *Sulphur,* may help in these cases. If there is much straining, *Sepia* will help better.

Capsicum, is very suitable when the tumours are much swollen, the blood discharged with burning pains, and mixed with slime, also when there is a *drawing pain in the back,* particularly in the small of the back, and *cutting pains in the bowels.*

Carbo Vegetablis, when much mucus is discharged or mucus and blood, with much burning in the anus, everything sours in the stomach, the patient is much troubled with wind, which is lodged in different parts of the belly, or becomes very weak. If it proves insufficient, follow with *Arsenicum Alb.*

Lycopodium follows, if *Sulphur* proves insufficient, when the piles always return after contipation, the patient is much troubled with wind, and has much pain under the short ribs.

Belladonna, for bleeding piles, with intense pain in the small of the back, as if it were breaking, if it proves insufficient give *Hepar Sulph.*, and if not completely cured in four or five days, give *Rhus Tox.*

Collinsonia, very useful in obstinate cases which bleed almost incessantly, with a sensation of sticks in the rectum, with constipation from inertia of the lower bowel. It should be used in mother tincture or 1 potency.

Aloes Soc., is indicated when the *piles protrude like a bunch of grapes,* bleeding often and profusely and are *greatly relieved by the application of cold water,* a very marked burning in the anus, the bowels feel as if scraped. There is a *tendency escape, to diarrhea, with a constant feeling as if stool would escape.*

9. WORMS AND ITCHING OF THE ANUS

An eminent physician writes, "When we consider how universally worms are found in all young animals, and how frequently they exist in the human body, without producing disease of any kind, it is natural to conclude that they serve some useful and necessary purpose in the animal economy." It has been testified that they exist, from the child's birth, in numbers sufficient of fulfil the end for which they were designed, and it is only when disease or hereditary habit of body favourable for their development exists, that worms show themselves in any quanntities, or by their presence produce any disturbance. Worm by themselves are not the *Causes* of diseases as is generally supposed, but the conditions of improper living, such as when children are allowed to eat too much of sugar, cakes and similar articles of a harmful nature, are the real causes which promote the formation of worms in large numbers. So, the

AFFECTIONS OF THE STOMACH AND ABDOMEN

proper method of removing, what are termed worm symptoms, is not by mere expulsion of the worms by mere worm powders or purgatives, but to remove the disordered condition of the system which is favourable for the development and support of the worms. The immediate effect of the worm powders which are poisons, and purgatives, is no doubt that the worms are killed in the process, but these poisons kill the children also, or affect the abdomen in such a manner that the consequences appear many years later. The effect of the purgatives is also to drive the worms from the faeces, which they naturally inhabit, to the mucous surface of the intestines, besides exciting a secretion, upon which they multiply and flourish. Children who have worms should avoid potatoes, heavy food of all kinds, sugar or articles made of sugar, as far as possible, also salt, but should be made to take light food, a good deal of ripe fruits, plenty of cold water and milk. Carrots are specially recommended as useful.

Cina 200 is one of the chief remedies for all complaints really arising from worms, especially when the following symptoms are present; boring with the fingers in the nose, picking the lips, changing of the color of the face, being at times pale and cold at others, red and hot, tongue coated, cross and fretful temper, bloated face, with dark circle around the eye, bloated abdomen, constipation or loose evacuations, fever, especially at night, with pain in the head, starting or talking in sleep, grinding of the teeth in sleep, itching of the anus, crawling out of thread worms.

Nux Vomica, when with worm symptoms, there is constipation, severs itching, burning, and pricking sensation at the anus, caused by little worms.

Aconitum Nap., is useful in the beginning when the child is restless, there is considerable fever with colic and distension of the abdomen, irritable temper and constant itching and burning at the anus. A dose may be given every two hours. If this proves insufficient, this may be followed by *Ignatia* after a few hours, and if this is also not sufficient give *Mercurius Sol.* If the trouble recurs, *Sulphur* may be given for four of five days in the morning at the time of *Full moon,* followed by *Silicea* in the same way during *New moon.*

For tape worms, give a dose of *Sulphur* in the mornings for two days during waning moon and at the next full moon, *Mercurius Sol.* in the same way, and eight days after, *Sulphur* again for two days. Sometimes a few doses of *Calcarea Carb.* taken daily for some days are enough of remove them.

For *small worms,* if the itching arises from small worms, and *Nux Vomica* is insufficient, and children are very uneasy with fever at nights, a few doses of *Aconitum Nap.* may be followed by *Ignatia* in the morning. *If they reccur at* New moon *or* full moon, give *Sulphur* or *Silicea* as indicated above.

Lycopodium Clav. is very useful when there is much itching at the anus, and may be followed by *Sulphur.*

10. PROLAPSUS OF THE ANUS

Definition : By prolapsus ani is understood a protrusion of falling down of the lower part of extremity of the bowels.

Causes : The most frequent cause of this accident is a natural laxity of structure. It also arises from habitual constipation, straining at stool, diarrhea, hemorrhoids (or piles), drastic purgatives, worms and other causes.

Treatment : If it occurs in children, the protruding membrane should be replaced by laying the child on its back. If the part is red or swollen, a weak solution of *Arnica tincture* should be applied to the parts and a dose of *Nux Vomica* should be given in watery solution every half hour.

Ignatia, is one of our principal remedies. It may be given daily for a week, and after a week's and after a week's interval, give *Sulphur* on alternate days, a few doses.

AFFECTIONS OF THE STOMACH AND ABDOMEN   207

Nux Vomica, when there is much pain and straining, especially in young children, and those subject to constipation. May be repeated in the evenings as in the case of *Ignatia.*

Sulphur, is an excellent remedy for both recent and chronic cases, may be given in alternation with *Nux Vomica (Nux Vomica* in the evenings followed by *Sulphur* in the mornings) for one week, and if after a week's interval there is no improvement, may be followed by *Calcarea Carb.* for some days.

Calcarea Carb. is an excellent remedy for chronic cases when other remedies have failed.

Mercurius Sol., when the protruded intestine is much swollen or is bluish, or bleeds and pains much at stool. This may be followed by *Ignatia. Doses* to be repeated as in the case of *Ignatia.*

11. HERNIA OR RUPTURE

Definition–varieties–frequency

The terms *"Hernia or Rupture"* means a swelling formed by the protrusion or escape of a portion of the intestine from the cavity of the abdomen. The places at which these swellings most frequently appear are the navel and the region of the groin. The region selected by the hernia gives it a particular name to express its position, as *Umbilical,* when it appears at the umbilicus or navel, *Inguinal,* when it appears in the groin.

There are several varieties of hernia, but only three are especially met with in children, namely, *Umbilical, Inguinal, and Oblique Inguinal.* The latter variety is where the intestines have intruded into the scrotum.

Hernia is termed *reducible,* when it can at any time by returned into the abdomen, and *irreducible,* when, without inflammation or obstruction to the passage of faeces, it cannot be returned to the cavity of the abdomen, either owing to adhesions or entanglement of the intestines. *Strangulated*, when the protrusion is not only incapable of being reduced, from constriction of the aperture through which they passed, but the circulation is arrested, the passage of the faeces throught the anus is cut off, inflammations sets in, the tumour becomes hard and tender to touch, pain, nausea, and vomiting occurs, accompanied by other alarming symptoms.

The first two varieties of hernia are not of uncommon occurrence in children of all ages.

Causes : Children whose muscular development is not compact, but, on the contrary, relaxed and flabby, leaving the natural outlets of the abdomen unusually large or capable of easy enlargement, are more prone of accidents of this nature than those who are robust and strong, having their muscular fibres closely and firmly knit together. The weakest parts are those at which the accident more frequently occurs. And in children, where there is general or local muscular debility, either from imperfect development or recent indisposition, the most trivial circumstance, as crying, coughing, or straining, may produce hernia, but in other cases, where no such predisposition exists, the protrusion only takes place under great bodily exertion, or in consequence of external injury.

Symptoms : *Umbilical hernia* need not be mistaken for any other tumour. Those appearing at the groin, however, are sometimes so closely caused by other diseases, that only physicians can recoginise its true nature, and so they should be consulted. The general symptoms of hernia are an indolent tumour upon some part of the abdomen, usually in children, at the navel or groin. The tumour appears suddenly, is developed above and descends. It is subject to changes is size, being smaller when the patient lies upon his back, and larger when he stands upright. The tumour diminishes when pressed upon, and grows larger when the pressure is removed. It is larger when he is coughing, sneezing or drawing a long breath.

AFFECTIONS OF THE STOMACH AND ABDOMEN

Vomiting, constipation, and colic are often, present in consequence of the unnatural situation of the bowels.

Treatment : This complaint is curable by internal remedies in the earlier stages, and especially in the case of children it is important that a cure should be effected during childhood, as otherwise, in after years, the individual will suffer great inconvenience and be unfitted for any kind of manual labour, and may any day be in danger of losing his life.

In every case of hernia, it is best ot consult a physician in order to ascertain its true nature.

Rupture at the navel is by far the most frequent form in which hernia appears in young children. It is generally first observed about two months after birth. It can be recognised by the unnatural protrusion of the navel. The navel, instead of closing, as it should have done, remains open, allowing a portion of the intestine, covered by the skin and integuments, to escape from the cavity of the abdomen.

The hernia, or swelling, thus formed varies in size from a bean to a lemon, always increasing in, size when he child strains, either by coughing or otherwise. It is ordinarily painless, unless it becomes very large. It is necessary in these cases to keep the intestines permanently within the cavity of the abdomen, so as to give nature an opportunity of closing the opening. This can best be accomplished by covering a piece of cork or card board with soft muslin, and then binding it over the opening with a broad bandage. It is best to obtain the help of a physician in order to do it properly.

The only medicines required are *Nux Vomica* or *Suiphuric acid*, one dose daily in the evening for a week, *Sulphuric acid* acts better in some cases.

Rupture at the groin is much more troublesome to treat than that at the umbilicus, as it is impossible to keep a truss, or any other mechanical device properly applied to the parts, especially with children under a year or eighteen months old. It is best to keep the parts bathed in cold water morning and evening and keep the child at rest.

Nux Vomica and Sulphur are the best remedies, not only for simple rupture, but also for the peculiar disposition or habit to the formation of hernia.

Sulphur, may be given every morning for four successive days and followed every evening by *Nux Vomica* for the same period. Then wait for eight days, and if there is no manifest improvement, repeat the remedies in the same way.

If there should be diarrhea, give a dose of *Chamomilla* every three hours till there is a change. When Hernia results from a fall, or injury of any kind, *Arnica Mont.* or *Rhus Tox.* will be the appropriate remedies, and may be given at intervals of two to four hours.

This treatment alone will be sufficient generally to effect a cure, long before the time arrives, when a truss can be usefully resorted to.

If there should be violent burning in the abdomen, as from a hot coal, with tenderness of the tumour, the least touch giving pain, sickness at the stomach, with bitter, billious vomitting, nervousness and cold perspiration, give *Aconitum Nap.*, a dose every half-hour. In case *Aconitum Nap.* only alleviates the symptoms for a short time, without any real relief, give *Veratrum Alb.*, in the same way for two hours. If your efforts should fail to reduce the hernia, if it is on the left side give *Allium Cepa*, if on the right side, *Rhus Tox.* If accompanied by *sour* vomiting instead of bitter, give *Sulphur,* and leave the patient to rest.

In all cases of *strangulated hernia,* the same medicines may be administered till an operation is performed.

12. DIARRHEA

Dulcamara, for diarrhea caused by taking cold, evacuations watery, worse at night, not much pain. It this does not relieve, give *Bryonia.*

Ipecac, for thin mucus, frothy, fermented evacuations, or small, yellow stools, with pain in the rectum, very offensive evacuations, with great weakness, dysenteric stools, with white *flocks* and subsequent pains, as though more would pass, great prostration, inclination to lie down, paleness of the face. *Continuous nausea with the characteristic vomiting of everything taken and violent colic is a strong indication for this remedy.*

When *Ipecac* gives but partial relief, follow it with *Rheum,* when the stools smell sour, it is better to give *Rheum* first.

Ipecac, given to nursing infants, when diarrhea arises from overloading the stomach, accompanied with nausea and vomiting, frequent crying, stool yellowish, or green and streaked with blood, and very offensive.

Chamomilla, especially for infants, evacuation slimy, green or yellowish, or of undigested matter, looking like chopped straw, and smelling like rotten eggs, distension of the belly, tongue coated, thirst, want of appetite, rumbling in the bowels. The child draws up it slegs, *cries very much and wants to be held or carried all the time.*

Convulsions, both legs move up and down alternately, grasping with the hands, mouth drawn to and fro, eyes staring, eyes and face distorted, stupor, cough with rattling in the chest, yawning and stretching. When *Chamomilla* is not enough in long standing cases, it should be followed by *Mercurius Sol.,* or *Sulphur* for a cure.

It is useful for adults, particularly when the stools are green, watery, hot and offensive, with bitter taste in the mouth, bitter eructations, bilious vomiting, fullness at the pit of the stomach, griping and headache.

Rheum, for sour-smelling evacuations, thin, slim fermented diarrhea, common to small children, sour smell proceeding from the child, which washing will not remove, diarrhea from acidity of the stomach, distension of the abdomen, colic, crying, both before and after an evacuation, ineffectual urging before and after stool. If *Rheum* does not give relief and the pain is very violent, give *Chamomilla* and if this is not sufficient, when the pain stops but weakness continues with distension of the abdomen, give *Sulphur.*

Pulsatilla, diarrhea *due to fat or rich food, ice cream or fruits, worse at night, after measles,* tongue coated white, bitter taste in the mouth and after food or drink, dryness in the mouth without thirst, vomiting of food or bile, aversion to fat, bread and milk, Rumbling, cutting stool, or when each stool is of a different color from the preceding one, *irresistible desire for fresh air, chilliness.*

Podophyllum, has an early morning diarrhea, stools are watery, yellow, profuse, forcible and *without pain,* at any time from 3 o'clock to 9 in the morning and a natural stool is apt to follow later, *stools very offensive, exhaustion and sense of weakness in the abdomen and rectum after the stool, most useful in diarrhea of children and may be one of the first to be* referred to.

Mercurius Sol., straining at stool is a prominent symptom, stools are green, slimy and bloody, watery and sour-smelling, accompanied *by a straining and tenesmus which produces a 'never-get-done' feeling, much soreness and pain in region of liver, flabby tongue taking imprint of the teeth,* and before the stool there is violent urging and sometimes chilliness, bad smell from the mouth, prolapsus of the rectum may follow the stool, great debility, perspiration on the last exertion, *restless sleep, oily,*

AFFECTIONS OF THE STOMACH AND ABDOMEN

offensive or sour smelling night sweat, particularly on the head, cold on the forehead.

Bryonia Alba, especially useful for *diarrhea occurring in hot weather, or whenever the weather becomes warmer,* if the prominent symptoms of this remedy are present viz., dry *mouth, with thirst for large quantities of water at long intervals, and a desire to lie down and remain quiet.*

Calcarea Carb., should be given more for the constitution and the prominent symptoms present than the character of the stool and diarrhea, and this is *one of the best remedies for chronic diarrhea, sour and undigested stools,* diarrhea in *fat children* with open fontanelles *during dentition,* in scrofulous and rachitic children i.e., children with pale and bloated or sunken face, emaciated, wrinkled and cold with swollen, distended abdomen like inverted saucer, with emaciation but with good appetite, who have *profuse sweat on the head when sleeping, especially on the back of the head, wetting the pillow, feet constantly cold and damp,* painful and difficult urination, the urine being usually clear, and *having a peculiar, strong, pungent, fetid odour.*

Calcarea Phos., should also be given according to the constitution. In scrofulous and rachitic children, who have disproportionately large heads, *the bones of the head very soft and thin, crackling like paper under pressure,* who are *greatly emaciated,* looking old and wrinkled, face pale, sallow, dirty white, brownish, sunken with blue rings around the eyes, *nose, chin, and tips of ears cold,* teeth develop slowly, abdomen sunken and flabby, curvature of the spine, spine so weak in the lumbar region that the child cannot sit upright unless the back is supported, slow in learning to walk on account of weak ankles, ravenous appetite, but with persistent vomiting of milk, *spluttering* diarrhea, forcibly expelled, but watery, greenish or undigested, extremely offensive.

Phosphorus, specially useful for chronic forms of diarrhea, *white, watery* discharge passing out *with great force as from a pipe,* watery stool with lumps of white mucus, or little grains like rice or sago, diarrhea *worse from warm food* and after eating, *better after cold food,* vomiting of what has been drunk, as soon as it has become warm in the stomach, vomiting relieved for a time by ice or very cold food or drink, weak, gone feeling in the abdomen, with burning between the shoulders, *anus constantly open.* Useful in chronic cases. It is better to give a dose of *Nux Vom.* 200 before giving *Phos.,* particularly in cases treated with allopathic medicines.

Argentum Nitricum, stools are green, after remaining on cloth, *expelled forcibly, with much spluttering* as in *Calcarea Phos.,* stools *worse from use of sugar or candy, or from drinking,* useful in sudden and sever attacks of cholera infantum in children who are very fond of sugar and have eaten too much of it, nausea with loud belching, also in diarrhea brought on by great mental excitement, emotional disturbances, etc.

China off., painless diarrhea of bad odour, slimy, bilious, blackish and mixed with undigested food, *worse at night, and after eating,* with rapid exhaustion and emaciation, *worse after fruit,* worse in summer, when there is much sour vomiting, after measles, *during* small-pox, *after severe acute diseases, desire to drink frequently* but little at a time, *distention of the abdomen, temporarily relieved* by belching, emission of large quantities of wind. It is useful in *chronic diarrhea of aged persons.*

Arsenic Album

The important characteristic are:
(*a*) Stools in small quantities
(*b*) The dark colour
(*c*) The offensive odour
(*d*) The great weakness following

The stools are dark yellow, undigested, slimy or bloody, often dark green and *very offensive, worse at night and after eating*

AFFECTIONS OF THE STOMACH AND ABDOMEN

or drinking, the mucus stools are not usually offensive, the watery ones are very much more offensive and often painless. Among the *principal causes are chilling of the stomach by cold food, ice water or ice cream, spoiled food and* what is called ptomaine-poisoning.

Veratrum Album

The important characteristics are :
- (a) A profuse watery stool, forcibly evacuated
- (b) Pain in the abdomen preceding stool
- (c) Great prostration following stool
- (d) Cold sweat, coldness, and blueness of the body generally.

The stools are watery and commonly called *rice water discharges,* severe pricking colic before the stool, and this pain continues during the stool, with nausea and vomiting and *cold sweat on the forehead* and after stool, great sinking and empty feeling in the abdomen. *Violent thirst for large quantities of very cold water and acid drinks* is an important general symptom. *Violent cramps of the extremities, Wrinkling of the skin of the hands and fingers. Skin cold, blue, remaining in folds when pinched.*

Aloes

The important characteristics are :
- (a) The lumpy, watery stool
- (b) The intense griping across the lower part of the abdomen before and during stool, leaving after stool
- (c) The extreme prostration and perspiration following
- (d) The feeling of the uneasiness, weakness and uncertainty about rectum-there is a *constant feeling as if the stool would escape, when passing flatus or urine.*

Worse, in hot and damp weather, early in the morning driving one out of bed, from 5 to 10 A. M., when walking or standing, after eating, or drinking, when passing urine.

It is useful in chronic diarrhea or dysentery.

Nux Vomica, after drastic medicines or prolonged drugging, after abuse of alcoholic spirit, after change of food (infants), after over-exertion of the mind. When there are *frequent but scanty evacuations,* accompanied with much straining and pressing down pain in the rectum, *backache, as if broken,* heat with red face and aversion to uncovering.

Sulphur, for green, slimy diarrhea which is so acrid as to occasion soreness of the part around the anus, or to produce military eruptions, *bloody in streaks,* frothy, sour, putrid, alternating with constipation, frequently accompanied by emaciation, or in children, with a hard, distended abdomen, when every fresh exposure renews the diarrhea. Diarrhea worse in the morning *early in bed,* in the evening and *after* midnight, in damp weather, *after taking milk, after suppressed eruptions,* in children, during dentition, *during sleep.* Expulsion sudden and involuntary. Sudden and violent urging (*driving one out of bed in the morning without pain*).

It will be useful after the failure of other remedies, and also in chronic cases for which it acts better in the 200th potency.

The following are the special indications for the several remedies for diarrhea.

AFTER A COLD–*Bryonia Alba, Dulc., Cham.*

AFTER MILK– Sulph., Calcarea Carb.

AFTER FRUIT– *Puls., China off..*

AFTER ICE–CREAM– *Arsenicum Alb., Puls., Carb Veg.*

AFTER FAT FOOD– *Puls.*

AFTER RANCID FOOD– *Arsenicum Alb.*

AFFECTIONS OF THE STOMACH AND ABDOMEN

AFTER DRUGGING– *Nux Vom.*

AFTER ABUSE OF SPIRITS– *Nux Vom.*

AFTER POTATOES–*Alumina.*

AFTER ABUSE OF MERCURIAL MEDICINES– *Hepar Sulp.*

IN AGED PERSONS– (when constipation and diarrhea come on alternately)–*Antimonium Crudum, Carb Veg., China off., Sulphur.*

IN FAT CHILDREN– *Calcarea Carb.*

IN SLENDER PERSONS–– *Phos.*

IN SCROFULOUS PERSONS– *Calcarea Carb., Calcarea Phos.*

AFTER TOBACCO– *Cham., Ign., Puls.*

AFTER SWEETS– *Argentum N., Mercurius Vivus.*

AFTER VACCINATION– *Thuja, Silicea.*

DURING SMALL–POX– *Arsenicum Alb., China.*

AFTER MEASLES– *China off., Puls.*

AFTER FRIGHT AND FEAR– *Gelsemium, Opium, Ignatia.*

AFTER GRIEF AND SORROW – *Phos. acid.*

VERY FETID SMELL, IN GENERAL– *Carbo Veg., China off., Arsenicum Alb., Psorinum, Podophyllum, Sulphur.*

SOUR SMELL– *Calcarea. Carb., Rheum, Sulphur, Hepar Sulp.*

WITH NAUSEA, inclination to vomit– *Ipec., Rhus T., Sulph.*

WITH VOMITING – *Antimonium. Crude, Arsenicum Alb., Ipecac, Sulph., Verat Alb.*

PAINLESS– *Podophyllum, Phos. acid., Hepar Sulp.*

CONSTANT OOZING – *Phos.*

GREAT WEARNESS AND PROSTRATION – *Arsenicum Alb., China, Phos., Verat Alb., Carb Veg.*

CHRONIC DIARRHEA generally – *Sulph., Calcarea Carb., Phos., Petrol.*

IN THE CASE OF PHTHISICAL PATIENTS– *Ferrum Met., Phos.*

AFTER TYPHOID, generally – *Phos.*

AFTER CHOLERA, principally– *Phos., Phos. Ac., Sulphur.*

13. DYSENTERY

Aconitum Nap., in the first stage of dysentery, *when the days are warm and the nights are cold,* the stools are frequent and scanty with tenesmus, the skin is hot and dry, with *restlessness, anxiety, fear of death and unquenchable thirst.*

Nux Vom., in the first stage of dysentery when there is *frequent urging to stool with tenesmus,* and the pains and tenesmus cease for a short time *after very stool,* but if the *pain and tenesmus* continue even *after the stool,* and there is a 'never-get-done feeling', *Mercurius Sol* is more suitable.

Mercurius Sol., this is by far the *most important remedy* for dysentery, severe tenesmus or painful constriction of the anus, urgent desire to evacuate, as if the intestine would force themselves out, after much straning, there is a discharge of light blood, sometimes streaked with mucus or greenish matter, violent straining both *before and after* an evacuation, frequent small mucus stools, great exhaustion and trembling, thirst for cold drink, aggravation of pains at night. It is useful in the dysentery of children when there is much crying and screaning.

The pains calling for *Mercurius Sol.,* are *increased* by an evacuation, while those of *Nux Vom.,* are relieved by a movement.

AFFECTIONS OF THE STOMACH AND ABDOMEN

The symptoms of *Mercurius Sol.* are worse during the afternoon and evening, while those of *Nux Vom.* are worse *after midnight* and in the *morning.*

Belladonna, more suitable for children and for severe cases of infantile dysentery with the following symptoms – *Head hot, while hands and feet are cold, rolling the head from side to side,* sleepiness with restlessness, *starting up suddenly,* moving during sleep with half-closed eyes, drowsiness with inability to sleep, great thirst for cold things. *Dry heat or hot sweat, quick, hard, small pulse.* Children cry much and are very cross, tongue dry, and red at the point and on edges, or has two white stripes on a red ground.

Rhus Tox., after getting wet all over, in rain or otherwise, while in heavy perspiration, especially if the discharge is bloody, slimy, brownish or greenish, and swims upon the water, *tearing pains down the thighs, has to change position to get relief, troublesome dreams, vivid, of hard work and difficulty-Frequently* applicable to dysentery in a later stage, when the disease shows a tendency to assume a typhoid type.

Mercuris Corrosivus, more violent form of dysentery with profuse bleeding and before, during and after stool, constant tenesmus and urging to stool and cutting colic, *tenesmus, something more than the never-get-done feeling of Merc. Sol.* It is an *intense painful tenesmus,* and at the same time the urine is hot, bloody, *retained or suppressed,* the stools are scanty, or mucus shreds and blood, and their is great burning at the anus.

Arsenicum Alb., scanty stools, burning in the rectum, thirst, and after the stool there is great prostration, stools which are undigested, slimy and bloody, blackish brown, horribly offensive stools, the tenesmus and burning of the anus and rectum continue after the stool. If *Arsenicum Alb.* is well indicated, its *characteristic thirst and restlessness must be present.*

Sulphur, is the remedy for persistent or chronic cases and when the other remedies do not give permanent relief, if tenesmus continues all the time, stools are slimy and there is frequent, sudden urging to stool, sometimes this condition is present without the tenesmus. In inflammatory dysentery, follows *Aconitum Nap.* well, when it has removed the acute symptoms, when the tenesmus has ceased, but blood is still discharged.

It is sufficient to give occasional doses.

14. CHOLERA

The subject divides itself under three heads -
(*a*)   Prophylactics, or preventive treatment.
(*b*)   Treatment of cholerine, or preventive treatment.
(*c*)   Treatment of cholera proper.

(a) Prophylactics

During the prevalence of cholera as an epidemic, Hahnemann recommended *Cuprum Met.30 and Veratrum Album* 30, to be taken in rotation every six or seven days, i.e., one dose of *Cuprum Met.* 30 is to be taken first, and after one week one dose of *Veratrum Album Met.* 30 is to be taken and again after another week *Cuprum Met.* 30 is to be repeated and to be followed again by *Veratrum Album* 30, and this is to be continued so long as the epidemic lasts. Where a whole family is to be protected, six globules may be dissolved in three ounces of water, and each member may be given one or two teaspoons as indicated above.

Hering recommended as the surest preventive that half a teaspoon of flowers of sulphur may be put into each of one's stocking before going out. This may be used in our country by tying a small quantity of sulphur or camphor in a piece of cloth into a knot which may be tied round the waist. As an alternative, the new copper quarter-anna coin may be tied in a string round the waist.

AFFECTIONS OF THE STOMACH AND ABDOMEN

In some epidemics, when diarrhea prevails at the same time as cholera, a dose of *Sulphur* 30 every week, will act as a preventive.

(b) Chlorine

During the prevalence of an epidemic of cholera, every diarrhea, however slight, should be regarded as being, possibly, as a preliminary to an attack of cholera, and should at once received careful attention. As soon as diarrhea occurs, the patient should go to bed and be warmly covered, but not so as to produce perspiration. The food should be light, but nutritious, and taken frequently in small quantities. The appropriate remedy should be taken without delay.

Sulphur, if the diarrhea comes on in the night, *after midnight,* the stools being yellow, pappy, and attended by great urgency, though the urging is often ineffectual, and if, at the same time, there are cramps in the soles of the feet, two globules of *Sulphur* 30 may be dissolved in one ounce of water, and two teaspoons may be given for a dose *every two hours* until relief is obtained. If the patient has begun to improve or continues to improve, no further doses should be repeated.

Phosphoric acid, if the evacuations are light coloured, liquid, copious and without pain, if the tongue is covered with a gluey mucus, and there are cramps in the arms, with a general sense of weakness, *Phosphoric acid* 30 should be given in the same way.

Arsenicum Album, if the evacuations are frequent, *small in quantity,* liquid, dark coloured, and quite offensive, attended by sharp pain very low in the abdomen and by burning in the rectum, and followed by great prostration of strength, if also, the patient has great thirst, *drinking but little at a time,* and is very restless in body and anxious in mind, *Arsenicum Album* 30 should be given as state above.

Croton Tiglinum, if the evacuations are sudden and very copious, consisting of a large quantity of yellow water, which passes *with a rush,* and if an evacuation occurs every time the patient drinks, *Croton Tiglinum* 30 is the remedy.

Veratrum Album, if the diarrhea is watery, copious, and very painful, and is accompanied by copious vomiting, which is repeated every time the patient drinks, and by coldness and blueness of face and hands, and cold sweat on the forehead, *Veratrum Album* 30 should be repeated every fifteen minutes till warmth returns, and water can be retained in the stomach.

(c) *Cholera Proper*

In true cholera, it attacks the patient suddenly and without warning, at once prostrating him and almost depriving him of vitality. The expression of the countenance in such cases is sunken and death-like, the pulse is feeble, almost imperceptible, the skin blue, cold, and shrivelled, and covered with a clammy sweat, cramps in the calves of the legs, fingers, and muscles of the abdomen, with stupidity or extreme anguish, vomiting and diarrhea, with rice-water discharges.

For sudden attacks and, in general, in the commencement, if the patient is attacked with cramps, nausea, excessive prostration, coldness and blueness of the surface, *Camphor Tincture* is the best remedy. *One drop* should be given in a lump of sugar, or a teaspoon of water, every *five, ten or fifteen minutes until* he gets warm and begins to perspire. In addition to the administration of Camphor, the patient's extremities should be vigorously rubbed, and bottles of hot water applied to them until the natural heat is restored. The room should be well ventilated, and cold water given freely if desired.

This is the first stage for which only *Camphor* is suitable and *Camphor* should not be continued after the patient gets sufficiently warm and perspires, as it is no longer useful. For the remaining

AFFECTIONS OF THE STOMACH AND ABDOMEN 223

symptoms, suitable remedies should be administered as indicated below. *Camphor Tincture* may be prepared by dissolving one gram of *Camphor*, in twelve drams of rectified spirit and stirred for some minutes. In emergencies, when *Camphor Tincture* is not readily available, pure camphor may be *finely* ground along with white sugar in a pestle and mortar, and a very small quantity of the size of a mustard seed may be put in a lump of sugar and administered every five minutes.

Carbo Vegetablis, sometimes the collapse is still more marked, even at the outset, the *tongue and very breath are cold,* the voice is extinct, there is no vomiting, diarrhea, spasm, or pain, the urine is suppressed. Give *Carbo Vegetablis* 30, 2 globules No. 10 dissolved in one ounce of water, and one teaspoon for a dose given every five minutes till warmth is restored. If reaction should ensue after the doses of *Carbo Vegetablis,* and the purging, vomiting and cramps return, the following remedies should be administered.

Veratrum Album, when the *evacuations are profuse,* both upward and downward, consisting of rice-water and frothy fluids, and great anguish in the abdomen, thirst for cold water, which is taken in large quantities, *but is vomited as soon as swallowed,* with contracted features, cold sweat on the forehead, hands and feet, moderate cramps in hands, feet and calves, with suppression of urine, *Veratrum Album* 30 should be given as above, a dose every five minutes until decided improvement is manifest.

In cases requiring *Camphor,* the *collapse* is the most prominent feature. In those which require *Veratrum Album,* the *evacuations and the coldness* are the most prominent symptoms. But in those cases which call for *Cuprum Met., the spasms or cramps* are most prominent.

Cuprum Metallicum, when the evacuations are not very copious, but the spasms in the chest and stomach are very painful, with great tenderness to touch, the spasms coming on in paroxysms, both in the stomach and in the extremities, the thirst is moderate, the vomiting is allayed for a time, by drinking water, the face is blue and cold, the respiration is short and laboured, voice husky, urine suppressed, give *Cuprum Metallicum* 30, as in the case of *Veratrum Album* every five minutes, for the first few doses, the interval being prolonged to half an hour or an hour as some improvement is noticed.

If too much of *Camphor Tincture* has been taken and terrible anguish and burning at the pit of the stomach are noticed, a few doses of *Phosphorus* 30 will antidote the effects of Camphor and relieve the patients

Carbo Vegetablis 30 is called for when the disease has reached the stage of *collapse, pulse imperceptible,* surface cold and bluish, *breath cold, and voice, extinct.*

Secale Cor. 30, especially for aged persons, and when there is rapid prostration of strength, violent thirst, cold dry, livid tongue, blueness and withered appearance of the skin.

Summary

Camphor Tincture should be given in *all* cases in the beginning.

When cholera is fully developed, *Veratrum Album* 30 is the principal remedy with the following characteristic symptoms-

(*i*) Sharp cutting pains in the abdomen.

(*ii*) Profuse watery stools like rice water, with nausea, vomiting, with a *cold blue surface, and cold sweat on the forehead and great weakness.*

(*iii*) Violent thirst for large quantities of very cold water and acid drinks, which is vomited soon after.

(*iv*) Great sinking and empty feeling in the abdomen, and great exhaustion after each stool.

(*v*) Moderate cramps in hands, feet and calves, with suppression of the urine.

AFFECTIONS OF THE STOMACH AND ABDOMEN

(*vi*)   Excessive coldness, skin withered and wrinkled.

Cuprum Met 30, after *Veratrum Album* when that remedy has not relieved the cramps, which are *very violent* and extend all over the body, cramps in the stomach, spasms or convulsions, in the chest and stomach are very painful, difficult respiration with husky voice.

Arsenicum Album 30, when the purging and vomiting become very frequent, the evacuations from the bowels being thin, watery and of a dark color and very offensive smell, or light colored and almost without smell, especially when accompanied by intense, burning pains or cramps in the stomach and bowels, with violent thirst, and great prostration of strength, also burning in the anus and rectum with tenesmus. It is *useful also in the last stage of the disease.*

Secale Cor., when the diarrhea produces great prostration of strength, especially in aged persons.

Carbo Vegetablis, when complete collapse is present, with coldness of breath *in the last stage.*

After-effects of Cholera and Convalscence

If cases have been badly treated or have been under allopathic treatment, the following remedies will be useful for the symptoms indicated-

Aconitum Nap. 30, hippocratic countenance, face bluish, lips black, expression of terror and imbecility, cold limbs with blue nails, collapse. *Aconitum Nap.* 30, 2 globules in one ounce of water, a teaspoon every two hours will improve the condition.

If *Aconitum Nap.* does not help, the following remedies will be necessary.

Carbo Vegetablis 30, attack often begins with hemorrhage from the bowels, collapse without stool, nose, cheeks and finger tips icy cold, lips bluish, cold breathe and tongue, respiration weak and laboured, *desire to be fanned,* cramps in legs and thighs, hiccough at every motion, vomiting, voice hoarse or lost, pulse thready, intermittent, scarcely perceptible, consciousness retained or coma, *Sopor, without vomiting, stool or cramps.*

Bryonia 30 or *Rhus Tox.* 30, if the affection takes the form of abdominal typhoid with delirium, these remedies may be given in watery solution, one teaspoon at intervals of 2 or 3 hours.

DURING CONVALESCENCE: *Sulphur 200, China off. 200,* or *Carbo Vegetablis* 200. Single doses at fortnightly intervals.

15. AFFECTIONS OF THE LIVER

Aconitum Nap., if the fever is high, with hot skin, much thirst, and whitish coated tongue, accompanied by moaning, great restlessness, and fear of death, shooting pains in the region of the liver.

Nux Vomica, when there are shooting or pulsative pains with great tenderness of the region of the liver when touched, nausea or vomiting, bitter or sour taste, shortness of breathe and sense of pressure under the ribs and about the stomach, pressive pain in the head, thirst, highly colored urine, giddiness and paroxysms of anguish, constipation. This remedy is especially called for in liver affections of those who have indulgled in alcoholic drinks to excess, highly seasoned foods, quinine, or those who have used too much of purgatives. It is the *first remedy in cirrhosis of the liver.*

Mercurius Sol., pains under the ribs of a pressive character, which do not *allow the patient to lie long on the right side,* bitter taste in the mouth, want of appetite, thirst, continued shivering, followed sometimes by clammy perspiration, *yellowness of the skin and of the whites of the eyes,* also in *enlargement* and *hardening of the liver.* The stools are either clay-colored from

AFFECTIONS OF THE STOMACH AND ABDOMEN

absence of bile, or yellowish, green bilious stools passed with a great deal of tenesmus. It is a splendid remedy for what is known as *'torpid liver'*

Belladonna, for *pains* in the *region of the liver which extend to the neck and shoulders,* particularly of the *right side,* swelling and tenseness at the pit of the stomach, oppressed and anxious respiration, congestion to the head with giddiness, dimness of vision and occasional fainting, great thirst, anxiety, restlessness and sleeplessness. It is often suitable after *Aconitum Nap., Merc Sol.* and *Lachesis.*

Lachesis, will be useful in cases where *Merc Sol.* and *Belladonna* appear to be indicated, but give only partial relief, and also in *obstinate chronic* cases in drunkards.

Bryonia Alba, when the *pains are pressive, with a feeling of tension in the region of the liver,* pains aggravated by respiration, coughing and movement, violent oppression of the chest with rapid and anxious respiration, thick yellowish coating on the tongue, constipation.

China off., when *worse every other day,* with *shooting and pressive pains in the region of the liver,* swelling and hardness below the ribs, pressive pain in the head, tongue thickly coated, yellowish, and bitter taste in the mouth.

Chelidonium, is perhaps our *greatest liver remedy* with very prominent symptoms, *soreness* and *stitching pains in the region of the liver,* and more prominently *a pain under the angle of the right shoulder blade,* which may extend to the chest, stomach, or hypochondrium, there is swelling of the liver, chilliness, fever, jaundice, yellow coated tongue, bitter taste and a *craving for acids and sour things,* such as lemon and pickles, the stools are profuse, bright yellow and diarrheic, they may also be clayey in colour.

Lycopodium Clav., the region of the liver is sensitive to the touch and there is a *feeling of tension in it, as if a cord were* tied round the waist, cirrhosis, the pains are dull and aching instead of sharp and lancinating as under 'Chelidonium', fullness of the stomach after eating a small quantity, pain in back and right side from congestion often yield to this remedy.

Sulphur, useful in chronic affections of the liver when other remedies have not helped, often completes a cure begun by *Nux Vomica,* liver complaints from abuse of mercurial medicines.

Special Indication in Liver Complaints

IF AFTER SUPPRESSION OF FEVER AND AGUE–*Arsenicum Alb., Sulph., Calcarea Carb.*

IF COMPLICATED WITH VERTIGO–*Bell., Nux Vom.*

WITH MUCH HEADACHE–*Bell., Nux Vom.*

WITH LOATHING OF FOOD–*Sulphur.*

CONSTIPATION–*Bryonia Alba, Nux Vomica, Sulphur.*

DIARRHEA–*Mercurius Sol., China off., Arsenicum Alb.*

COUGH–*China off., Sulphur.*

LASSITUDE–*Nux Vom., Sulph.*

BURNING PAINS–*Mercurius Sol., Arsenicum Alb., Bryonia Alba.*

ACHING, DULL PAINS–*Bryonia Alba, Sulphur, Lycopodium, Mercurius Sol., Nux Vom.*

ULCERATIVE PAINS AND THROBBING–*China off., Nux Vom.*

IF LIVER SIMPLY PAINFUL WITHOUT SWELLING–*Bell., Bryonia Alba, China off., Nux Vom., Sulphur, Lycop.*

SWOLLEN LIVER AND HARDNESS–*Sulphur, Nux Vom., Mercurius Sol., Bell., Arsenicum Alb., Chelidonium.*

TEARING PAIN–*Mercurius Sol.*

STINGING, LANCING PAINS–*Bryonia Alba, China off., Mercurius Sol., Nux Vom., Sulphur, Chelidonium.*

FEELING OF WEIGHT AND FULLNESS–*Nux Vom., Sulphur.*

IN RHEUMATIC INDIVIDUALS, AND THOSE SUBJECT TO ARTHRITIS–*Calcarea Carb., Lycopodium.*

16. JAUNDICE

Definition : It is characterised by yellowness of the eyes and skin, whitish stool, urine having the color of saffron, and communicating a yellow tinge to white liver, deranged digestion, and sometimes pain in the region of the liver.

Causes-duration : Jaundice depends upon various and very different internal causes. It may arise from inflammation of the liver, obstruction of the gall-duct, from diseases of the bowels, and from fevers. And frequently we cannot ascertain at all even in the simplest cases, the precise cause of the trouble. The most frequently recognised, exciting causes are, severe mental emotions, as rage, fright, grief, anger, despondency and irritable temper, also particular kinds of food, the excessive use of strong coffee, acids, unripe fruit, and indeed any error in diet which has a tendency to dirange the digestive apparatus. It is not infrequently caused by the excessive use of quinine, calomel or other purgative medicines.

Its duration depends to a large extent on the exciting cause, the constitution of the patient, and the treatment which he is under. It may last for a few days, or a week or even longer, if improperly treated, for years.

Symptoms : This disease is generally caused by or accompanied with, great languor, depression of spirit, slight chills, or rigors, or flushes of fever, loss of appetite, giddiness, constipation, flatulence, sour eurctations, and sometimes there is nausea and vomiting, there is also a sense of weight and uneasiness about the chest and abdomen, with some pain in the region of the liver. There is frequently a disagreeable itching or tingling sensation in the skin before the discoloration appears. The yellow tinge begins in the eyes and extends to the temples, brow and face, then to the neck, chest, and whole surface of the body. In some spots, the color is deeper than in others, especially so in the folds, and wrinkles of the skin. The color varies from a slight yellow to a deep lemon or a greenish-brown. Constipation is generally present, the evacuations are scanty, and of a pale-yellow colour, indicating an absence of bile. The urine is commonly high-coloured, at first yellow, afterwards of a deep saffron colour. Bilious sweat sometimes occurs, staining the patient's cloth yellow.

The characteristic yellow colour of the skin is owing, no doubt, to the presence of bile, or its coloring matter in the blood, and the deep tint of the urine is derived from the same source.

In milder forms, there will be, but little fever, but in bad cases there is frequently a high fever accompanied with a stupid sleep from which it is difficult to arouse the patient. This latter symptom appears to be caused by the retained bile which acts upon the nervous system as a narcotic poison, and is regarded as dangerous.

Treatment : *Mercurius Sol.* is the best remedy in most cases, if the patient had not already taken calomel or other mercurial medicines, A dose may be given every four hours (4 doses per day), for three or four days, and if not better, give *Hepar Sulph.,* or *Sulphur* in the same manner.

If calomel or other mercurial medicines had been used, it will be better to begin with *China off.,* which may be followed in obstinate cases by *Hepar Sulph., Sulphur* or *Lachesis.*

Mercurius Sol. is especially useful when the disease is caused by a derangement of the digestive system.

Nux Vomica, followed by *Chamomilla*, when it is due to fits of passion, *Nux Vomica,* also useful in cases caused by indolence

AFFECTIONS OF THE STOMACH AND ABDOMEN

or sedentary habits, or is accompanied by constipation or by constipation alternating with diarrhea.

Sulphur and lachesis are most suitable for very irritable persons in whom the symptoms of jaundice appear even upon very trifling causes, or to eradicate the trouble in those susceptible to the disease.

When the trouble arises from abuse of Quinine, give *Mercurius Sol., Belladonna, Calcarea Carb., Nux Vomica,* when it is due to abuse of purgatives give *Chamomilla* or *Mercurius Sol.*

When bilious symptoms appear, with yellowness of the skin, in persons who have taken much calomel, given *China off.* or *Hepar Sulph.* One dose morning and night for a few days.

Jaundice of Infants

This occurs occasionally in infants and may be recognised by the yellowness of the whites of the eyes and urine in the commencement, and afterwards of the skin of the whole body. The bowels are at times constipated, and at others loose, and the stools are generally light or clay-coloured. This may arise from exposure to cold, or from the injurious habit of administering castor oil immediately after birth and other causes.

Chamomilla, may be given first, one dose of one or two drops of the solution, every four hours and this will be enough in many cases to effect a cure. If this is not enough, *Mercurius Sol* may follow in the same way. *China off.,* for the remaining symptoms.

Nux Vomica, if the child is extremely irritable and if, in addition, there is constipation.

17. AFFECTIONS OF THE SPLEEN

Ceanothus Americana has been found very useful in the 6th potency, for enlarged spleen. Its indications are deep seated pain the splenic region, deep stitches, *worse in damp weather*, with enlarged spleen. Chronic pains in the spleen. Pain in whole left side, with shortness of breath.

China off., has congestion, pain and stitches in the region of the spleen, with swelling of the spleen. Dull aching in region of the spleen. Nervous system is sensitive, physical or mental effort aggravates.

Capsicum, Jahr considers this as one of our most efficient remedies for sensitive, swollen and enlarged spleen.

Arnica Mont., swelling of the spleen due to injury, the patient is dull and apathetic. It is also useful in the typhoid patient with dull or even acute pain in the spleen.

Natrium Muriaticum, produces *stitches, pressures* and *congestion in the spleen, swollen spleens resulting from malarial fevers.* Patient anemic, upper part of the body emaciated, inclined to catch cold, has taken large quantities of quinine, and craves salt.

Arsenicum Alb. and Sulphur, in chronic splenitis, but if the spleen in simply very sensitive, and also if it is *swollen* and hardened, *particularly after fever and ague.*

18. URINARY DISORDERS

(a) *Retention of Urine in Infants*

New born infants generally discharge the contents of the rectum and bladder shortly after birth, occasionally it happens that the urine is retained for a longer period, and the infant is uneasy, nervous of the bladder, there is usually more or less fever, and the child twists its body and draws up its legs. If relief is not soon afforded, convulsions and other dangerous symptoms follow.

Treatment : *Aconitum Nap.* is the principal remedy and should be given in *one drop* doses of the solution every hour till there is relief.

If *Aconitum Nap.* does not afford relief, *Pulsatilla* should be given in the same way.

When spasmodic symptoms develop themselves, give *Ipecac.*

(b) Difficult and Painful Urination in Children and Adults

Aconitum Nap., for the most common cases with painful urging, for children if they put their hands to the parts and scream, when no urine or very little passes, sometimes only in single drops with great pain, the discharge is very red, dark and turbid, particularly for women and children. If *Aconitum Nap.* does not give relief, give *Cantharis.*

Pulsatilla, if there are pressing, cutting pains or redness and heat in the region of the bladder, especially for women, when the menses are suppressed or are scanty, also for less pain but much uring.

Arnica Mont., if due to a blow or fall on the bladder or back, or a sudden fall of the whole body.

Nux Vomica, for after-effects of the *use of liquor or some strong medicines*, after suppressed piles, with burning, pressing and tension in the back, and the region between the ribs and hip-bones.

Belladonna, if the pains are more percing, extending from the back to the bladder, in spells, with great anxiety, restlessness and colic. If *Belladonna* gives only temporary relief, give *Hepar Sulph.*

Mercurius Sol., when there is very violent, constant desire to urinate, the stream being very small, with perspiration at the same time, urine dark red, soon becoming turbid and offensive.

(c) Frequent Urination–Involuntary Urination

WETTING THE BED.

Sulphur, is the most important remedy in all cases, and may be given to start with, *one dose* on alternate days, or eight days, and may be allowed to act for some time. If this does not help, then the following remedies may be given according to special indications.

FOR LITTLE BOYS–*Causticum*

SMALL AND FAT CHILDREN–*Calcarea Carb.*

FOR YOUNG GIRLS–*Sepia, Belladonna, Pulsatilla.*

SCROFULOUS INDIVIDUALS, *(*thin, pale children with protruding stomachs*)*–*Belladonna, Sulphur, or Calcarea Carb.*

When urine is passed in large quantities and is pale and watery–*Belladonna*

If wetting occurs during the first part of the night–*Sepia* (for girls), *Causticum* (for boys).

If children wet themselves involuntarily day and night–*Belladonna or Causticum.*

Arsenicum Alb., when the urine is hot, and has a putrid smell, and if the child lies upon its back with the arms over the head.

Silicea, especially for children, in whom the slightest scratch becomes a sore, not disposed to heal.

Causticum, for children when the urine is burning, and with *frequent desire to urinate both day and night,* and for adults, an inability to retain the urine caused by a sort of paralysis of the neck of the bladder. In the case of adults for this trouble, *Arnica Mont., Rhus Tox.* and *Ruta,* also useful.

China 200, when it is due to worms.

CHAPTER XII

DIABETES

1. DIABETES MELLITUS, GLYCOSURIA

This disease is characterised by the presence of sugar in the urine.

Exciting Causes : *Mechanical injuries,* especially concussions of the whole body or of the brain and spinal cord in particular, *diseases of the nerve-centres,* such as inflammations, degeneration, softenings and tremors of the brain, violent *mental emotions* such as fright, anxiety, anger, grief, solicitude, care, immoderate mental strain, *errors in diet, exposure to cold and moisture,* severe bodily exertions, *sexual excesses,* also the introduction into the system of some chemical substances such as amyl nitrate, corrosive sublimate, turpentine, morphia, strychnine, etc.

Symptoms : Increase of the urinary excertion and of thirst.

Treatment

FOR DEBILITY, *Phos., Phos ac., Arsenicum Alb., China off.*

FOR HEPATIC SYMPTOMS, *Kalium Bich., Mercurius Sol., Hepar Sulp., Sulph.* when there is diminished bile in the faeces. *Mercurius cor., Podo., Nit ac.,* when there is increased flow of bile. *Nux Vom., Lycopodium, Mercurius Cor., Chel.* when there is headache, vertigo languor, weariness in limbs, uneasiness in liver, loss of appetite, flatulence, great depressions and irritability of temper, *Colch., Nux Vom., Kali Iod.* in gouty disposition. *Kalium Iod.* in symphilitic taint.

FOR URINARY AND SEXUAL SYMPTOMS, *Arsenicum Alb., Kalium Bich.*, when there is rapid decrease in the secretion of urine with stranguary, or excessive itching in the vagina.

FOR PULMONARY AFFECTION, *Phos., Arsenicum Alb., Hep Sulp.*

FOR NERVOUS SYMPTOMS, *Phos., Argentum Nit., Aurum* if cerebral, *Nux Vom., Silicea, Phos.* if spinal.

FOR CARBUNCLES, *Arnica Mont., Phos., Arsenicum Alb., Sil., Hep Sulph.*

Argentum Met., the urine is profuse, turbid and of sweet odour. Micturition frequent and copious especially at night. Scorotum and feet edematously swollen. Anxiety and pressure in the pit of the stomach and want of breath.

Arsenicum Alb., in a drunkard, horrible thirst, emaciation and exhaustion with odd hallucinations, eruptions on the skin and tendency to boils, teeth loose, skin dry and mealy, kidneys affected, edema of the legs.

Lactic acid, an exceedingly good remedy in the gastrohepatic variety of diabetes. The symptoms are, urinates copiously and freely, urine light yellow and saccharine thirst, nausea, debility, voracious appetite and costive bowels. Dry skin, dry tongue, gastralgia.

Lycopodium Clav, excessive micturition in gushes, fluor albus drops out in clots, drawing pains in the right groin on rising from the seat, better after motion, sexual desire and power gone, pulmonary phthisis, with hetic fever, gouty lithemia.

Natrium Mur., despondency, excessive dryness of mouth, no sweat, skin cool, sallow complexion, constipation, with sensation of contraction of the anus.

Natrium Sulph., it has polyuria, intense itching of the skin, especially upon the upper surface of the thighs.

DIABETES

Phosphorus, useful in diabetes and pancreatic diseases, especially in those of a tuberculous or gouty diathesis. Sudden and extreme dryness of the mouth and marked physical restlessness are also guiding symptoms to this remedy, especially with a dark watery stool.

Phosphoric acid, corresponds to diabetes of nervous origin, the urine is increased, perhaps milky in color and containing much sugar. It suits cases due to grief. worry and anxiety, those who are indifferent and apathetic, poor in mental and physical force. It is unquestionably curative of diabetes in the early stages, great debility and bruised feeling in the muscles. There will be loss of appetite, sometimes unquenchable thirst and perhaps the patient will be troubled by boils. When patients pass large quantities of pale colorless urine or where there is much phosphatic deposit in the urine, it is the remedy.

Plumbum, it is considered one of the most *important* remedies in this form of disease. Lowness of spirits, anguish and melancholy, diminution of sight, dryness of mouth, dry cracked tongue, suppuration of lungs, hectic fever, impotence, dryness and brittleness of skin, gangrene.

Uranium Nitrate, considered useful in diabetes *orignating in dyspepsia.* It has polyuria (excessive secretion of urine), excessive thirst, dryness of the mouth and skin. Its strong characteristics are that the disease is due to assimilative derangements such as defective digestion, languor, debility and much sugar in the urine, enormous appetite and thirst, yet the patient continues to emaciate. It should be used in the 3 x trituration.

Insulin, has been prepared as a Homeopathic remedy for use in diabetes. It is useful in acne, carbuncles, erythema with itching eczema, in the gouty, transitory glyosuria when skin manifestations are presistent. Give three times daily after food. It is indicated in persistent cases of skin irritation, boils or varicose ulcertion with polyuria.

Dose. 3 x 30 x (tincture), 5 to 10 drops in water *for one day.* Care should be taken not to overdose.

2. DIABETES INSIPIDUS, POLYURIA

Definition : Also known under the name of *polyuria, hyperuresis, urine profluxio, polydipsia* is applied to every chronic, morbidly increased excretion of urine, free from sugar, which is caused by no profound structural changes of the kidney, and which constitutes either the sole or at least the most prominent and primary morbid phenomenon.

Exciting Causes : Injuries of the skull, violent and sudden emotions of chronic diseases of the brain and spinal cord, and a single excessive ingestion of cold beverages or other fluids.

The remedies recommended are :

Apis Mell., Argentum Met., Phos. acid, Squilla.

CHAPTER – XIII

DISEASES OF THE KIDNEYS

NEPHRITIS–INFLAMMATION OF THE KIDNEYS

The main remedies with their indications are given :

Aconitum Nap., incipient inflammation of the kidneys, stinging and pressing pains in kidney region. Kidneys act but slightly, urine contains albumen and fragments of casts. Urine hot dark, red with white faeces, red and clear bloody urine. Also, urine *suppressed* or retained. Renal region sensitive, with shooting pains. Painful urging to urinate. *Aconitum* has *fear*, tosses about with anxiety. Attacks are sudden violent. Ailments from fright, vexation, chill, cold winds (*Bryonia, Nux Vom., Hepar Sulp*).

Apis Mell., Pain in both kidneys (Bright's disease) renal pains, soreness, pressure on stoping. Pain left kidney *(Benzoic Acid, Thuja, Kalium Ars.) suppression* of urine. Acute inflamatory affection of kidneys, with albuminuria as in scarlet fever or diphtheria, or, after these, as a sequel to acute disease. It may be of use in any form of Bright's disease with dull pains in the kidneys, scanty urine and frequent micturition, the urine is heavily charged with albumen and contains blood corpuscles. Typical Apis is thirstless, intolerant of heat.

Arnica Mont., in inflammations of kidneys, bladder, even pneumonia, its mental state and the sore bruised feeling all over the body would enable you to do astonishing work. Does not want to be touched, horrors in the night *(Aconitum Nap.).* Horror of instant death. Chill followed by pains in the kidneys, nausea and vomiting. Piercing pains in the kidneys, nausea and vomiting. Piercing pains *as from knives* plunged into kidneys, chilly and inclined to vomit.

Urine difficult, scanty, dark with thick brown sediment, *suppression of urine.*

Terebinthinum, congestive kidneys with dull aching and smoky-looking urine. Violent *burning* and drawing pains in kidneys and bladder and urethra. Pressure in kidneys when sitting, relieved by motion. Stiff all over, heaviness and pains in region of kidneys. Renal disease producing dropsy, rapid attack with lumbar pain, urine greatly diminished, loaded with albumen, contains casts and blood, *suppressed,* urine smoky, with 'coffee grounds' or thick slimy sediment, *smells of violets.* Early scarlatinal nephritis. Tongue smooth, glossy, red *(Crot Hor. Pyrog.),* or a coating which peels in patches *Tereb.* has purpuric conditions, ecchymoses *(Arnica Mont.).* Hemorrhages from all outlets, especially in connection with urinary or kidney troubles (Comp. *Phos., Crot Hor.).* Ascites with anasarca, in organic lesions of kidneys.

Belladonna, stinging, *burning* pain, from region of kidneys down into bladder. *Suppression. No remedy has a greater irritation in the bladder and along the urinary tract. Bell.* pains, clutch, come and go suddenly. *Bell.,* typically, has redness, great heat to touch, dilated pupils–it comes midway between *Aconite Nap.* and *Arsenicum Alb.*

Helonias, burning sensation, kidneys, can trace their outlines by the burning. Congestion and pain in the kidneys with albuminuria, right kidney extremely sensitive, albuminuria acute or chronic, usually tired but knows no reason. Burning, scalding pain when urinating *(Canth.).* Affects the female genital organs.

Eryngium Aquat, must urinate every five minutes, urine dripping away all the time, burning like fire.

Cantharis, the whole urinary organs and genitalia are in a state of inflammation and irritation. Discharge of bloody urine burns like fire. *Intensity and rapidity are the features of this remedy.* Dull pressing or paroxysmal *cutting* or *burning* pains in both

DISEASES OF THE KIDNEYS

kidneys, very sensitive to lightest touch, urging to urinate. Painful evacuations by drops of bloody urine or pure blood. Intolerable urging before, during and after urination, *suppression*, violently acute inflammation or rapidly destructive. (comp. *Mercurius Cor.*).

Mercuris Cor., tenesmus vesicae with intense burning. Urine *suppressed* or hot urine passed drop by drop with much pain (*Canth.*). Urine hot, burning, bloody, contains filaments or flesh-like pieces of mucus, albuminous, shows granular fatty tubulic, with epithelial cells on their surface also in a state of granular fatty degenerations (*Ars Alb. Phos.*). Patient looks pinched, shrivelled melancholy. A drug of violence, of inflammations with *burning* (*Canth.*) of *desperate tenesmus*, the 'never-get-done' remedy in dysentery. Useful in syphilitic complications.

Mercurius Sol., nephritis with diminished secretion of urine with great desire to pass it. Urine saturated with albumen, dark brown mixed with blood, with dirty white sediment. Hematuria, with violent and frequent urging to urinate. Urine dark red, becomes turbid and fetid, smells sour and pungent *(Benzoic)* mixed with blood, white flakes or as if containing pus, flesh-like lumps of mucus, as if flour had been stirred in, scanty, fiery-red, very dark, with burning and scalding sensation during urination as from raw surfaces (*Canth.*), Worse at night, worse hot and cold, profuse, oily sweat, which does not ameliorate.

Chelidonium Majus, violent paroxysms of pain in kidneys, with intense headache, vertigo and syncope. Pain and tenderness in kidney regions, sensitive to pressure even of clothing, *(Argentum Nit., Hep Sulph.)*-(Compare *Lach.*). Urine reddish, turbid contains fibrin flakes and sand. *Characteristics are, pain under right shoulder angle.* A great liver medicine, a righ-sided medicine.

Colchicum, pain in the region of kidneys, hyperemia, nephritis, bloody, ink-like, albuminous urine. Dropsy after scarlatina urine like ink, after scarlatina (comp. *Lach., Kalium chlor.*). Urine burns when it passes. *Suppression,* retension, chiefly in acute form of Bright's disease.

Characteristics, small painfully acute, nausea and faintness from smell of cooking *(Arsenicum Alb. Sep.).* Loathing of food, sight and smell of it, urine contains clots of putrid decomposed blood, albumen sugar.

Helleborus Niger, post scarlet fever nephritis. Congestion of kidneys with extensive effusion of serum in abdominal cavity and tissue of lower extremities. Dropsy after scarlet fever with albumen and fibrin casts in urine. *Suppression* of urine or urine highly albuminous, dark, no sediment, *breathes easier lying down,* acute dropsies. Urine scanty, dark, or smoky with decomposed blood with floating dark specks, like coffee grounds, albuminous, scanty, top part clear. A great remedy in meningitis and hydrocephalus, chewing motions, boring head into pillow, automatic motion of one arm and leg. Staring eyes wide open, insensible to light.

Allium Cepa, pains in renal regions and region of bladder, very sensitive. Burning pressure in bladder, then in sacrum, pain in kidney region more left side. Urine frothy and iridescent *(Hep Sulp.),* red.

Berberis Vulg., soreness lumbar region and kidneys. Can bear no pressure, no jar, has to step down carefully, jar or jolt intolerable *(Bell.). Burning stitches,* loins and kidneys. Sore kidneys with urinary disturbances, and excessive deposits. Little calculi form, start down ureter, pains run up kidney and down to bladder. *Berb Vulg.* has bubbling sensations and pains that radiate from a point. *Pain in back a chief indication for Berb Vulg.*

Sabina, nephritis with retention or discharge by drops with burning *(Canth.).* Urine bloody and albuminous. *Pain from lumbar region to pubis.* Burning pain during micturition in rheumatic subjects. Metrorrhagia from plethora.

DISEASES OF THE KIDNEYS

Benzoic Acid, kidney pain which penetrate the chest on taking a deep breath. Sore pain back, *burning in left kidney,* with drawing pain when stooping, dull pain in kidneys, loins stiff. *Urine of a very repulsive odour (Ocimum Can., Calc Carb., Ars Alb.),* pungent *(Mercurius Sol.),* from time or first passing urine on clothing scents the room, contains mucus and pus, strong, hot, dark-brown urine.

Ocimum Canum, (Brazilian Alfavaca) *important* remedy for diseases of the kidneys, bladder and urethra, used widely in Brazil as a specific for these troubles. Crampy pain in kidneys, urine turbid thick, purulent, bloody, *brick dust red or yellow sediment,* formation of spike crystals of uric acid. Urine with *intolerable odour* like musk.

Phos., "Bright's disease, with sensations of weakness and emptiness." Albumen and exudation cells in urine, "fatty degeneration *(Mercurius Cor., Arsenicum Alb.)* of kidneys, liver and heart with anemia." Urine contains epithelial, fatty or waxy casts. Dropsy accompanied by diarrhea. Uremia with acute atrophy of brain and medulla. Hematuria, general dissolution of blood. Thirst, craves ice, worse lying on left side, fears thunder, dark, *Phos.,* is a profuse, easy bleeder (comp. *Crot Hor., Terebinth.),* blood bright.

Hepar Sulph., pain, kidneys with incessant, painful urging and voiding a few drops of *purulent urine.* Emaciation, renal region sensitive to slightest touch *(Argenicum Nit.).* Violent fever with unquenchable thirst, diarrhea and night sweats. Croupous nephritis, suppurative stage, fever chills alternating with burning heat, has to wait for urine to pass never able to finish urinating, some remains in the bladder. Urine dark red and hot, acrid, scalding, brown-red, last drops mixed with blood, on standing, turbid and thick with greasy pellicle, or iridiscent *(All Cepa). Hepar Sulph. is characteristically chilly, with hyperaethesia, mental and physical.*

Silicea, suppuration of kidneys, abscesses. "Old inveterate catarrhs of bladder, with pus and blood in the urine." Bloody, purulent discharge, thick or curdy. *Sil.* is chilly, worse cold damp weather.

Sensitive to noise, pain, cold, every hurt festers. *Silica headaches need heat*, and wraping up. Foot-sweats, especially foul, ailments from susppressed foot-sweat.

Arsenicum Alb., nephritis with stitiches in renal region, on breathing and *abscess of kidney (Merc Sol., Hep Sulph., Sil., Crot Hor.)*, Uremia, with vomiting, colic. Urine dark-brown, dark-yellow, turbid mixed with blood and pus, greenish. Urine like thick beer, rotten smell *(Benzoic Ac.). Suppression of urine*. Albuminuria, fatty degeneration *(Mercurius Cor., Phos.)*. Extreme restlessness, anxiety, prostration.

Crotalus Hor., nephritis albuminosa, in toxemia, or pregnancy. Urine dark, smoky from admixture of fluid blood. Hematuria. *Urine extremely scanty*, dark red with blood, jelly like, green-yellow from much bile. One of our greatest remedies for *sepsis*. Black water fever, urine like dark bloody jelly. Skin may be yellow to green yellow colour of eyes. May have hemorrhage from any and every part of body *(Tereb.)* dark thin blood. Putridity. Even the most rapid and desperate cases.

Lachesis, stitches in kidneys, extending through ureters. Urine almost black, frequent, foamy, dark *(Kalium Ars.)*. Like coffee grounds, black, scanty after scarlatina *(Colch.)*, loaded with albumen, *suppressed*, no urine, no stool. *Lach.* is cyanosed, extremely sensitive to heat and *touch*, especially about neck and abdomen. Sleeps into an aggravation. Typically, loquacious, suspicious and jealous.

Kalium Ars., tensive pain in left kidney. Edema left foot, extending to right and over whole body. Blackish urine *(Lach.)*, foams on shaking, on standing leaves a thick, reddish slime. Stitches, dull or sharp in both renal regions. Urine, the more he presses the less the flow.

Kalium Chlor., nephritis, frequent urging, could only pass a few drops of bloody urine *(Canth.)*. Urine black and albuminous, greenish-black. Prostration, coldness and easy hemorrhage.

DISEASES OF THE KIDNEYS

Argentum Nit., touching the kidney region increases the pain to the highest degree *(Hep Sulph., Chel.)*. Acute pain, kidneys, extends down ureters to bladder *(Lach.)*, worse slightest touch or motion, even deep inspiration. Typical *Argentum Nit.* has apprehension, gets diarrhea from anticipation *(Gels.)*. Craves sweets, which disagree. Is nervous, hurried, walks fast *(Lil Tig.)*.

Cannabis Indica, constant pain right kidney, sharp stitches both kidneys. Aching, *burning*, in kidneys keep him awaked at night. Pain in kidneys when laughing. *Cann Ind.* has the *most extravagant mental symptoms,* with exaggerations of time and space.

Cannabis Sativa, ulcerative pain in kidney regions. Sensation of soreness kidneys and bladder. Gonorrheal cases *(Thuja)*.

Aurum Met., kidneys hyperemic, with pressure round waist, and increase of urine. *(Cardiac Hypertrophy)*. *Supprression* or retention of urine. Hematuria. In *Aur.*, all the natural healthy affections are perverted, he loathes life, is weary of life, longs to die, is suicidal. Absolute loss of enjoyment in everything.

Eupatorium Per., chronic nephritis. Dull, deep pain kidneys, cutting pain, *suppression* of urine.

Sarsaparilla, neuralgia, attacks of most excruciating pain from right kidney downwards. Chronic nephritis. Renal colic and passage of gravel. Much pain at conclusion of passing water, almost unbearable. *Lyc.* has red sand with clear urine, *Sars.* has white sand with scanty, slimy or flaky urine. Urine dribbles while sitting.

Lycopodium Clav., nephritis with characterisitc *Lyc Clav.* symptoms. One of the *'suppression of urine'* drugs, 4 to 8 P.M. aggravation of symptoms. Desire for hot drinks, sweets, *Characteristics,* red sand in urine, urine reddens and causes eruptions if allowed to remain in contact (esp. babies). A *(Lyc.)* symptom-polyuria at night only.

Bryonia Alba, inflammation and pain kidneys. Pinkish urinary deposits, uric acid crystals. Whenever he *strains himself, lifting,* or unusual motion, pain in kidneys, rousing up of congestion and long-lasting pain. After overheating or over exertion, he gets pain in the back.

Sulphur, violent pain in kidney region *after long stooping.* Chronic nephritis. Secretions burn and redden orifices, eye-lids, anus, etc., 11 A.M. emptiness and hunger. Burning soles at night, puts them out. Theorizing, 'the ragged philosopher'.

Nux Vom., nephritis from *stagnation of portal circulation.* Bloating abdomen. Pressure, heat, *burning* in loins and kidneys. Pains in small of back as if bruised, so violent, he cannot move. Hemoturia, after abuse of alcoholic stimulants or drugs, suppression of Hemorrhoidal or menstrual discharges. Pressure and distension in abdomen, loins and kidneys. Spasmodic retention of urine, discharge drop by drop. Stranguary after beer. *Nux Vom.,* is irritable and chilly with hyperaesthsia mental and physical *(Hep Sulp.).*

Rhus Tox., tearing pains in kidneys, edema, *after exposure to wet.* After exposure to much dampness, edema of face, feet, developing into general anasarca, urine full of albumen. Tearing pains small of back, urine contains blood and albumen. Urine voided slowly, paralytic weakness of bladder. *Rhus Tox.* is worse for *cold, wet (Dulc.),* washing, chills kand draught, *worse* for first moving, but better for continued motion.

Natrium Mur., in cases with previous history of *malaria* and quinine. Tension and heat in renal regions. Polyuria with violent desire to urinate, inability to retain urine. *Curious* symptom, *unable to pass urine unless alone.*

Thuja, kidneys inflamed, feet swollen. Urine profuse, light yellow, contain sugar, foams, scanty, exceedingly dark, deposits brown mucus. *Pain left kidney to epigastrium.* Especially useful in gonorrheal or 'vaccinosis' cases.

TYPHLITIS, PERITYPHLITIS, AND APPENDICITIS 247

Laurocerasus, urinary difficulties, with palpitation and gasping for breath, coming on by spells. Suppressed urine, retension from paralysis of bladder. Involuntary urination.

Stramonium, kidneys secrete less urine or none, in acute disease, in children, in eruptive fevers, etc., great desire to urinate, though secretion is suppressed. Urine dribbles away very slowly and feebly. Retention, sensation as if urine could not be passed, because of narrowness of urethra. After straining, a few drops are passed. Better after drinking vinegar.

CHAPTER – XIV

Typhlitis, Peerityphlitis and Appendicitis

As *Appendicitis* is commonly spoken of as a very dangerous disease which may atttack any one, of any age, and at any time, irrespective of any distinctions as regards locality, climate, food habits or health, and when any person has the misfortune of falling a victim to this dire disease, it is considered most urgent and important that an immediate surgical operation is necessary to save his life. This has been the case ever since this new disease was discovered some years ago, and the same method of diagnosis and treatment has been in operation all these years. In this connection, it will be interesting to ascertain what homeopathy can offer for the treatment of this dangerous disease, and so this subject has been included in this hand book for the information of all those interested in homeopathy. While allopathy insists on an immediate surgical operation in all cases, irrespective of the nature of the complaint and the condition of the patient so long as it is diagnosed as 'appendicitis' and labelled as such, homeopathy, on the other hand, bases its diagnosis on the symptoms presented by the patient, in the form of sensations, such as, pain, etc., their nature, their locations and the forms in which they trouble the patient most, the origin or the cause of the trouble, if it could be ascertained, and how it developed from stage to stage to bring about the present serious condition. All the relevant facts which could be ascertained, and the most prominent or outstanding symptoms of suffering, presented by the patient, will enable the intelligent homeopathic physician to choose the appropriate remedies to migrate the immediate suffering of the patient, and to fix upon a course of treatment to be followed in order to give him relief. The course of treatment to be followed will be mainly constitutional, unless the case is too far advanced, and the affected parts are too much deteriorated, so that no medicines could have any effect on them, or repiar the damage, in which case it may be necessary to remove the diseased parts by a surgical operation and thus save the patient. Thus, homeopathy tries, by a course of internal medicines, to ease the sufferings of the patient as a first step and then to improve the general condition of the patient, as a whole, so as to restore him to normal health. Even in the advanced cases where an operation is necessary, and is performed, the patient can be given suitable constitutional treatment to avoid complications, and to bring him to normal health. Homeopathy has thus saved a very large number of patients from the troubles and the risks involved in surgical operations during all these years.

Definition: Although *Typhlitis, Perityphlitis* and *Appendicitis* are three distinct forms of diseases, yet, considering them in a diagnostic point of view, their symptoms during life are so intimately interwoven that a differential diagnosis among them is rarely possible.

Typhllitis is an inflammation, or cattarrh of the mucous membrane of the caecum, in consequence either of cold, or acumulation of hardened faeces, or foreign bodies, such as cherry-stones, plum stones and the like. It may spread over a considerable portion of the colon ascendens, and to the vermiform process, it may spread to the muscular layer of the gut, cause ulceration and even perforation of these parts, and terminate in peritonitis, inflammation of the loose areolar tissue around the caecum, and formation of abscesses in the right iliac fossa.

Perityphlitis is an inflammation of the loose areolar tissue around the caecum, either in consequence of typhlitis, or starting here independently, it is attended with a feeling of numbness and formication in the right limb and but little meteorism. It terminates, if not checked, in the formation of abscesses in the right iliac fossa, which either discharge into the neighbouring viscera or break through the abdominal particles mostly in the neighbourhood of

Poupart's ligament. As such absesses, if not originally caused by perforation of the caecum from within, mostly perforate the posterior wall of this organ. It occasionally happens that the abscess, when it discharges exteriorly, contains faecal matter also.

Appendicitis may be caused like *typhlitis* by hardened faecal matter, or foreign bodies. It terminates either in obiliteration of this process, or, when its opening gets closed, in an accumulation of a slimy, serous fluid, by which its wall become distended, forming the so-called dropsy of the appendix, or in the formation of abscesses in the right iliac fossa, or, lastly, in more or less extended peretonitis.

Symptoms : The symptoms of the three pathological states may be summed up under the following heads :

(*i*) *External swelling* in the right ilio-caecal or ilioinguinal region of the abdomen. It is felt directly under the abdominal wall, which is movable upon it, except where a perforation to the outside is imminent, and shows considerable heat and redness.

(*ii*) *Pain,* it usually commences suddenly, is sharp, lancinating, or boring, and increase on motion, worse from touch, and is confined either to the right iliac fossa alone, or extending over a larger surface, according to the extent of the inflammation.

(*iii*) *Obstinate constipation,* which may last for days, though interrupted sometimes.

(*iv*) *By an intercurrent diarrhea* of a slimy, watery substace. This is not a favourable sign, only faecal discharge gives relief.

(*v*) *Vomiting* may take place at any stage of the disease, but does so most frequently, at its height.

(*vi*) *Belching* and *meteoristic distension* of the stomach and upper part of the abdomen.

TYPHLITIS, PERITYPHLITIS, AND APPENDICITIS

(*vii*) *Singultus* or *hiccough* is a frequent sign, and very distressing to the patient, preventing all rest and sleep.

(*viii*) *Pain in the genitals,* erections of the penis, drawing up of the testicles, difficulty in urinating, numbness of the right leg, are consequences of the swelling pressing upon the corresponding nerves.

(*ix*) The *edematous swelling* of the right leg is the consequence of its pressure upon the crural, and iliacal veins, such a desperate condition of things must necessarily involve the whole system.

(*x*) *In fever,* which is more or less violent, according to the extent of inflammation

Therapeutic Hints

Belladonna, great pain in the ilio-caecal region, cannot bear the slightest touch, not even the bed-cover, nausea, vomiting, necessity of lying motionless on his back, high fever, increasing during the afternoon, with red or pale face, slight perspiration during the fever, it comes after the chill of the *Aconitum Nap.* state has passed off, and the inflammation has localised itself. Much pain contra-indicates *Aconitum Nap.*

Bryonia Alba, has throbbing and sharp, stitching pains confined to a limited spot, and the patient is constipated. The ilio-caecal region is very sore and senstive to touch. Any movement is painful and the patient lies perfectly still and on the painful side. The febrile disturbances of the drug will be present.

Ginsen, stinging pain and swelling and gurgling noise in the ilio-caecal region, dry tongue, heat and delirium when going to sleep.

Hepar Sulph., after the abuse of mercury, ilio-caecal region swollen, deep, in a circumscribed lump, lying on the back, with the right knee drawn up, as easiest position, frequent urging to stool and urination.

Dioscorea, its indications are-bowels filled with gas and griping, twisting pains, the pains are *constant,* the patient never being entirely free from pains. One peculiarity about the pains is, that they are relieved by stretching the body rather than bending double, or by bending backwards. It is best given in tincture in doses of 20 to 40 drops in 4 ounces of *hot water preferably,* a tea spoonful every 30 minutes to two hours.

Lachesis, great sensitiveness to contact of the abdomen, swelling in the ilio-caecal region, painful stiffness from the loins down to the sacrum and thighs, constipation, scanty urine with red sediment, stranguary, only possible position is that on the back with the knees drawn up (comp. *Hepar Sulp.).* Fever increases towards 3 P.M, patient feels worse after sleep.

Mercurius Sol., painful, hard, hot, and red swelling in the iliocaecal region, painful to touch, face red or pale, sickly, thirst, red, dry tongue, constipation, or frequent slimy discharge with straining, sweat without relief.

Plumbum Met., large, hard swelling in the ilio-caecal region, painful to the touch and least motion, or when sneezing or coughing, the whole abdomen sensitive, *the navel drawn in,* frequent sour belching, nausea, retching, constipation, anxious countenance, dry tongue, red on the edges, brown coating in the middle, great thirst, lame feeling in the legs, eructations of gas and vomiting, both have a faecal odour.

Rhus Tox., hard, painful swelling of nearly the entire right side of the abdomen, pain worse when sitting, or when stretching the right leg, impossibility of lying on the left side, bettter when lying on the back, with right leg drawn up, and when gently pressing the swelling from below upwards, pale, anxious face, burning of the palms of the hands, profuse sweat at night, small, frequent pulse, after taking cold by getting wet.

TYPHLITIS, PERITYPHLITIS, AND APPENDICITIS

Thuja, only those parts of the body perspire which are uncovered, those covered are hot and dry.

Arsenicum Alb., when the condition points to sepsis. There are chills, hectic symptoms, diarrhea and restlessness, and sudden sinking of strength. *It relieves vomiting in these conditions more quickly than any other remedy.*

Echinacea, very useful in septic conditions, with characterisitic tiredness. It should be used in $1x$ and $3x$ (tincture).

Arnica Mont. in septic cases after operations.

Ignatia, useful for those who become exceedingly nervous from any abdominal pain, also for the nervous symptoms of the disease, and may also be used in cases where operation has been performed, and no relief resulted. It very often happens that many cases of simple colic are diagnosed as appendicitis and operated upon. It is, therefore, advisable that, in such cases, *Colocynth* 30 and *Magnesia Phos. 30* should be given in watery solution every hour or two, to start with even in operable cases. If the patient is habitually constipated, *Bryonia Alba* 30 may be used in the same way. The following remedies will be useful :

For the smell as of faeces of the vomit :
Asaf., Mercurius Sol., Opium, Plumb.

For already formed abscess in the right iliac fossa :
Hepar Sulp., Iod., Kalium Carb., Lach., Lycop, Mercurius Sol., Silic.

Dr. William Howard Hay, M.D., an eminent surgeon of U.S.A., who wrote, *'A New Health Era'* some time ago says, that diseases of the human body are caused by the development of acid end-products by eating wrong types of foods, or the wrong combination of event the right types, and that the best way of treating them is to regulate the intake of such foods, and their correct combination so as to leave an alkaline residue. Anything that depletes our alkaline reserve depletes our functional activities. He says even so-called surgical cases are developed through the same causes, and that thought he had operated many surgical cases during his thirty years, experience as a surgeon, he had done wrong in operating them and that they were really unnecessary and should have been treated by means of correct dieting. As regards the treatment of Appendicitis, he says-

"No case of *Appendicitis* requires operation. Every case recovered simply through emptying the colon, withholding every thing from the digestive tract, and application of the ice-bag.

"To lose the tonsils or the appendix is to place on the body a permanent handicap, not such as will terminate life, but, such, as interfere with function in some, or many ways, so long as you live. Constipation follows the removal of the appendix, as effect follows cause, also, the absence of tonsils opens the way for all sorts of infections later on, as witness the sore throats, the catarrhs, the sinus involvement, the frequent colds, bronchitis following removal of tonsils. Remember that nature creates nothing without purpose and to remove any of the body organs is a vandalism against the future function of a body that should be conserved in all its parts and members, if it is to continue to function as originally intended."

So, his advice is, that the patient should be given enemas to empty the colon, should be given fresh fruit or vegetable juices only, till he gets normal. The ice-bag will help to empty the colon and relieve the pains.

CHAPTER – XV

CANCER–CARCINOMA

Cancer is a malignant tumor with the production of epitheliod cells. These tumors consist of morbid growth in the connective and epithelial tissues of the blood-vessels and their sheaths, which either retain the character of the affected tissue, or become altered by modification of the newly formed elements and by changes in their relations to the connective tissue and vascular distribution. They may appear in any part of the body and may be due to a variety of causes, but primarily they seem to be a hereditary pre-disposition, abuses of spirituous liquors, blows and falls of all kinds, and tuberculosis.

Cancer cases fall into three groups–

(*a*) Those in the pre-cancer stage,
(*b*) Those in the early or incipient stage,
(*c*) Those in the late or advanced stage.

In the pre-cancer stage, Homeopathy offers a wide field of constitutional treatment. That stage embraces all the countless manifestations of chronic disease, such as diabetes, epilepsy, psoriosis, eczema, arthritis in its many forms, asthma, hay fever and numerous tubercular affections, as well as the venereal diseases, together with the numerous abnormal mental and emotional afflictions which harasse mankind today. All these are further aggravated by the numerous drugs, serums, vaccines, etc., which are employed on a large scale in the treatment of the various diseases. If a true scientific Homeopathic treatment is given over a course of a few years, even persons with a history of cancer in their families, and who had inherited tendencies need not develop cancer.

Dr. A. H. Grimmer, M.D. of Chicago has treated numerous cases of cancer falling under the three groups, and has reported that he was able to cure at least ninety-five percent of cases following under the first group, about seventy-five percent of cases falling under the second group, and only about 10 per cent of those falling under the third.

The small percentage of cures under the third group was due to the prevalent radium and X-ray treatment in the earlier stages, which was intended to destroy the bacillae in the affected organs, but, which in this process of destruction of the germs, had destroyed or deteriorated also tissues, and thus devitalised the patients to such an extent that they were unable to respond readily to the action of Homeopathic remedies, and it took a long time before those remedies could produce any appreciable impression on them. In spite of these drawbacks, a number of cases have been cured after these drawbacks, a number of cases have been cured after prolonged and careful treatment with a number of remedies extending over 2 or 3 years, according to the severity of the case.

The leading indications of some of the more important remedies useful in the common types of cancer falling under the second and third groups are given. In detailing the symptoms under each head, only those relating to the parts of the body affected are given. In choosing the appropriate remedy for each case, the leading characteristics of the remedy as given in the Materia Media (See Appendix II, and a text book of Materia Medica for those not included therein), and the conditions of aggravation and amelioration should also be taken into account.

1. CANCER OF THE TONGUE

Symptoms, It is of the epithelial kind and commences usually at the edge near the tip of the tongue, as a small hard lump, which after a while, forms an ulcer of a roundish shape, with raised eges and uneven bottom. It distinguishes itself from every other ulcer by its continuous encroachments, by its hard, lardaceous bottom, by the viscid, milky juice, which can be squeezed out by pressure, upon its edges, and by the lancinating, boring, burning pains with which it is attended, robbing the patient of rest at night, and not infrequently leading him to suicide. By-and-by the adjacent parts of the tongue begin to swell, and the cancer itself spreads either upon the superior or inferior surface of the tongue. The disease is slow, lasting from one to three years.

Therapeutic Hints

Alumen, hardening of tissues of tongue, ulcers with indurated base, scirrhus of the tongue.

Arsenicum Alb., violent burning on tongue. Swelling about root and tongue, externally and internally. Tongue, *dry, and morbidly red, with paipllae considerably raised at the tip, lead coloured. Edge of tongue red, takes imprint of teeth, gangerene of tongue, sports on tongue, burning like fire.*

Carbo An., knotty indurations in the tongue. Burning blisters on tip and edges of the tongue. Burning on tip of tongue and rawness in mouth. Taste bitter, especially morning, sour.

Carbo Veg., glossitis, when tongue becomes indurated, tongue heavy, with difficult speech, tip of tongue raw and dry, tongue turns black. Bitter taste, before and after eating, salty taste.

Causticum, speechless, from paralysis of the organs of speech, painful vesicle on the tip of the tongue, stuttering, difficult, indistinct speech. Tongue coated white on both sides, red in the middle.

Conium Mac., speech difficult, from lingual paralysis, tongue swollen, painful, stiff, taste bitter.

Hydrastis Cand., tongue swollen, shows marks of the teeth, as if burned or scalded, later a vesicle forms on tip. Taste flat, peppery.

Lachesis, tongue, trembles when protruded, or catches behind the teeth, swollen, coated white, papillae enlarged, dry, red, cracked, mapped, dry, black and stiff blisters mostly about the tip.

Muriatic Acid, cancer of tongue, deep ulcer, with black base, and inverted edges, hard lump on side of tongue, growing into a deep, wasty ulcer, so that speaking is difficult.

Nitritum Ac., tongue, sensitive, even mild food causes smarting, white, dry, morning, coated green, with ptyalism, dry, fissured, deep, irregular shaped ulcer on the edge of the tongue. Ulceration of tongue, with tough, ropy mucus.

Phytolacca, tongue, fiery red at tip, coated yellow and dry, thickly coated at back part. Tongue, hot, rough, tender and smarting at tip, also small ulcers, like those caused by mercury, thick, protruding. Burnt feeling on back part of tongue.

Sepia, tongue painful, as if sore or scalded. Vesicles, white coated. Taste, bitter, saltish, putrid or offensive, food taste too salty.

Silicea, taste, of blood, of soap suds, bitter, with thick mucus in throat, of rotten eggs. Sensation of hair in fore-part of tongue. One-sided swelling of tongue. Ulcer on right border of tongue, eating into it, and discharging much pus.

Sulphur, taste, sour, bitter, sweetish, foul when awaking in morning. Tongue, white, or yellow, brown and dry, fured in morning but wears off during day.

2. CANCER OF THE LOWER LIP

Therapeutic Hints

Arsenicum Alb., cancerous growth of the skin of the face, rapidly progressing ulceration, thin, bloody, offensive

CANCER–CARCINOMA

discharge, sharp, burning pains and extreme sensitiveness to cold air. Severe pains along right inferior maxillary nerve. Bites tumbler when drinking. *Sore lips and ulcers in the mouth. Eruptions on the lips.* Contractive quivering or jerking on one side of upper lip, especially when falling asleep.

Aurum Met., cancer of nose and lip, tongue swollen with scirrhus-like hardness, ulcers on tongue, with foul breathe, painful swelling of submaxillary glands.

Condurango, most efficacious in *open cancer of concerous ulcers,* where it effectually moderates the severity of the pain, epithelial cancer of lower eye-lid, on left side of nose, carcinoma of lip, an unclean and sinuous ulcer, with surrounding hardness and swelling, burning pains, lip inverted, *painful cracks at the angle of the mouth,* ulcer on chin, perforating the gums, lumps on chin, cancer of tongue.

Conium Mac., induration of lymphatics of lip after contusion. *Cancer of lip from pressure of tobacco pipe.*

Kali Mur. Epithelioma of lip, ulcertion of mouth, has perforated cheeks and threatens to become cancer of the face, discharge ichorous and foetid, scurvy in cachetic people.

Kreosotum, burning pain on face, worse, talking or exertion, better, lying on the unaffected side, nervous, excitable. Peeling off and cracking of cubicle of upper lip. Wants to moisten the lips frequently, without being thirsty. Tumor, size of a pea, on lower lip, with acrid, watery ichor, making the surrounding parts sore.

Lachesis, Cancer of lower lip, dry, cracked, bleeding.

Lycopodium Clav., swelling of lower lip, with a large ulcer on the vermillion border of the lower lip.

Sepia, suspicious tubercle on lip of a cartilaginous appearance, sometimes bleeding and having a scirrhous appearance, with a broad base. *Epithelial Cancer of Lower Lip,* with a burning pain and pricking as form a splinter of wood, of ulcers covered with large, thick, scurfs, corrosive ichor oozes from under the scabs, complexion yellow and earthy.

Silicea, scirrhous induration of the upper lip and face. Cancer of lower lip, ulcer greyish, superficil, excruciatingly painful.

3. CANCER OF THE ESOPHAGUS

The only remedy suitable for this trouble is *Spigelia.*

Spigelia, cancer of esophagus, pylorus, or rectum, narrowing the lumen of the canal, with constant, severe and pressing pains, passing through to the bck and shooting down into the thighs.

4. CANCER OF THE STOMACH

According to pathological researches, there are three different forms of cancer of the stomach.

a. *Scirrhous*, a fibrous growth in which the connective tissue stroma predominates over the cell formation, generally orginates in the sub-cutaneous cellular tissue.

b. *Carcinoma Medullaris,* is a narrow growth in which the cancer-cells predominate over the stroma, forms round isolated lumps in the mucous membrane of the stomach, and spreads sponge-like upon the inner surface of the stomach.

c. *Carcinoma Alveolaris,* a jelly-like growth, in which we observe a colloid degeneration of the cancer-cells, invests at first the sub-mucous cellular tissue, but penetrates frequently to the peritoneum, and forms large tumors on it.

All these kinds of cancer may often be seen together, and they mostly invest the pylorus, sometimes of the lesser curvature, still rarer the cardia, and most rarely the other parts of the stomach.

CANCER–CARCINOMA

The inner cavity of the stomch is much changed by this disease. It becomes greatly *enlarged* by stricture of the pylorus, or much diminished by the stricture of the cardia, there is cancerous degenertion of the coatings of the stomach. The mucous membrane in the neighbourhood of the cancer exhibits chronic catarrhal inflammation, which is sometimes spread all over it, and in the further progress of the disease, ulceration and erosion of smaller or larger blood-vessels with consecutive hemorrhage obtain.

The causes of carcinoma of the stomach are not known, but heredity appears to deserve some consideration. The disease has been observed most frequently between the years of fifty and seventy.

Symptoms

(a) GENERAL CANCER CACHEXIA, emaciation, paleness of the skin and the mucous membranes, ash-coloured or yellow colour of the face, brittle, dry, harsh and wrinkled skin, peeling off of branny scales, especially from the lower extremities. The expression of the face is sad, the eyes are sunken, the malar bones stick out, the ankles are edematous.

(b) TUMOR IN THE PIT OF THE STOMACH, this is present, however, only when the cancer invests the pylorus.

(c) THE STRICTURE OF THE PYLORUS causes, further, *a sinking in of the abdomen*, the intestines are empty, because the food is prevented from going through the pylorus. When there is a stricture of the cardia, the *epigastric region is fallen in,* because not sufficient nourishment is allowed to enter the stomach, the intestines are likewise empty, only the ribs protrude.

(d) VOMITING, this happens if there is a stricture of the pylorus, generally from four to five hours after eating. The masses that are thrown up are digested. In case of stricture of the cardia, the vomiting takes place immediately after or even during eating, without nausea or exertion, it is only a throwing out of the swallowed food. If widenings of the esophagus exist at the same time, the vomiting follows a little latler. If the cancer is located in another part of the stomach, the vomiting may be entirely absent, or it may, after having been regular for a time, slacken off and cease altogether.

(e) HEMORRHAGE FROM THE STOMACH, the blood is thrown up either decomposed as a brownish, chocolate-like mass, or when larger blood-vessels have been destroyed, as clear blood.

(f) THE PAIN IN THE EPIGASTRIUM, which has its seat generally in the cancerous tumor, is worse from eating, usually of a lancinating or burning character, and never extending to the spine, it may be absent altogehter.

(g) The appetite is generally diminished, in some cases, however, it is increased, but the patients are afraid to eat because of the following pain and vomiting.

(h) The stool is usually retarded, but when the cancerous growth softens and dissolves, we observe colliquative diarrhea, and when there is hemorrhage in the stomach, bloody evacuations.

As regards the nature of the cancer, a very slow progress of the disease, together with additional ascites make it probable that it is a jelly-like cancer-*Carcinoma Alveolaris*. An acute progress and rapid growth of tumor with frequent and large hemorrhages point to *Carcinoma Medullaris*. A slow progress and considerable hardness and considerable hardness and modulated appearance of the tumor indicates a *Scirrhous*. This latter is by far of the most frequent recurrence.

Whatever the kind of cancer, a proper study of the indications will lead to the selection of an appropriate remedy.

Therapeutic Hints

Acetic Ac., this remedy is praised highly. Scirrhous of pylorus, cancer of stomach, ulcerative gnawing pain at one spot in stomach, with agony, and depression, preventing sleep, *intense and constant thirst*, severe burning pain in stomach and abdomen, vomiting after every meal of yellow, yeast-like matter or blood, pale, waxen skin, tongue pale and flabby, marked debility, copious pale urine.

Animal food is absolutely prohibited for this disease.

Arsenicum Alb., burning pain in the stomach, excessive thirst, desire for acids, worse from cold drinks and cold diet, better from hot drinks vomiting of all he takes, vomiting of black substances, terrible sensation of weakness and exhaustion, with anxiety in region of stomach, and restlessness.

Arsenicum Iod., violent burning in stomach.

Belladonna, cutting, clawing pain, nausea, gagging and vomiting, staring eyes, dryness in mouth and throat, fainting. cancerous ulcers, burning when touched, black crusts of blood at the bottom of the ulcer, scanty pus.

Bismuth, violent, crampy pains, burning and stinging in the region of the stomach, stomach enlarged, hanging down to the crest of the ilium, hard lump between the navel and the edges of the lower ribs on the right side, Scirrhous of the pylorus, abdomen bloated in ridges, with great rumbling of wind along the colon, which is rarely passed off, but then gives relief, vomiting, only at intervals of several days, when the stomach has become filled with blood, and then of enormous quantities, and lasting a whole day, vomits all fluids.

Carbo Veg., burning pain, extending from the pit of the stomach into the small of the back, anxiety, cold extremities, cold, sticky sweat, intermitting pulse.

Carbo An, saltish water rises from the stomach and runs out of the mouth, accompanied by retching, and followed by violent empty eructations, cold feet and hiccough, pressure, clawing, griping and burning in the stomach, scanty, hard stools in lumps, copper coloured eruption on the face.

Cadmium Sulph., soreness in pit of stomach on pressure. Violent *nausea,* retching. *Black vomit.* Vomiting of mucus, green slime, blood, with great prostration, and great tenderness over the stomach. Burning and cutting pain in stomach. Carcinoma, helps the persistent vomiting. Coffee ground vomiting. This remedy acts will in the case of drunkards.

Conium, vomiting of chocolate-colored masses, sour and acrid, pressing, burning, squeezing pain, extending from the pit of the stomach into the back and shoulder, swelling in pyloric region, hardness of the abdomen from swelling of mesenteric glands.

Condurango, severe pains, vomiting of coffee ground masses, hard, knotty, large swelling in pylorus, complete loss of appetite, emaciation, cachetic look, constipation, stricture of esophagus, with burning pains behind sternum, where food seems to stick. Vomiting of food, and indurations in left hypochondium with constant burning pain.

Hydrastis Can., vomits everything, except water with milk, pain in pit of stomach, emaciation. Cannot eat bread or vegetables. Atonic dyspepsia, gastritis.

Kreosote, painful, hard spot on the left side of the stomach.

Lachesis, gnawing pressure, relieved after eating, but coming on again in a few hours, and the more violent, the emptier the stomach, great sensitiveness to contact, especially to that of his clothes, drunkards.

Lycopodium Clav., after eating or drinking, vomiting of dark, greenish masses, bloatedness of the stomach and bowels, rumbling in the bowels, obstinate constiation, hard swelling in the epigastric region as from a hoop, great emaciation and internal debility. Perforating ulcer, worse sitting bent, *better* walking about and when warm in bed. Vomitting of bile, pus and coagulated blood.

Mezereum, great emaciation, the muscles of the face are tensely drawn, like strings, constant vomiting of chocolate-colored masses, with great burning in the throat, violent retching, accompanied with the agony of death, sleeplessness and exhaustion, obstinate constipation, hard lumps in the epigastric region. Burning and uneasiness in stomach, relieved by eating, canine hunger at noon and evening.

Phosphorus, epigastric region sensitive to touch, constant nausea and fullness in the stomach, after eating, or drinking even a swallow of water, vomiting of a sour, foul smelling fluid, which looks as though it had been a mixture of water, ink and coffee-grounds. In the sunken abdomen, a circumscribed, hard swelling, pale, earthy complexion, great emaciation, sleepiness, peevishness, fine gurgling noise in the abdomen, urine scanty, red or brown, with reddish or yellowish red sediment, bowels constipated, dry, rumbling stools.

Sepia, sour taste after eating, vomiting of mucus, caused by taking even the simplest food, the pain in the stomach increases by vomiting, and extends to the back, with anxiety, oppression of the chest and cold perspiration, hard places in the region of the pylorus, constipation. Twisting in the stomach, and rising in throat, tongue becomes stiff, speechless, afterwards the body may become rigid.

Silicea, burning or throbbing in pit of stomach. Sensitiveness of pit of stomach to pressure. Pressure as after eating too much. Induration of pylorus. Anguish in pit of stomach, attack of melancholy.

Staphysagria, sensation as if stomach were hanging down, relaxed.

Sulphur, sensitiveness to touch in region of stomach. Marked weakness about 11 A.M, empty, gone or gaint feeling, pressure at stomach, also after eating.

5. CANCER OF THE INTESTINES

Cancer of the intestines appears in any of the 3 forms mentioned under part 4. It originates primarily in the submucous and mucous coats of the intestines, or reaches over secondarily from a cancer of the stomach, or of the peritoneum, the liver, ovaries, uterus, or other neighbouring organs.

Symptoms: The presence of an uneven potato-like tumor, the slow but steady development of intestinal obstruction, the peculiar dry and ash-coloured skin, the fast wasting away in strength and flesh, and the age of the patient, as cancer very rarely appears before the age of forty.

6. CANCER OF THE RECTUM

In the beginning of its development, when it causes a pressure upon, and a consecutive swelling of the hemorrhoidal veins with occasional bloody discharges, and pain from the sacrum down into the thighs, it is most easily confounded with hemorrhoids. Later, however, the obstruction of the rectum becomes more apparent by the form of the discharged feces, which appear pressed, flattened, angular, or pass off in small, hard nuts, like sheep dung. Manual examination reveals now a knotted tumor, which encircles the gut like a ring. In still further advanced stage, this tumor suppurates, and the bursting of blood-vessels may occasion profuse hemorrhages.

Therapeutic Hints

Alumen, constipation of the most aggravated kind. No desire for stool for days. Violent ineffectual urging to stool. No ability to expel stool. *Marble-like masses pass, but rectum still feels full*. Long-lasting pain and smarting in the rectum after stool. Hemorrhage from bowels.

Apis Mell., *soreness of the bowels and abdominal* walls felt when pressing upon them, or sneezing. Burning, stinging in the bowels.

Peritonitis, with exudation, urine scanty, dark.

Arsenicum Alb., gnawing, burning pains like coals of fire, relieved by heat. Violent pains in abdomen, with great anguish, has no rest anywhere, rolls about on floor and despairs of life. Painful spasmodic protrusion of rectum. *Burning* pain and pressure in rectum and anus.

Belladonna, distended, hot, colic, as if a spot in the abdomen were seized with the nails, a griping, clutching, clawing, great pain in the right ileocaecal region, cannnot bear the slightest touch, not even the bed clothes. Violent, cutting pressure in hypogastrium now here, noe there.

Carbo An., abdomen greatly distended, much annoyed with flatus, painful sensation in right, lower abdomen, as if something would be squeezed through. Soreness in abdomen while coughing.

Carbo Veg., colic from flatulence, abdomen full to bursting, pain worse from least food, better from passing flatus, or hard stool. Burning, lancinting pain in epigastrium and deep in abdomen, worse from eating, with anguish, flatulency, diarrhea.

Clematis, lancinating pains, from belly to chest, aggravated by breathing, also during urination. Increased sensitiveness of both inguinal regions. Swelling and induration of the inguinal gland, with jerking pains.

Condurango. See part 4.

Graphites, cramp in the lower abdomen. Colic, immediately after eating. Griping, digging pains in the abdomen. Pain in the belly in the left side, when lying on the right, and *vice versa*. Burning pains radiating through abdomen, in gastralgia. Large blisters on raised base, from navel to spine. Pain in the inguinal regions. Glandular swelling in the groins, painful pressing toward the groin and anus. Chronic diarrhea, stools brownish, liquid, undigested, *offensive*. Very fetid gas preceded by colic. Varices of the rectum. Fissure of anus.

Hepar Sulp., pain in the abdomen. Fermentation above the navel, with eructation of hot air. Colic, with dry, rough cough. Rumbling in the abdomen. Swelling and suppuration of the inguinal glands.

Hydrastis Can., burning in the region of the navel, with 'goneness', faintness, in the epigastrium. Loud rumbling with dull aching in the hypogastrium and small of back, worse moving, cutting, colicky pains, with heat and faintness, constiption, better after passing flatus. Sharp pain in the caecal region. Sharp pain in the region of the spleen, with dull groins, cutting pains extending into testicles.

Kreosote, ulcerative pain in abdomen. Pain in region of umblicus. Abdomen distended and tense, like a drum, without being hard or painful. Burning in the bowels. Sore pain in abdomen during deep inhalation. Painful sensation of coldness in abdomen, icy-coldness in epigastrium, dyspepsia. Violent abdominal spasms, worse in the groins.

Lachesis, painful distension, flatulence, can bear no pressure. Burning like fire in hypogastric and lumbar region, cutting in right side of abdomen, causing fainting attacks. Abdomen hot, sensitive, painfully stiff from loins down the thighs, pus formed. Peritonitis.

Phosphorus, very sensitive abdomen, painful to touch, rolling and rumbling in abdomen, during and after drinking. Painful feeling of weakness across whole abdomen, worse in hypogastric region after a short walk, must lie down. Shooting in the abdomen, with empty feeling, sensation of coldness in the abdomen. Abdomen flaccid, with chronic loose bowels. Tympanitis, mostly about the caecum and transverse colon.

Phosphoricum Acid, rumbling in abdomen, and noise as from water. Meteoristic distension of the abdomen, rumbling and gurgling, painless stool.

Rhus Tox., soreness as if beaten, in hypochondria and still more in abdomen, worse on the side lain on, when turning, and when beginning to move. Abdomen bloated, especially after eating. Sensation as if something was torn off in abdomen. Visible contractions of abdomen above navel.

Sepia, colic, with great distension and sensitiveness. Rumbling in abdomen, especially after eating. Colicky pains in lower abdomen, with straining and increased pain during stool. Abdominal pains relieved by warmth. Inguinal gland inflamed.

Sulphur, intestines feel as if strung in knots, worse from bending forward. Painful sensitiveness of abdomen to touch, as if internally raw and sore. Painful swelling of inguinal glands.

Thuja, while sitting, stitching in abdomen as from needles. Spasmodic stricture, as if something alive was pushing out. Soreness of the navel. Painful swelling of inguinal glands.

7. CANCER OF THE BREAST

The scirrhous form is the most frequent, it appears either deep in the gland or nearer the surface, as a round tumor, which draws the region of nipple inward, causing a navel-like depression by its gradual contraction and its adhesion to the external skin.

Its development is, in most cases, slow, often intermitting, making halts for a long time. Finally, it perforates the skin and appears as an open cancer, making rapid strides to final destruction.

It is generally found in one breast at a time, sometimes in both, and often combined with scirrhous degeneration in other parts of the system. It causes the most intense burning, stinging, lancinating pains, which deprive the patient of sleep and rest. The open ulcer discharges profusely an offensive ichor, or it bleeds easily and profusely when, by erosion, blood vessels become destroyed. The nutritive action of the system is completely prostrated and we see the patient gradually lose strength and sink, with symptoms of marasums, edema of the lower extremities, colliquative diarrhea or a sudden profuse hemorrhage from the ulcer.

Therapeutic Hints

Apis Mell, when there is *stinging, burning* pain, whether in scirrhous tumors or in open cancers, pain in the ovarian region, with bearing down, scanty, dark urine, edema of the lower extremities.

Arsenicum Alb., nightly, burning pain like fire, with great restlessness, loss of strength and emaciation, the pains grow better from the external application of warmth.

Arsenicum Iod., with swelling of gland in axilla.

Asterias rubens, cancer, around nipples, which is sunk in, skin adherent and smooth, livid red spot which ulcerates, discharging very fetid ichor, edges pale, hard, everted, arterial skin swollen and painful, axillary glands swollen, hard and knotted, nocturnal lancinating pains in tumor.

Belladonna, scirrhous tumors, with erysipelatous inflammation and stitching pains, frequent bearing down in the genital organs.

Bromium, scirrhous mammae, great depression of spirits, suppression of menses, stitches from mammae, firmly adhering to its surroundings, with lancinating pains, worse from pressure and at night, gray, earthy complexion, oldish look, emaciation, swelling and induration of glands.

CANCER–CARCINOMA

Calcarea Carb., indurations of the breast, too early and too profuse menstruation soreness and swelling of breast before the menses.

Calcarea ox., has more than any other remedy relieved the terrible pains in open cancers.

Carbo An., scirrhus tumor, hard and uneven, the skin over it is loose, on places, of a dirty, blue red appearance, the pains are burning and drawing toward and axilla, oppression of the chest, nightly perspiration of the thighs only, desponding.

Clematis, scirrhous mammae, with stitches in shoulder and gland, very painful during increasing moon, or when the whole gland is very painful, worse in cold weather and during the night, while perspiring, she cannot bear to be uncovered.

Conium Mac., *scirrhus cancer of mammae,* hard as cartilage and uneven, sharp, shooting pains and occasional twings and *concealed cancer of bones,* effects of contusions and bruise, it acts best in the first stage of scirrhous.

Graphites, when the tumor grown out of old cicatrices, which have been formed by repeated gathering of the breast.

Hydrastis Can., scirrhous tumor, hard, heavy, and adherent to the skin, which is dark, mottled and very much puckered, the nipple being retracted, pains like knives thrust into the part, cachetic appearance of the face.

Lachesis, tumor in the left breast, with lancinating pain, in consequence of pressure upon the tumor the pain extends into the left shoulder and down the arm, there is a constant painful feeling of weakness and lameness in the left shoulder and which is aggravated by using the arm. In open cancer, when it has a dark, bluish-red appearance, with blackish streaks of coagulated and decomposed blood, chronic leucorrhea, painful menstruation on the first day.

Lapis Alba, mammary and uterine cancer in scrofulous women, with burning, shooting, stinging pains, glandular tumors, cancer, as long as ulceration has not set in.

Lycopodium Clav., hard tumors with stitching or cramping pain, circumscribed redness of the face, worse from 4 P.M, during the paroxysms of pain, she is obliged to walk about and to weep, she feels better in the open air.

Phosphorus, when the ulcer bleeds easily.

Sepia, induration in the breast and ovaries, yellow, spotted face, chronic leucorrhea.

Silicea, with great itching of the swollen gland.

Tarentula Cub., atrocious pains in cancer or carbuncle, when the surface is dark and bluish.

8. CANCER OF THE WOMB

The degeneration begins almost always at the vaginal portion, rarely extends to the fundus, is, however, very apt to spread down the vagina, over to the baldder and rectum, causing, at the period of its decay, a most horrid destruction of these parts.

Symptoms: Its most important symptoms are-pain in the small of the back, loins and groins, which grow more and more violent, hemorrhages, at first only during the menstrual periods, later at any time, and leucorrhea, which becomes more and more watery, corroding and offensive.

The cauliflower exerescence, is a canceroid hypertophy of the papellae in the mouth of the womb, which sometimes attains to an enormous size in the shape of cauliflowers. It looks bright red, bleeds easily and is prone to cancerous degeneration, in which state it undermines the general constitution by pain and loss of blood, like cancer of the womb, to which it is similar in all its symptoms.

CANCER–CARCINOMA

A differential diagnosis, between the two can be gained only by an examination with the speculum.

Therapeutic Hints

Apis Mell. ovarian affections with drawn-in nipples of mammae, scirrhous or open cancer of the breast, with stinging, burning pains, following old cases of mastitis, weak, faint sensation in epigastrium, with loss of appetite, morbid irritability of urinary organs.

Arsenicum Alb., great exhaustion, restlessness and fits of anguish, with terrible, sharp, burning pains, all worse about midnight, acrid, corroding and burning discharges, watery, light or dark colored, often very offensive *(Ars Iod.).*

Aurum Mur, stinging, cutting, pressive pains in the uterine region, very offensive discharges, belching up of wind, craves nothing but sour things, the mind constantly dwelling on suicide.

Belladonna, painful bearing down in the pelvis, as though everything would fall out of the genitals, a similar pain in the small of the back, frequent, transient stitches in the region of the womb, hemorrhages from the womb, profuse, often very offensive.

Calcarea Carb., burning soreness in the genital organs, aching in the vagina, profuse menstruation, flow of blood between the monthly periods, cold feeling on the top of the head, great sensitiveness to cold air and liability to catch cold, scrofulous diathesis.

Carbo An., burning in the abdomen, extending into the thighs, labor-like pain in the pelvis and small of the back extending into the thighs, with discharge of slimy, discolored blood, irregular menses, uterus swollen and hard, cachetic appearance of the face, earthy colour of the skin, great weakness.

Carbo Veg., paroxysmal spells of burning in the uterine region, varicose veins on the external genital organs, cold knees in bed.

Conium Mac., stitching pain in the womb, accompanied by such symptoms as accompany pregnancy, nausea and vomiting, craving sour or salt things, pain and swelling of the mammae during the menses, dejection of spirits, etc.

Graphites, cauliflower excrescence, burning, stitching pains like electrical shocks, through the womb, extending into the thighs, great heaviness in the abdomen when standing, with increased pains and faintness, menses only every six weeks, with discharge of black, clotted, offensive blood, and an increase of all the sufferings, constipation, earthy color of the face, frequent chilliness, sad, desponding.

Iodium, cutting in the abdomen, with pains in the loins and small of the back, uterine hemorrhage at every stool, indurations of the uterus, painfulness and feeling of heaviness in both mammae, they hang down, relaxed and lose their fat, dwindling and falling away of the mammae, the patient feels worse from external warmth, after abuse of merucury.

Kreosote, cauliflower excrescence, awfull burning as of red-hot coal in the pelvis, with discharge of clots of blood having a foul smell, bearing down and sense of weight in the pelvis, drawing pains in the small of the back and uterine region, extending to the thighs, intermingled with stitching pains, the vagina is swollen and burning hot, long-standing leucorrhea becoming more and more watery, acrid, bloody and ichorous all the time, frequent hemorrhages from the womb, dwindling and falling away of the mammae, with small, hard, painful lumps in them, wretched complexion, great debility, sleeplessness.

Lachesis, pain in the parts as if swollen, they do not bear contact, and have to be relieved of all pressure, coughing or sneezing causes stitching pains in the affected parts, tenacious and acrid menstrual flow with labor-like pains, discharge of a few drops of blood from the nose before menses, which are scanty and delaying,

CANCER–CARCINOMA

especially indicated during the climacteric period, with frequent uterine hemorrhages.

Lycopodium Clav., drawing in the groin, burning and gnawing, chronic dryness of the vagina, pressing through the vagina on stooping, discharge of wind through the vagina, pain in the small of the back, extending down to the feet, incarcerated flatulence, with rumbling in the left hypochondriac region, red sand in the urine, jerking of single limbs awake or asleep, feels worse in general from 4 to 8 P.M.

Magnesium Mur., scirrhous indurtion of the womb, uterine spasms extending to the thighs and occasioning leucorrhea, discharge of black clots of menstrual blood, more when sitting than when walking, large, hard, difficult stools which crumble off as if they are expelled.

Mercurius Sol., syphilitic taint, prolapsus of the vagina, swelling of inguinal glands.

Murex purp., a lively, affectionate disposition has turned to melancholy from the effects of the disease, frequenty profuse menstruation, and strong sexual desire, soreness in the region of the cervix, or a feeling as though something was pressing on a sore spot in the pelvis, with pain in the right side of the uterus going into the abdomen or thorax, watery greenish leucorrhea, irritating the parts, dragging and relaxation in the perineum, pains in the hips, loins, and down the thighs, worse from exertion.

Nitricum Acid, irregular menstruation in shorter or longer intervals, during the intervals, a profuse, discolored, brownish and offensive leucorrhea, great debility, nervousness, and depression of spirits, hemorrhoidal tendency, great pain in the rectum after stools, lasting for hours, even worse after a diarrheic evacuation, the urine is very offensive. During a ride in the carriage, they feel much better.

Natrium Carb., induration of the neck of the womb, the os uteris is out of shape, pressing in the hypogastrium towards the genital organs, as if everything would come out, metrorrhgia, putrid leucorrhea, headache in the sun and from mental labour, she gets nervous from playing on the piano, and feels great anxiety during a thunder-storm.

Phosphorus, frequent and profuse metrorrhagia, pouring out freely and then ceasing for a short time, heat in the back, chlorotic appearance, instead of menses, watery, slimy or acrid discharge, causing blisters.

Phytol, menses too frequent and too copious, mammae painful, sterility, constipation, syphilitic taint.

Rhus Tox., great soreness in vagina, preventing an embrace, the menstrual flow being profuse, protracted and of a light color, causes biting pain in the vulva.

Sepia, induration colli-uteri or vagina, painful stiffness in the uterus, pressing from above downwards, oppressing the breathing, must cross her thighs in order to get relief, pot-belliedness, yellow saddle across the bridge of the nose, feels worse while riding in a carriage. Menses scanty, aversion to coitus, sad and indifferent.

Silicea, she feels nauseated during an embrace, diarrhea or else, great costiveness before the menses, profuse menses with repeated paroxysms of icy coldness over the whole body at the time of their appearance, indurations of the mammae, most of the symptoms appear about new moon.

Tarantuta Cub., cancerous ulcer of os, indurtion of neck and fundus, chronic vaginitis with granulations.

Thuja, cauliflower excrescences. Dr. A. H. Grimmer, M.D., has listed the following remedies which are able to cope with cancer in the advanced stages.

AFFECTIONS OF THE HEAD

Anti Iod., Ant Ars., Anatherum.

Arg Met., Alum. Sil., Benzoquinone.

Bellis per., Cadm Met., Chad Chrome., Conium Mac., Calcarea flour., Hydrastis Can., Kali bi., Lapis Alba., Nat Hexametaphos, Phytol, Metastatic melanoma, Schirrhinum, Scorphularia Nod., and Symphytum, and also the *Cadmium* combinations.

CHAPTER – XVI

FEVERS

1. ORDINARY FEVERS

Leading Indications

DUE TO EXPOSURE TO DRY COLD AIR, *Aconitum Nap.*,
DUE TO EXPOSURE TO COLD GENERALLY, *Nux Vomica*.
DUE TO GETTING WET IN RAIN, OR AFTER HEAVY PERSPIRATION, *Rhus Tox*.
DUE TO OVEREATING, OR EXESSIVE USE OF COFFEE OR TOBACCO, OR HEAVY SPICED FOODS OR ALCOHOL, *Nux Vomica*.
DURING SUMMER, *Bryonia Alba*.
WITH CONSTIPATION, HEAVINESS OF HEAD AND HEADACHE, *Nux Vomica, Bryonia Alba*.
WITH THROAT SYMPTOMS AND HEADACHE, *Belladonna*.

Detailed Treatment

Aconitum Nap., fever generally brought on by *exposure to dry cold* winds, or chilling of the body after overheating, especially when warm and sweaty, *frequent chilliness*, redness of the face, great heat and often outward pressing headache, *anxiety and restlessness*, dry skin, violent thirst, full bounding pulse and sweating relieves.

Nux Vomica, generally brought on by *exposure to cold of any kind*, starting with *stopping of the nose*, great heat, the whole body burning hot, the face is especially red and hot, yet the *patient feels chilly when unconvering,* heaviness of the head, with *constipation due to overeating,* or as a result of *excessive use of coffee, tobacco, highly spiced foods or alcoholic beverages.*

Belladonna, general dry heat with chills, little or no thirst, in fact, the patient may have a dread of water, *cold extremities* and *throbbing headache.* The fever is *worse at night, eyes red and glistening,* the skin is hot and burning, the heat seems to steam out from the body, it may be followed by profuse sweat which brings no relief.

Bryonia Alba, the patient lies quiet as *any movement makes him worse,* there is *extreme pain in the whole body,* with intense headache and a sensation as if the head would burst at the temples, sharp pains over the eyes, faintness on rising up, *dry mouth* and a *tongue coated white in the middle,* there is much thirst for *large quantities of water at long* intervals, and severe constipation.

Sulphur, an excellent fever remedy coming in after *Aconite Nap.,* when the skin is dry and hot and thre is no sweat, the fever seems to burn the patient up, the tongue is dry and red, and the patient at first is sleepless and restless, but soon becomes drowsy.

2. INFLUENZA

- Feverish symptoms with *severe bone pains–Eupatorium perf.,*
- with *severe muscular pains and great prostration, Gelsemium,*
- with *severe aching pains all over the body* and *worse on motion,* and severe constipation–*Bryonia Alba.*

Detailed Treatment

Eupatorium Perf, deep seated bone pains especially in the back, wrists and ankles, eye balls sore on turning, nausea or vomiting and debility.

Gelsemium, severe bodily pain *with great general prostration,* the patient wanting to lie perfectly still, and *trembling* from weakness with the least exertion, *fever with no thirst,* and the tongue *trembles when protruding it.*

Bryonia, severe pain in the whole of the body, wanting to lie quiet, and worse on the least motion, mouth and throat *dry with great thirst,* headache and severe constipation.

Nux Vomica. "*After drinking, immediately shivering and chilliness.* Chilliness on the least movement. On the slightest exposure to the open air, shivering and chilliness for an hour, dreads to go into open air. He cannot get warm. Attack, as of fever. Shivering and drawing in the limbs."

"Serious ailments from catching cold are often removed by it"-Hahnemann.

Rhus Tox., especially useful in cases brought on by exposure to dampness, or getting wet in rain, or bathing in cold well water or river water, influenza with severe aching in all the bones, sneezing and coughing, cough worse in the evenings, there is much prostration and depression, *aching pains and nightly restlessness are important symptoms.*

Arsenicum Alb., especially when there is a copious flow from the nose, with great weakness and prostration.

Causticum, has a tired, sore, bruised sensation all over the body and soreness in the chest when coughing, with the additional symptom of involuntary urination when coughing.

After Influenza, badly recovered from, Gelsemium, a temperature of about 99°F, *not ill, not well.* If they are chilly, with sweat and chills, if they feel a weakness and heaviness of limbs and eyelids. *Gels* quickly puts them right.

China off., continued deibility, with chilliness. Anemic, worse on alternate days. Weariness of limbs with desire to stretch, move or change position.

Sulphur, partially recovers and relapses. Frequently flusheds of heat. Uneasiness in blood.

Psorinum 200, for quick convalescence.

3. MEASLES

Definition : This disease is characterized by inflammatory fever, by catarrhal symptoms, hoarseness, dry cough, sneezing, drownsines and an eruption. The eruption appears generally on the fourth day, in the shape of small, red dots, like flea-bites, which as they increase, unite together into irregular circles or horse-shoe shapes, leaving the intermediate portions of the skin, of their natural color. These red points are slightly elevated, and can readily be felt by passing the hand over the surface.

It has its period of incubation, its introductory fever, its peculiar rash, it occurs but once to the same person, and is contagious.

Causes : The causes of measles are epidemic influences and contagion. The former is by far the most active. The average period of incubation or time required to develop the disease after exposure, is from seven to twenty days.

Symptoms : As a general rule, the first symptoms complained of are lassitude, irritability, aching in the back and limbs, and shivering, which is soon followed by fever, thirst and headache, and by irritation of the mucous membrane of the eyes, nose, mouth and larynx.

The symptoms preceding an attack are those of a cold in the head, with sneezing and watering of the eyes, copious flow from the nose, soreness of the throat and a dry, hoarse, peculiar cough. This lasts generally for three days, and on the fourth day the eruption makes its appearance. The rash takes two or three days in coming out. During this period, the fever and other symptoms are at their height. When the eruption reaches the highest point of intensity, the fever gradually begins to decrease and the other symptoms also begin to disappear gradually. About the seventh or eighth day of the attack, the disease begins to subside. After the eruption passes away, the parts covered by the eruptions are covered with dry, small bran-like scales. This lasts for six or seven days, and during this period great care is necessary not to expose the patient to chill or cold.

During an epidemic, as a prophylatic, *Pulsatilla* 30 or *Morbillinum* 30 may be given once every week, or every two or three days on the first appearance of catarrhal symptoms.

LEADING INDICATIONS:

HOT, DRY SKIN AND THIRST, *Aconitum Nap.*

RASH, WEAKNESS OF THE EYES, LOOSE COUGH, *Pulsatilla.*

THROAT SYMPTOMS, *Bell.*

INFLAMMATION OF THE EYES, *Bell.*

ROUGH, HOARSE COUGH, *Hepar Sulp.*

IF ERUPTIONS LATE IN COMING, *Sulphur, Belladonna, Pulsatilla.*

GASTRIC DERANGEMENTS, *Ipec., Puls.*

Detailed Treatment

Aconitum Nap., one of the first remedies called for when the fever is violent, with hot, dry skin, heat in the head, giddiness, redness of the eyes, with dread of light, short, dry, hollow and great weakness. A few doses will be enough to control these symptoms.

Euphrasia, when the catarrhal symptoms predominate, burning tears come out of the eyes which are red and swollen, cough is dry and very harse, and there is intense throbbing headache. A wonderful medicine in measles.

Pulsatilla, comes later when the fever subsides or stops : there is coryza and profuse flowing of tears, when the eruption is slow in coming out. If it does not reduce the symptoms, *Sulphur* should be given.

Arsenicum Alb., in malignant types of black measles, or measles with tendency to bleeding, with sinking of strength, diarrhea, delirium, restlessness and debility, and the stools are prticularly offensive and exhausting.

Bryonia Alba, when the rash appears late, or runs an irregular course, and when the cough is dry and painful, and there is soreness of the limbs and body, pains or stitches in the chest.

Atriplex Portensis, rash goes in and brain symptoms appear. Stupor with stinging pains, extorting cries. Thirstless, worse from heat, hot room, hot fire. Better cool air. Urine scanty. *A great remedy for edema and effusions.*

Cuprum Met., symptoms violent. Starts from sleep, spasms, cramps, convulsion. Cramps of fingers and toes, or start there.

Helleborus Nig., when entire sensorial life is suspended and child lies in profound stupor.

Sulphur, when the skin is dusty, and the rash does not come out. Convalescence makes tardy progress, and the patient is weak and prostrate.

Belladonna, when sore throat is present and there is mental excitement, when the eruption does not appear and there is headache and great inflammation of the eyes.

Ipecac., for arresting vomiting, and also when there is oppression of the chest.

Hepar Sulph., dry or loose cough, with little or no expectoration.

Morbillinum, said to be prophylactic.

After-effects of Measles

COUGH–*Bryonia Alba, Sulphur, Causticum, Drosera.*

DIARRHEA–*Puls., Sulphur.*

INFLAMMATION OF, OR THE DISCHARGE FROM THE EARS, AND DEAFNESS–*Puls., Mercurius Sol., Hep Sulph., Sulphur.*

SKIN AFFECTIONS WITH ITCHING AND BURNING–*Sulphur, Arsenicum Alb.*

TENDERNESS OF SKIN–*Mercurius Sol.*

SWELLING OF THE GLANDS OF THE NECK–*Arnica Mont., Dulcamara, Mercurius Sol.*

4. CHICKEN–POX

Definition : Chicken-pox, or varicella, as it is technically called, is a contagious, eruptive, febrile disease characterised by more or less numerous transparent vesicles, which appear first as a small red dot and gradually change into vesicles about the size of a small pea, containing a watery, sometimes a milky fluid. It is propagated by contagion and by epidemic influences.

Symptoms : As precursory symptoms, we have chills followed by heat, hurried pulse, loss of appetite, nausea, and sometimes vomiting. After which, the eruption makes its appearance gradually. Very often, the premonitory symptoms are entirely absent and the appearance of the eruption is the first indication of the presence of the malady.

The eruption is usually accompanied by a sensation of heat and itching, which cause much uneasiness.

Treatment

Aconitum Nap., is required when fever is present.

Belladonna, when there is much headache, or congestion to the head.

Pulsatilla, if the eruptions are slow in coming, and gastric symptoms are present. The duration of the disease may be shortened by the use of this remedy.

It may also be used as a preventive, during an epidemic, and may be given once in 3 or 4 days.

If the eruption is considerable, *Antimonium Tart.* or *Mercurius Sol.* will be helpful.

Sulphur, when there is itching and burning.

5. SMALL-POX

Definition : Small-pox is an epidemic and contagious, eruptive, febrile disease, characterized by an initial fever, which upon the third or fourth day is followed by an eruption of red pimples. In the course of two or three days, these pimples are gradually changed into small vesicles, which contain a drop of transparent fluid. From the fourth to the sixth day, these are changed into pustules, for the suppuration process now commences, converting the serum or transparent fluid, contained in the vesicles, into pus or matter, after which the pustules dry up, and are converted into scabs, which fall off between the fifteenth and twentieth day.

Causes : Small-pox is a contagious and epidemic disease. The principal cause of the disease is contagion. The period of incubation after one is exposed to the disease varies from nine to twelve or fourteen days.

Symptoms : First or Febrile Stage

This commences from nine to twelve or fourteen days after exposure to the contagion. The patient first complains of pains in the bones and loins, accompanied with headache and soon followed by fever, dry, hot skin and great thirst. Nausea and vomiting often exist from the beginning of the attack, there are at the same time loss of appetite, oppression in the stomach, and constipation, more or less obstinate, tongue red and dry. The principal symptoms, during this stage of the disease, is *the pain in the loins,* which though varying much in degree, *is always severe.*

In some cases, the head symptoms are severe, consisting of restlessness and irritability, light hurts the eyes, there is swimming in the head, the mind wanders, the patient is uneasy, and there are convulsions sometimes. These symptoms continue till the eruption makes its appearance, which is usually from forty-eight to seventy-two hours.

Treatment

Aconitum Nap., is especially called for during the chill and first few hours of the fever, and when there is severe pain in the head full bounding pulse, thirst, intolerance of light, and delirium.

Belladonna may follow *Aconitum Nap.,* especially when there is severe headache and delirium, also when there is intolerance of noise.

Bryonia Alba, for the severe backache, pains in the bones, soreness of the chest, and constipation.

Antimonium Tart. 30 and *Thuja 30,* if given at this stage are said to arrest, or mitigate the eruption.

Variolinum 30, probably the most potent of all, having the complete picture of the disease from which it is prepared. Dullness of head. Severe pains in back and limbs, which become quite numb. Chills followed by high fever. Violent headache. White-coated tongue. Great thirst. Severe pains and distress in epigastric region with nausea and vomiting, mostly of greenish water. In many cases, profuse diarrhea. In some, despondency. Small-pox pustules on different parts of the body, mostly abdomen and back. Pustules perfectly formed, some umbilicated, some purulent. Given steadily, the disease will run a milder course. It changes imperfect pustules into regular ones, which soon dry up. Promotes suppuration and desiccation. Prevents pitting.

Malandrinum 30, a very effectual protection against infection with small-pox and vaccination.

Second or Eruptive Stage

If in spite of the use of *Antimonium Tart.* and *Thuja,* the further progress of the disease is not arrested, and if the eruptions are slow in appearing, and there is constipation, headache and pain in the back, *Bryonia Alba* should be given.

If during this stage, there is hoarse rattling cough, *Antimonium Tart.* or *Ipecac* should be used.

As soon as the vesicles begin to form, *Variolinum 30* is the *most important remedy* and should be given to avoid complications, and facilitate an even course of the sisease.

Third or Suppuration Stage

At this point, the eruption changes from vesicular to pustular, that is, the serous fluid in the vesicles is converted into pus. This change takes place from the fourth to the sixth day of the eruption, or about the eighth or the ninth day of the disease.

If there are no special symptoms calling for any other remedy, *Variolinum 30* may be continued during this stage, and will help towards the stage of decline of the disease.

Mercurius Sol. is called for when there is sore throat and considerable fever.

Arsenicum Alb. should be given when the skin between the pustules becomes dark, livid or brown, and the patients are very restless, anxious and the belly bloats and is very sensitive to touch and diarrhea sets in, should the pox itself become black, and typhoid symptoms set in, *Muriatic acid* should be given. For stupor during this stage, give *Opium.* For diarrhea, *China off..*

Fourth or Stage of Decline

When the disease has run its even course and this stage is reached, *Sulphur* 30, given daily for 3 or 4 days in the morning, will complete the cure.

Prophylactic : *Variolinum* 200 or *Malandrinum* 30 given *weekly,* during an epidemic, acts as a preventive of the disease.

Summary : As a prophylactic during an epidemic, give *Variolinum 200* or *Malandrinum* 30 weekly. If this is given as a precaution, the regular attack may be avoided in most cases. If, however, an attack appears in any case, it will be mild and can be managed with a few remedies and complications will rarely occur.

If it starts with fever, even after the use of *Variolinum 200, Aconitum Nap. 30, Belladonna 30* or *Bryonia Alba 30* may be given according to the symptoms and if it is followed by *Antimonium Tart. 30,* if there is nausea and vomiting, or *Thuja 30* if there are no special symptoms, further development may be arrested or mitigated. If, however, the eruptions appear, *Variolinum 30,* if continued for a few days, will reduce the trouble completely.

6. AGUE AND INTERMITTENT FEVER–MALARIA

In this class of fevers, the *accessory symptoms* and the *time of appearance of the fever,* constitute the *chief* indications for the selection of the appropriate remedy, and the succession of chill, heat and sweat, *when* the patient is thirsty, and *what* he feels between the attacks from the subsidiary symptoms which to confirm the selection. It is also important that the indicated medicine should not be given *during the height of the fever,* as it will only aggravate the symptoms, but should be given during the *decline* of the fever, or *when the fever is absent.*

FEVERS

There are three classes of patients we have to deal with in this connection, viz., (a) those who live in marshy places or malarial tracts who are always exposed to this infection, (b) those who have contracted this fever while living in those places, and continue to get periodic attacks of the fever even after removing to other places, and those who have got this fever in a chronic form, and (c) also those who have developed other troubles consequent on the continued use of quinine and other suppressive treatment.

Treatment

(*a*) FOR THOSE WHO LIVE IN MARSHY PLACES OR MALARIAL TRACTS.

As soon as the patient feels unwell, he should take a dose of *China off. 30,* if not better in twelve hours, a dose of *Ipecac 30,* after another twelve hours, another dose of *China off. 30.* If this does not prevent the fever from coming, one of the following remedies should be selected according to the symptoms.

(*b*) FOR THOSE SUBJECT TO PERIODICAL ATTACKS.

Ipecacuanha is one of the most important remedies and is useful in most cases, When no other remedy is clearly indicated, it is best to commence the treatment with this medicine. Two globules (No. 10) may be dissolved in an ounce of water, and one teaspoon may be given for a dose every three hours, *as soon as the chill commences,* and in this way it is possible to prevent the fever from developing. The same plan may be followed a few hours before the expected attack on the following or any other day.

When there is any doubt in regard to the choice of a remedy, especially at the commencement of the disease, this remedy may be given. *Ipecac is specifically indicated if large doses of quinine had been given,* or if the fever commences with an internal chill which gets worse in the warmth, little or no thirst in the cold stage, but a great deal during the hot stage, clean or slightly coated tongue, nausea and vomiting, and oppression of the chest immediately before the attack, or during the cold and hot stages.

If *Ipecac.* does not always help altogether, it alters the character of the fever, so that other remedies are indicated.

Nux Vomica, very frequently after *Ipecac,* more particularly if, at the onset of the paroxysm, the extremities feel as if paralysed and *chill and heat are mingled,* one being felt externally, the other internally, *with dread of being uncovered in the least even during the hot and sweating stages,* external warmth affords no relief, giddiness with a feeling as if drunk, cramps in the muscles of the abdomen or calves of the legs, stitches in the sides, heat and pain in the head, buzzing in the ears, thirst and anxiety during the hot stage, constipation.

Arsenicum Alb. is always useful in all cases suppressed by large quantities of quinine.

Time of fever– 1 to 2 p.m., or 12 to 2 a.m.

In this remedy, the different stages are not distinctly marked, but the chilliness, heat and sweat occur simultaneously, or when there are frequent changes from chilliness to heat, and *vice versa,* or internal chilliness with external heat, also when the paroxysm is imperfectly developed, when there is little or no sweating, or at least not for some time after the heat has subsided, great prostration of strength, burning pains in the stomach, insupportable pains in the limbs, or all over the body, *anxiety and restlessness, excessive thirst, drinking often but little at a time,* uneasiness about the heart, or oppression and spasms of the chest, *nausea* or *sickness and vomiting,* bitter taste in the mouth, violent headache, continuing after the hot stage, buzzing in the ears during the sweating. *All the sufferings* of the patient, as, the headache, pain in the limbs, etc., *are increased during the attack.*

It anitdotes the effects of quinine, and if it is given in the *30th* potency at weekly intervals for a few doses, and then in the *200th* potency, fortnightly or at longer intervals, effects a radical cure of the complaint in several cases.

China off., the paroxysm *begins generally towards midday, with intense thirst* long before the chill, but *no thirst* as *chill increases or during heat,* and thirst begins after the fever subsides, and *increases when the sweat begins, exhausting sweat,* after the fever subsides, *exhausting night sweats* followed by ringing of the ears, with sensitiveness in the regions of the liver and spleen, scanty urine, loss of appetite, and bloated abdomen are present as the after-effects of the fever.

The important difference between *Arsenicum Alb.* and *China off.* is that all the three stages, viz., chill, heat and sweat are present in the latter, while the chill and heat stages only are present in *Arsenicum Alb.* In the case of *China,* the *fever never comes at night,* and the symptoms of thirst are guiding.

Natrium Muriaticum, is one of the best remedies in intermittent fever, is useful in all cases badly treated with preparations of quinine and *Arsenicum Alb.*, and should be used in the *30th* potency in ordinary, and *200th* potency in chronic cases. The chill is hard and severe, and *begins between* 10 and 11 *a.m.* *with great thirst, which continues through all the stages,* but is *more during the heat stage, headache is present from the beginning,* but becomes *most violent during the heat stage,* the sweat is profuse and sour and gradually relieves all pains except headache, drink refreshes the thirst, *chaps* and *fissures on the lips,* particularly at the corners of the mouth, are *characteristic.*

Its effects last for some days and so the *medicine should not be repeated too soon,* and is better given at long intervals.

Apis Mell., 3 p.m. fever. Chill begins with thirst and is *worse in warm room, and external heat,* chilliness with heat of hands and feet, no thirst with heat or sweat, burning oppression, smothering sensation in the chest with chill and heat, sweat with urticaria.

Apis Mell., is useful in acute or chronic cases of malaria, occurring as the sequelae of eruptive disease, such as measles, urticaria or nettle rash. In old cases, badly treated with quinine, *Natrium Mur.* follows well, if *Apis Mell.* does not cure.

Arnica Mont., is indicated in cases maltreated with quinine or patent ague cures, and in acute cases when the fever relapses every four or five days. The following symptoms should be present– Frequent suppression of urine, thirst, drawing pains in the bones before the chill, chill begins with thirst, bruised, sore feeling, great weakness, and so must lie down, but the bed feels hard and the frequent change of position necessary, during the heat, motion or slightest uncovering makes the patient chilly, *heat intolerable*, sweat is sour and offensive. *Arnica Mont.* will remove the bad effects of quinine and in chronic cases, should be followed by *Arsenicum Alb.* or *Natrium Mur.* according to indications.

Sulphur, if the indications for any remedy are not clear, *Sulphur* will clear up the case for another suitable remedy, or will complete the cure. It will also prevent the tendency to relapse. it is also useful after the suppression of eruptions on the skin in eruptive fevers, and after the abuse of quinine.

Sulphur, worn next to the skin in the form of flowers of sulphur is an effective antidote to the malarial poison.

Veratum Alb., when there is *external coldness with internal heat*, cold clammy sweat, particularly on the forehead, and general coldness of the whole body or chilliness without heat, or chilliness and heat by turns, giddiness, constipation of the bowels, or diarrhea, sometimes nausea, or vomiting, and pains in the back and loins.

Mercurius Sol., in quickly *alternating chills and heat*, with restlessness, thirst, palpitation of the heart, *profuse, offensive, sour perspiration*.

Belladonna, has been found useful when two or more attacks occur in the twenty-four hours, the cold stage slight, and the hot stage violent, or the reverse, violent chill and slight heat, *great sensitiveness,* and inclination to shed tears, constipation, or loose and scanty chalk-like stools, sometimes attended with *violent congestion to the head, a red face, severe pain in the head, and dullness or stupor.*

Pulsatilla, particularly when the slightest disorder of the stomach brings on a relpase. It is particularly indicated by absence of thirst during the entire fit, or thirst only during the hot stage, *heat and chillness* at the same time, bitter taste in the mouth, bitter or sour vomiting of phlegm or bile, the *attacks come on in the afternoon or evening,* and the patient complains of chilliness all the time.

Rhus Tox., the attacks usually come on in the later part of the day, and consist of *heat, preceded and followed by chills, coldness of some parts of the body, and heat of others,* perspiration after midnight, or towards morning, *the heat accompanied by a rash,* pain in the bowels and diarrhea, pressure at the pit of the stomach, palpitation of the heart, and anxiety.

Carbo Vegetablis, when the attack is preceded or attended by pains in the teeth and limbs, *thirst, only in the cold stage,* with vertigo, redness of the face, and sick stomach during the hot stage.

Calcarea Carb., when there are alternate chills and heat, external coldness and internal heat, heat in the head and face with coldness of the limbs, sometimes cold up to the abdomen, giddiness, feeling of heaviness in the head and limbs, violent pains in the small of the back and anxiety. (Compare *Sulphur* and *Veratum Alb.*).

Antimonium Crudum, is indicated when the tongue is very much coated, bitter and nauseous taste, belching, sickness of the stomach, vomiting, little or no thirst, and constipation or diarrhea (See *Pulsatilla).*

Bryonia Alba, for symptoms similar to *Antimonium Crudum,* but attended with much thirst, or the *heat before the chills,* red cheeks in the cold stage, yawning, and stitches in the side during the heat, more *coldness and chills than heat,* and constipation or diarrhea.

(*c*) FOR THOSE WHO HAVE CONTRACTED OTHER TROUBLES DUE TO THE ABUSE OF QUININE.

Next to opium and mercury which are largely used in the preparation of allopathic medicines, quinine is the main remedy used in different forms for all fevers. It leaves very serious effects on the constitution and causes incurable diseases. It is more difficult to expel quinine from the system than mercury, and any amount of purgatives will not remove the effects which remain in the blood and all the fluids in the body.

Homeopathic remedies by their deep and powerful action are capable of removing these ill-effects, if they are tried persistently and given continuously and with patience for a long time.

The following remedies are indicated for the several complaints which are the after-effects of the abuse of quinine in its several forms :

(*i*)   For *Rheumatic pains,* heaviness, prostration, soreness in all the limbs, drawing pain in the bones, great sensitiveness of every part of the body, when exercise, speaking or blowing the nose or loud sounds aggravate the pains– *Arnica Mont.*

(*ii*)   When the body is cold, with cold perspiration, constipation or diarrhea– *Veratrum alb.*

(*iii*)   For Jaundice– *Mercurius Sol. and then Belladonna.*

(*iv*)   For het in the face, rush of blood to the head, much pain in the head, face and teeth–*Belladonna.*

(*v*)   For earache–*Pulsatilla.*

FEVERS

(vi) For ulcers of the legs, dropsy, short cough and shortness of breath–*Arsenicum Alb.*

(vii) For dropsy and other swellings–*Rhus Tox.*

(viii) If after suppression of fever, earache, toothache, headache and pains in the limbs appear–*Pulsatilla* and then *Calcarea Carb.*

(ix) For affections of the stomach– *Ipecac., Pulsatilla, Nux Vomica, Sulphur, Calcarea Carb., Carbo Vegetablis, Arsenicum Alb., China, Antimonium Crud., Bryonia Alba.*

(x) If the fever continues in spite of the use of quinine– first *Ipecac,* and then according to indications, *Arsenicum Alb.* or *Carbo Veg.,* also *Arnica mont.* or *Veratrum Alb., Belladonna, Mercurius, Sulphur* or *Calcarea Carb.*

7. TYPHOID FEVER

Many cases begin with the following symptoms, great weakness, pains in the head, back and the limbs, worse on moving, white coated tongue, dry, parched lips and mouth, with or without thirst for water in large quantities at a time, loss of appetite, empty belching and constipation, the patient does not want to move as he feels worse by doing so, the patient gets sick and faint when rising up from lying position. When these symptoms are present, two globules of *Bryonia Alba 30* may be dissolved in two oz. of water, and given as 4 doses once in 2 or 3 hours, and no more medicine need be given for 24 hours. If there is relief at the end of this period, no other medicine will be necessary. If there is no relief, further medicine will be necessary according to symptoms. If there is *extreme muscular and nervous prostration with general trembling,* i.e., if the patient attempts to walk, the legs tremble, or the hands tremble when he tries to lift them, or the tongue trembles when he protrudes it, with inclination to drowsiness, or he sleeps frequently with incoherent muttering, head feels heavy with giddiness and dimness of vision, tongue slightly coated, speech indistinct, little or no thirst, no constipation or diarrhea, *Gelsemium 30* may be given. *Drooping of the eyelids is very characteristic indicating the general prostration.*

If there is *great prostration and soreness as if bruised* in whatever position the patient lies, *the parts rested upon feel sore and bruised,* stupor, face flushed, dusky, dark red, with a *stupid, drunken expression, tongue coated with a streak down the middle,* at first white but soon turns brown with red edges, sometimes tongue is large and flabby with a red dry tip, nervous, and cannot go to sleep, *Baptisia 30* may be given.

These three remedies are ordinarily enough in the early stages of typhoid, either to abort it or prevent its getting complicated. The following further points of difference between the three remedies may be noted in order that the appropriate remedy may be selected in the beginning. *Muscular soreness and prostration,* present in all three remedies, *soreness most prominently, under 'Baptisia Tinct.', prostration most, under 'Gelsemuium', drowsiness with red face, Gelsemium* and *Baptisia Tinct.* with *Baptisia Tinct.* the mind being more clouded.

Gelsemium and *Bryonia Alba* want to be still, the former on account of *much weakness,* and the latter on account of *much* pain. *Bryonia Alba is constipated, Baptisia tinct.* is diarrhoeic, *Gelsemium,* neither. Tongue of *Bryonia is white, with parched lips and thirst.* Tongue of *Gelsemium is thinly coated or not at all,* and *trembles when protruded,* and *there is no thirst.* Tongue of *Baptisia Tinct.* turns dark with a streak through the middle. Urine of *Bryonia Alba* is scanty and high colored, that of *Gelsemium* may be profuse and of *Baptisia Tinct,* scanty, dark and offensive.

In typhoid, *Baptisia Tinct.* vies with *Pryogen* and *Arnica Mont.*

Frequently, the disease is cut short in the beginning by homeopthic medicines. If the indicated remedy is given right from

FEVERS

the beginning and continued till there is a change, all complications can be avoided and the disease will run an even course towards a cure. *Bryonia Alba,* more than either of *Gelsemium* or *Baptisia Tinct.,* is liable to be the *remedy* all through the case. As long as the white or yellowish tongue, parched lips and thirst. Constipation, pain in the head and delirium in mild form, *about the business of the day and dread of motion* continues, *Bryonia Alba must be continued.* For those who had been injected with anti-typhoid serum, it is better to commence the treatment with *Baptisia Tinct 30* to antidote its effect.

Attention to the food, giving mainly a milk diet from the beginning, *and no solid's whatever,* is of the utmost importance. Good nursing and proper feeding are indispensable agents in its treatment, and more so than in any other disease.

The following remedies may also be required in some causes.

Rhus Tox., if diarrhea supervenes, the tongue becomes dry as a board and especially is *red at the tip in the shape of a triangle,* pointing backward, again if the delirium and stupor increase, with low form of muttering much of the time, and the patient *cannot lie still* but must *toss and change position* every little while, as if temporarily relieved of suffering by so doing, *Bryonia Alba* is not suitable, but *Rhus Tox.* must be given and follows well.

Pyrogen, bed feels hard *(Bapt Tinct.)* Great restlessness, must constantly move *(Rhus tox.),* to relieve soreness of parts *(Arn.),* tongue (typically) clean, smooth, fiery-red, or dry and cracked.

Horribly offensive diarrhea *(Bapt Tinct.)* Pulse quick, or out of proportion to temperature.

Phosphoric acid, the ptient lies on his back very still, with a *stupid, indifferent* or *apathetic condition,* does not want to talk and answers slowly, there is also diarrhea, actual or threatened, with *excessive meteorisitic distension of the abdomen,* with great rumbling and noise as from water, if there is diarrhea, it is painless, yellow, watery, or very *light coloured,* even white.

Arnica Mont, has an apathetic condition, or indifference, similar to *Phosphoric acid,* but the *Arnica Mont depression is more profound,* as is also that of *Baptisia,* for they both *go to sleep in the midst of answering a question,* but are similar only as regards the stupor.

Lachesis, is one of our best remedies in typhoid, muttering stupor, even almost complete insensibility, sleeps with mouth open, *dry, red* or *black tongue,* which on attemtping to protrude, *trembles and catches on the lower teeth* (thus indicating great weakness), stools *very offensive,* whether formed or not and if there is hemorrhage, it is of dark decomposed blood, with sometimes an appearance of flakes of *charred straw* in it, the throat seems full, with loud breathing, and the patient, though stupid, is very restless, seems to feel suffocated and *does not like to have anything about the throat or chest,* throws off the covers therefrom, but, unlike other remedies, *if he does get any real sleep all his sufferings are greatly aggravated-the more he sleeps the worse he feels.* The 200th potency is more useful in such cases.

If the case grows from bad to worse, then the following remedies will be required.

Arsenicum Alb., when the powers of life seem to be greatly exhausted, great *restlessness* and anxiety, which is manifested by constantly moving head and limbs, while the trunk lies still on account of too great weakness, tongue either red, dry, cracked or balck and stiff. *Excessive thrist* for little water at a time, burning in stomach or bowels, or both, meteoristic distension of the abdomen, diarrhea, watery, bownish, or bloody and *offensive, also worse at midnight, especially about one o'clock.*

After *Arsenicum Alb.* has done all it can, then if the case is still sorse, *Carbo Vegetablis* and *Muriatic acid* can help.

Carbo Vegetablis, it is the stage of collapse, dissolution of the blood, and paralytic conditions, there is almost total obliviousness to everything, the face if *deathly pale,* sunken, hippocratic, cold, there may be hemorrhages from the nose, mouth or anus, one or all at a time, and always with that *deathly paleness,* abdomen meteoristic, with rumbling and gurgling of wind, diarrhea of cadaverous smell and often involuntary, rattling breathing in bronchi, filled with mucus,the circulation becomes so weak that the blood *stagnates in the capillaries,* with cyanotic blueness of face, lips and tongue, the nose and breath grow cold, as do also the *extremities* which are covered with cold sweat, and under the extremely weak heart action, the breathing becomes so difficult htat the patient craves for fresh air and desires to be fanned. In this condition, *Carbo Vegetablis* will help the patient wonderfully and may save his life. *If Carbo Vegetablis* helps to some extent, and the case required further help, *China off.* is the best remedy and will do the rest to save the patient.

Muriatic acid is another remedy, which vies with *Carbo Vegetablis* in such extreme cases, with the following sysmptoms-half open eyes, face *dark red and bloated, stertorous breathing,* involuntary stools and retained urine. This stage may alternate with wild delirium, with loud talking, laughing or singing and attempt to escape, but the leading indications are those relating to the *stupid state.*

8. RHEUMATIC FEVERS–ACUTE RHEUMATISM

This fever very often sets in with heaviness and weariness in the limbs, vertigo and a violent headache, which sometimes exhausts the patient a good deal, and very often a dry cough and congestion of the lungs supervene, attended with dryness of the mucous membrane of the nose and eyes, which are sometimes very painful.

These fevers occur most frequently during wet or rainy weather, and sometimes during the prevalence of influenza.

Aconitum Nap., if there is high fever, dry, hot skin, thirst and redness of the cheeks, violent, shooting or tearing pains, worse at night, redness, or shining swelling of the part affected, the pains are aggravated by the touch, extreme irritability of temper, disposition to uncover the parts, and relief from doing so.

Belladonna, when the pains are chiefly in the joints, shooting or burning, worse at night and on movement, excessive swelling, and shining redness of the affected parts, fever with redness of the face, hot, moist skin and thirst.

Arnica Mont., when the joints feel as if bruised or sprained hard, red and shining swelling, sensation as if the limbs were resting on some hard substance, feeling as if lame, and swelling in the affected part of the pains are aggravated by the motion, great fear of persons approaching, because they might touch the affected part.

Bryonia Alba, if there are shooting tearing or tensive pains, shifting *pains which affect the muscles rather than the bones* red and shining swelling and rigidity of the parts affected, *the pains are worse at night, and on the least movement,* profuse perspiration or coldness and shivering, much heat, with headache and derangement of the stomach, peevish or passionate temper.

Chamomilla, when there are drawing or tearing pains, with a sensations of numbness or lameness in the parts affected, the pains are aggravated at night, fever with burning, partial heat preceded by chilliness, hot perspiration, desire to remain lying down, great agitation and tossing about.

Mercurius Sol., for *shooting*, tearing, or *burning* pains, which are *aggravated at night*, especially towards morning, and *in the warm bed*, or by exposure to damp, or cold air, puffy swelling of the affected parts, the *pains seem to be seated in the bones or joints,* profuse perspirtion without relief.

Lachesis, may follow, if *Mercurius Sol.* is not sufficient.

FEVERS

Rhus Tox., for *tearing, burning* or *wrenching* pains, with a sensation of weakness and crawling in the affected limb, red and shining swelling of the joints, with rigidity and shootings, when touched, the *pains are worse during rest, and in cold or damp weather. Rhus Tox. is* often suitable after *Aconite Nap., Arnica Mont.* or *Bryonia.*

Pulsatilla is serviceable when the pains are *aggravated in the evening or at night in bed, or in a warm room,* or on changing the position, *pains which pass quickly from on joint to another, sensation of numbness in the parts affected,* the pains are *relieved by cool air,* for patients with a pale face and disposed to shiver and be chilly.

China off., for pains which are *aggravated by the slightest touch, profuse perspiration, great debility,* especially *from weakening causes, as loss of blood or other fluids.*

Hepar Sulph. and Lachesis, are frequently useful, when other remedies though indicated fail to give much relief.

Administration of the Remedies : It is always best to commence the treatment with *Aconite Nap. 30* in watery solution in teaspoon doses (two globules in one ounce of water every three or four hours and if it is not sufficient to give relief, it paves the way for *Bryonia Alb.* 30, *Rhus Tox.* 30 or *China off.* 30, which are generally useful at this stage, or other remedies indicated according to the symptoms. If the disease becomes protracted, it is better to administer the remedies dry on the tongue, *two globules No.* 10 and allow each remedy to act for at least 48 hours before making a change.

9. GASTRIC AND BILIOUS FEVER

The following are the leading indications for the different remedies:

IF THERE IS MUCH FEBRILE HEAT–*Aconitum Nap.*

IF THERE IS MUCH VERTIGO–*Nux Vom., Bryonia Alba, Bell.*

FOR VIOLENT HEADACHE–*Bryonia Alba, Nux Vom.*

SEVERE PAINS IN THE STOMACH–*Bryonia Alba, Arsenicum Alb., Nux Vom.*

CONSTIPATION, TORPID STOOL–*Bryonia Alba, Nux Vom., Arsenicum Alb.*

DIARRHEA OR MORE FREQUENT STOOLS–*Puls., Chamomilla, Mercurius Sol., Arsenicum Alb.*

COLICKY PAINS–*Chamomilla, Mercurius Sol.*

SLEEPLESSNESS OR BAD SLEEP–*Bell., Nux Vom., Chamomilla, Arsenicum Alb.*

CHILLINESS–*Puls., Nux Vom., Mercurius Sol., Bryonia Alba.*

BURNING DRY HEAT–*Aconitum Nap., Bryonia Alba, Camomilla.*

ABSENCE OF THIRST–*Puls.*

INTENSE THIRST–*Aconitum Nap., Arsenicum Alb., Chamomilla.*

IF THE FEVER IS CAUSED BY EXCITEMENT–*Chamomilla, Bryonia Alba.*

10. FILARIAL FEVER-FILARIASIS

For this fever with the attendant symptoms, chill, glandular swellings, painful swelling on the calves of the legs, high fever, *Mercurius Sulphuricus* acts as a sepcific. For the acute symptoms, this remedy may be given in the *30th* potency in watery solution every three or four hours.

After the fever subsides, *Mercurius Sulphuricus 30* may be given in single doses dry on the tongue, once in four days, for 2 or 3 doses and then at weekly intervals.

It may then be given in the *two 200th potency,* at fortnightly intervals, to prevent a recurrence of the trouble.

In chronic cases, when the fever recurs periodically, it may be given in the *200th potency* fortnightly. For chronic swellings of the legs which remain after the fever, the remedy should be given in 1 *M and higher potencies* at long intervals.

As this is a troublesome complaint, prolonged treatment with the very high potencies is necessary for a cure which is possible in recent cases.

CHAPTER XVII

DISEASES OF WOMEN

1. DELAYED AND OBSTRUCTED MENSTRUATION

Definition : When the menses do not appear at the period of life, at which they may be naturally expected, we call it *delayed* or *retained* menstruation. This delay may be owing to a disordered condition of the general system, or to functional inactivity, or weakness of the uterine organs themselves. By *obstructed* menstruation is meant an actual impediment to the flow. In such cases, there is periodically an evident effort on the part of Nature to produce the change, the patient having all the premonitory signs-the pains, aches, etc., the ovaries and womb perform their part, but still the flow does not appear, there is an obstruction, either at the mouth of the womb or somewhere within the vagina. This obstruction may be congenital-that is having existed from birth, or it may be the result of some former disease,-inflammation, perhaps of the parts.

Causes : Among the causes of delayed menstruation, have been mentioned above, an imperfect or late development of the uterine organs, functional inactivity, weakness or disorder of the uterus or ovaries, or an entire absence of these two organs. Perhaps, in the majority of cases, the direct or immediate cause lies in some peculiar condition of the ovaries. It is most frequently met with in those who lead indolent and sedentary lives, who indulge in luxurious and gross diets and who have been accustomed to hot rooms, soft beds and much sleep. It may also be due to over-texation of the mental faculties, want of exercise in the open air, badly lighted,

DISEASES OF WOMEN

cold and damp dwellings, and sudden and extreme atmospheric changes. The disease is not unfrequently a mere symptomatic or sympathetic condition, dependent upon some disease existing in a distant part or organ of the body.

The cause of *obstructed* menstruation are also an imperfect formation, or development of the parts.

Pulsatilla, is the first remedy for menstrual suppression and is indicated when the menses flow by fits and starts, or when it is due to sweating and coldness of the feet, also in delayed first menses in girls, in patients who are disinclined to exertion, with poor appetite, long for acids and are apt to faint easily and suffer from anxiety. If no improvement follows after a week or ten days, give *Sulphur.*

Calcarea Carbonica, when the first menses are delayed and there is apt to be congestion to the head or chest, giving rise to lung troubles, in fleshy scrofulous girls with fair complexion, perspiring easily on the head and subject to acidity of the stomach. Palpitation of the heart, short breath, worse ascending, cold damp feet.

Sepia, in delay of first menses and there is leucorrhea instead.

Bryonia Alba, has nose bleed instead of menses, frequently accompanied with bursting headache. Palpitation of the heart and constipation. *Lycopodium* is suitable for similar symptoms.

Phosphorus, in women of a delicate constitution, with slight form, weak chest, of lively disposition, and predisposed to lung diseases, when, in place of menstruation, expectoration of blood in small quantities occurs, with hacking cough and pains in the chest.

Arsenicum Alb., is applicable to cases attended with great weakness, also in swelling of the face, especially around the eyes, with paleness of the complexion, more in the morning, swelling of the feet and ankles in the evening and a feeling of heat or burning in the veins.

Sulphur after *Pulsatilla,* when the latter has been insufficient, and also after any of the above remedies, especially if the patient complains of heat in the head, giddiness, palpitation of the heart, and shortness of breath, particularly on going upstairs, loss of appetite, sickness at the stomach after eating, emaciation, and depression of mind.

Administration of Remedies : Give one of the remedies, according to the indications, a dose in the 30th potency, every morning for a week, if the symptoms abate, wait for one week without medicine, and afterwards give one dose of *Sulphur 30 for three days in the mornings,* and if there is no improvement after waiting for a week, select some other remedy.

2. SUPPRESSION OF THE MENSES

Definition : By suppression of the menses is understood a disappearance of the same, after having been regularly established for a longer or shorter period, independent of pregnancy, or old age.

Causes : Among the causes of acute suppression, may be cold caught during the flow, by exposure to damp night air, by wet feet, etc., by fear, bodily shocks, or by sudden violent mental emotions, either just previous to, or during the menstrual discharge. Fevers, inflammations or almost any acute disease, occurring before the period, will have the same effect.

Chronic suppression is commonly a consequence of the acute, or it may arise from the gradual supervention of delicate heath, or from disease of the ovaries or womb.

Treatment : When the suppression of the menses is caused by the presence of some other disease in the system, the cure of such disease must first be effected by appropriate treatment, before we can expect the return of the flow. If, however, the suppresssion

DISEASES OF WOMEN

is sudden-the result of cold, or fright, or other morbific cause, we should try to remove this trouble by suitable medicines.

Aconitum Nap., when a sudden suppression of the menses is occasioned by fright, and especially, if there is a congestion of blood to the head and chest, with redness of the face, pains in the head, giddiness, nausea, and faintness. When the suppression is due to fright, this remedy should be administered *immediately,* and if there is no speedy relief, or if the relief is only partial or temporary, it may be followed with benefit by *Opium* or *Veratrum.*

Bryonia Alba, is most suitable for unmarried women, when the suppression is followed by a sensation of swimming in the head, with heaviness and pressure towards the forehead, *aggravated* by *stooping* and by *motion,* pains in the chest, dry cough, bleeding of the nose, bitter or sour eructations, pain in the pit of the stomach after eating, rising of food, pains in the small of the back, and also pains of a drawing character in the lower part of the abdomen, constiption.

Belladonna, will be serviceable after *Aconitum Nap.,* in plethoric subjects, when there is congestion to the head, bleeding of the nose, and for most of the symptoms mentioned under *Aconitum Nap.,* when that remedy is insufficient.

Pulsatilla, is the chief remedy in this affection, and will give relief in the majority of cases, *especially* when the *suppression* is the *result of the effects of cold* or a *chill* by exposure to dampness, and the patient suffers from headache, chiefly confined to one side, with shooting pains extending to the face, ears and teeth, palpitation of the heart, feeling of suffocation, flushes of heat, nausea or vomiting, disposition to *diarrhea,* pressure in the lower part of the abdomen, frequent desire to pass urine, and *whites.* It is best adapted to those of a *mild, easy disposition,* with inclination to *melancholy and tears.*

Veratrum Alb., for nervous headache, *hysterical affection*, frequent nausea and vomiting, pale, earthy colour of the face, *coldness of the hands and feet,* or *nose, great weakness,* with *fainting fits.*

Sulphur, for pressing headache, chiefly in the back part of the head, extending to the nape of the neck, or one-sided headache, or pain over the eyes, with heat and throbbing in the hand, heaviness of the head, confusion of the head, giddiness, dimness of vision, bluish circles round the eyes, pimples on the forehead and around the mouth, and red spots on the cheeks, voracious appetite, sour stomach, sour and burning eructations, fullness and heaviness in the stomach and abdomen, constipation, with ineffectual efforts to evacuate, disposition to piles, sometimes loose, slimy stools, cramps in the abdomen, whites, numbness of the limbs, great disposition to take cold, difficulty of breathing, pain in the loins, great depression after talking, fatigue and weakness of the limbs, irritability of temper or disposition to melancholy and tears.

In *chronic* or long standing cases, especially occurring in debiliated persons, *China off., Causticum, Natrium Mur., Graphites* and *Arsenicum Alb.* will be useful.

3. MENORRHAGIA–PROFUSE MENSTRUATION

Too frequent and of too long duration.

Definition : By the term *Menorrhagia* is meant an immoderate flow of the menses.

Causes : Some women are hereditarily pre-disposed to uterine hemorrhages, with a weak condition, or a relaxed or flabby state of the uterus, or the same condition may be induced by the frequent child-bearing, by abortions, by prolonged or too frequent suckling, by rich living, indolence, hot rooms, and soft beds.

Among the exciting cuases are over-exertion, lifting heavy weights, running up and down the stairs, local injuries, falls, the use

DISEASES OF WOMEN

of drastic medicines, irritating purgatives, exposure to cold, and mental excitement and moral emotions.

Symptoms : The discharge is excessive, or continues longer than usual and is attended by pains in the back, loins and abdomen, which resemble those of labour, the patient is also troubled with leucorrhea or whites.

Treatment : Rest in the horizontal position is in most cases imperative. If the flow is *excessive,* clothes wrung out of *vinegar* (or lemon juice) and water may be applied to the lower bowels.

Crocus Sat is a *most important* remedy, especially in cases where the menses have returned too soon and the discharge, which is copius, consists of *dark-coloured clots.*

Ipecac., for too great a flow, and also for *flooding after labour,* especially when there is a profuse discharge of *bright red blood,* may be allowed by *Sabina.*

Belladonna, when the menses return too soon, are accompanied with bearing down pains, and pressing outward, also severe headache, with flushed face and cold extremities.

Chamomilla, when with the symptoms calling for *Corcus Sat.,* there are also griping pains through the abdomen, severe colic, or pains like those of labour, extending from the back forwards towards the abdomen, great thirst, and paleness of the face.

Platina, in cases where the discharge is too great, and consists chiefly of *dark-colored blood* and is attended with bearing-down pains, sexual and general excitability.

Nux Vomica, when the menstruation is too copious, and returns before the usual time, when it continues too long, or stops and returns again. It is *particularly adapted* to women who made *too free use of coffee,* wine or *other stimulants,* all of which should be strictly prohibited for several months.

Ignatia, is most serviceable in cases in which the discharge continues too long, and is frequently attended by *yawning* and *hysterical symptoms.*

China off., in cases of great debility in consequence of too copious or too long continued menstrual discharge. It *should be given after other remedies have controlled* the discharge, and the patient *suffers from the weakness only.*

Sabina, menstruation too profuse, too early, flow by spells, with colic and labour-like pains, pain from back to front, *flow increased by motion.*

Sulphur, given during the intervals, two or three times, allowing a week between the doses, will often be beneficial when other remedies have failed.

Calcarea Carb., administered in the same manner will also be useful. It is especially adapted to persons of relaxed muscular fibre, to weak or scrofulous subjects.

4. DYSMENORRHEA (Painful Menstruation)

Menstrual Colic

Definition and Causes : The term *Dysmenorrhea* signifies a difficult monthly flow. The menstrual discharge is preceded by severe pains through the loins and in the lower part of the abdomen. These pains are sometimes so intense as to be almost insupportable, compelling the patient to go to bed, forcing from her tears and groans, as she writhes under the agonising pain. The pain is in the nerves of the womb, and perhaps may be fairly attributed to the compression which they receive from the congested state of the organ which exists during the period of menstruation. The pains may also be neuralgic or rheumatic in their character.

The most common exciting causes are exposure to cold, sudden fright, or shocks or violent mental emotions. Indeed, any

DISEASES OF WOMEN

cause which would excite inflammation, or produce a suppression of the menses, would be sufficient to cause dysmenorrhea.

The *neuralgic* variety of dysmenorrhea occurs chiefly in unmarried females, and in the married who have not borne children. It is most confined to women of irritable, hysterical and nervous temperament. The *inflammatory variety* of the disease most freqeuntly attacks those of a full habit and of a sanguine temperament, married or unmarried, whether they have borne children or not.

Symptoms : The pain commences usually in the region of the sacrum–the lower portion of the backbone–and extends round and through the lower part of the bowels, and down the thighs. The amount of suffering varies, but it is some times very severe, the forcing or bearing-down sensation, which is often present, is frequently so great, that it seems as though the whole contents of the pelvis would be forced out. In some instances, the torture is so extreme, that the patient cannot lie still, but constantly keeps rolling about, lies or presses upon the abdomen, endeavouring to get ease from her sufferings. Nausea, sickness at the stomach, and severe retching are not uncommon.

As a general rule, the discharge appears slowly, and is at first scanty, or it may appear in slight gushes.

Belladonna, where there is severe pain in the back, and strong bearing-down in the lower part of the abdomen, as if the parts would fall out, accompanied with violent congestion of blood to the head, confusion of slight, frightful visions, screaming, redness and bloated appearance of the face and frequent, ineffectual efforts to stool with much straining.

Chamomilla, for pains resemblilng labour pains, commencing in the small of the back, and extending around to the front and lower part of the abdomen, menses premature and too profuse, attended with violent abdominal cramps, great sensitiveness of the abdomen, discharges of dark, coagulated clots.

Coffea, when there is great nervous excitement, wringing of the hands, grinding the teeth, screaming, great restlessness, twisting of the whole body, distressing colic, fulness and pressure in the abdomen, as if it would burst, coldness of the body numbness and stiffness. May be given in alternation with *Pulsatilla,* or may be followed by *Cocculus.*

Pulsatilla, for abdominal spasms with discharge of dark clots, or of pale blood, weight in the bowels, as from a stone, pressing pain in the abdomen and the small of the back, pains in the sides, nausea and vomiting, frequent inclination to pass water, and ineffectual efforts to evacuate the bowels, the flow will be fitful, and more severe the pains are, the more chilly the patient will get, the pains change from place to place.

It is more useful when given *between* the periods.

Cocculus Ind., a most useful remedy in dysmenorrhea, and scanty, irregular menstruation. Uterine cramps. Profuse discharge of clotted blood and severe headache accompanied by nausea, a heaving up and down of the stomach as in sea-sickness. It also has a dark flow. It has a pain as if sharp stones were rubbed against each other in the abdomen, and distension of the abdomen from accumulation of flatus, the pains are worse at night, awakes the patient and make her irritable.

Nux Vomica is most useful in relieving writhing pains in the abdomen, accompanied by nausea, or pains in the back and loins, as if dislocated, feeling as if bruised of the bones of the pubis, spasms and pricking in the lower part of the abdomen, paroxysms of pressing and drawing pains, frequent desire to make water and sensation in the bowels as if they would burst.

Veratrum Alb., for menstrual colic, with nervous headache, nausea and vomiting, coldness of the hands, feet or nose, great weakness, fainting fits and diarrhea.

Platina, leucorrhea before and after the menses. The menses

DISEASES OF WOMEN

are too frequent, too profuse, last too long, and are accompanied by cramp, colic and forcing pain.

Sulphur, abdominal cramps and colic during the menses. The menses are preceded by headache.

Cimicifuga, it is especially useful in *rheumatic* and *neuralgic* cases, and in congestive cases it may be considered along with *Belladonna.* The characteristic indication in dysmenorrhea is *pain flying across the pelvic region from one side to the other.* Headache preceding menses, during menses, sharp pains across abdomen, has to double up, labour-like pains, and during menstrual interval, *debility* and perhaps a scanty flow. The pains of *Cimicifuga* are *not so severe and intense,* nor felt with such acuteness, as are those of *Chamomilla.*

Caulophyllum, the dysmenorrhea of the remedy is *spasmodic* in charcter, the pains are bearing down in character. The spasmodic, intermittent pains are in the groins, broad ligaments or even chest and limbs. It produces a continued spasm of the uterus, similar to the first stage of labour, the flow is mostly normal in quantity. Hysterical convulsions with dysmenorrhea, pains shoot to various parts of the body. It is a useful remedy to be given *between* the periods.

Magnesia Phosphorica, the pains calling for it are *neuralgic* and *crampy,* preceding the flow, *relief from warmth and aggravation from motion* are characteristic.

The remedies to be made use of, *between the periods,* are *Sulphur, Pulsatilla, Nux Vomica* and *Caulophyllum.* One dose in the 30th potency every *fourth* evening, or later in the 200th potency *fortnightly.*

5. TARDY AND SCANTY MENSTRUATION

Definition : After menstruation has once become established, it may show itself less frequently than at the regular periods, that is, instead of returning once in 28 days, it may be delayed to five, six or more weeks. And besides, the discharge, when it does appear, is not free, and does not afford relief, which regular, healthy menstruation does. This is especially the case in young females.

Elderly females, those who are about to experience a 'change of life', are almost always subject to intermissions and delays in their menstrual periods. In their case, the discharge, when it makes its appearace, is apt to be very excessive.

Treatment : For irregular menstruation, whether it is too late or too early, too scanty or too profuse, *Pulsatilla* is most generally the appropriate remedy. It is especially adapted to females of mild and easy disposition, and partcularly for the following symptoms, pain low down in the abdomen and through the small of the back, nausea and vomiting, shivering, pale face, alternate crying and laughing, sadness and melancholy, giddiness, fullness about the head, semi-lateral headaches, roaring in the ears, drawing pains, extending to the face, tendency to diarrhea and leucorrhea. All the symptoms are *worse* in the afternoon and in the evening, the pains frequently change from place to place, and are *relieved* by the patient being *in the open air.*

Natrium Muricaticum, menses too late and too scanty with rush of blood to the head.

Sepia, delayed menses, with violent colic, fits of fainting, leucorrhea and pressure in the abdomen, uterine cramps, face bloated, and marked with yellow spots, especially across the cheeks and nose.

Belladonna, if there is a rush of blood to the head, nose-bleed, redness of the eyes, intolerance to light and giddiness, especially after stooping, the menses delayed, but when they to appear, too profuse.

Bryonia Alba, if, instead of menstruation, there is bleeding from the nose, with congestion of the head and chest.

Causticum, menses delayed, but profuse, pains in the sides, yellow complexion.

Cocculus Ind., scanty discharge of dark clots, excessive nervousness, contracting, pinching pains in the pelvis.

Graphites, menses too late, too little, and too pale. During the menses, spasms and violent cutting pains in the abdomen, labour-like pains, nausea and violent headache.

Lachesis, especially applicable during the 'critical period'. Short and scanty menses, before the discharge, vertigo and headache, colic and leucorrhea.

Phosphorus, for females of a delicate constitution, those predisposed to lung difficulties, and when in place of regular menstruation, there is spitting of blood, or menses too soon and too profuse. During the menses, there is weariness, shivering, headache, pain in the back.

Sulphur, when other remedies have not been sufficient, or when there is great heat in the head, giddiness, palpitation of the heart, shortness of breath, abdominal cramps, pains in the sides amd bowels, loss of appetite, sickness at the stomach, emaciation, and depression of spirits.

6. CHLOROSIS OR GREEN SICKNESS

This disease is almost exclusively peculiar to young ladies at about the period of puberty, and is characterized by a pale, yellowish-green countenance, deficient warmth, perverted appetite, with occasional nausea or sickness, great physical and mental weakness, impaired digestion, palpitation of the heart and general derangement of the sexual function.

A similar condition may, however, be induced in females of a more advanced age, and of delicate constitution, by excessive loss of blood or other fluids, sedentary occupation, exposure to dampness and cold, insufficient food and clothing, mental emotions of an unpleasant kind, etc.

Pulsatilla, especially for females of a mild, easy disposition, given to sadness and tears. The symptoms indicating this remedy are, sallow complexion, alternating with redness and flushes of heat, frequent palpitation of the heart, great difficulty of breathing, with a sensation of suffocation after the least exertion, weariness, and heaviness of the legs, cold hands and feet, looseness of the bowels, pressure and heaviness in the abdomen, nausea, vomitting, chilliness, swelling of the feet, frequent headache, especially upon one side, buzzing in the ears, with pains which extend to the teeth, and frequently fly from one side of the face to the other, acrid, burning or thick, painless leucorrhea, like cream.

Bryonia Alba, may be given in alternation with *Pulsatilla,* when there is frequent congestion of the chest, bleeding from the nose, constipation, coated tongue, flushes of heat, chilliness, cough, with expectoration of clots, dark, coagulated blood, and especially, when *Pulsatilla* affords but partial relief.

Sulphur, for obstinate cases, and especially, though apparently well indicated, if the above remedies fail to afford relief, also, when the following symptoms are present, humming in the ears, great depression after talking, difficulty of breathing with sense of weight in the chest, constant drowsiness in the day-time, pressure in the abdomen, voracious appetite, sour eructations, emaciation, constipation of the bowels, with hard stool, sensitiveness to the open air. Suitable for irritable persons, or those inclined to sadness and crying.

Calcarea Carb., this remedy is suitable after *Sulphur,* especially when the difficulty of breathing is very great, and there

DISEASES OF WOMEN

is excessive emaciation, weariness and heaviness of the body, palpitation, nausea, and vomiting, desire for wines, salt things and dainties.

Lycopodium Clav., especially when *Calcarea Carb.* affords only partial relief, also, when there is obstinate constipation, extreme languor and cough, with tendency to consumption.

Ferrum Met., will be serviceable after *Calcarea Carb.*, when the sallowness continues, with great debility, want of appetite, nausea, etc. When the complexion is very pale, the lips bloodless, and the heart's action palpitating, irregular.

Belladonna, when there is a pressing or bearing-down pain, as though the internal parts would fall out, with or without leucorrhea, scanty and painful menses, preceded by colic.

China off., when the disease occurs after a severe fit of sickness, or after hemorrhages.

7. CHANGE OF LIFE–CESSATION OF MENSES

Definition: By the pharse, "Change of Life", or the 'Critical Period', is understood the final cessation of menstruation. This change usually takes place at *about* the forty-fifth year, though in some cases it takes place some years earlier, and in others it may be postponed till the fiftieth year, and even later.

Women of delicate constitutions, and those who have been 'living high,' and whose habits have been sedentary, generally experience the change earlier than those of a robust constitution or those who live temperately and who lead active lives.

As the change approaches, the menses gradually becomes irregular both in regard to their time of recurrence and the quantity discharged. They may also return 'too soon' or be delayed beyond the usual time. The quantity discharged is at times much less than common. Sometimes the discharge returns every two weeks, then ceases for several weeks, or even months, and afterwards recurs for a few periods as regularly as ever, and then altogether ceases.

In the majority of women while this change, which lasts usually from a year to a year and a half, is in progress, there is more or less disturbance of the general health. And not unfrequently it is difficult, sometimes quite impossible, to say exactly what is the matter with the patient, except that she is generally out of health. A host of symptoms present themselves, the patient complains of headahce, vertigo, billiousness, indigestion, flatulency, acidity of the stomach, diarrhea, costiveness, irregularity in the urinary discharge, piles, pruritis, (violent itching of the private parts), cramps and colics in the abdomen, palpitation of the heart, hysterics, nervousness, pains in the back and loins, swelling of the abdomen, swelling of the extremities, paleness and general debility.

The remedies called for during the change, or those which we most frequently have to use are *Pulsatilla, Lachesis, Bryonia Alba, Cocculus Ind., Ignatia,* and *Sulphur.* As a rule, treatment may commence with *Pulsatilla* and *Lachesis.* One dose, two globules No.10 of *Pulsatilla* 30 may be given for four days, then after an interval of four days without medicine, give *Lachesis 30* in the same way. If the symptoms abate, wait as long as the improvement continues, if they do not abate, repeat the remedies as before, or select a new one.

It is very important in these cases to pay strict attention to the diet and exercise. The diet should be light and easily digested. Every thing of a stimulating nature, such as coffee, tea, spices, etc. should be rigidly avoided. Life in the open air and activity of some kind will be found beneficial.

8. PROLAPSUS OF THE UTERUS OR FALLING OF THE WOMB

Definition : Prolapsus of the uterus, or as it is commonly called, 'falling of the womb', is in reality a descent or sinking down of the organ. In some cases, the displacement is but slight, scarcely noticeable, while in others it is so great as to permit the uterus to protrude through the external parts. Among the causes of this disorder, may be mentioned–menorrhagia, or a debilitating leucorrhea, if allowed to continue for a long time, the too early getting up after delivery or abortion, of too early resumption of household duties, frequent child-bearing, miscarriages, or difficult labours, the incessant running up and down, long flights of stairs by females of a delicate constitution, the weakening effects of purgatives and other drugs-such as large doses of ergot and other allopathic drugs.

Symptoms

There is generally more or less bearing down, or dragging sensation in the lower part of the abdomen, drawing from the small of the back and around the loins and hips, presssure low-down toward the lower parts, with a desire to make water, sometimes without ability to do so a sense of faintness and occasonally a variety of nervous or hysterical feeling and alarms which almost overwhelm the patient.

Treatment

In order to help patients suffering suffering intense pain from the prolapse, a *pessary* is recommended and applied, but this gives only a temporary protection and does not give real relief to the patient. Homeopathic remedies have, on the other hand, the specific power to give prompt and perfect cures.

The remedies are *Aurum Met., Belladonna, Calcarea Carb., Nux Vomica, Platina, Sepia.*

Belladonna, when the following symptoms are present—pressure, as from a load in the lower abdomen, or, as if the contents of the abdomen would fall out, heaviness even in the thighs, crampy pains through the abdomen and pelvis, also extending down to extreme point of spinal column, great sensibility and irritability, also when accompanied by leucorrhea and menorrhagia.

Nux Vomica, for congestion of the womb, with pressure downwards, especially when walking, or after walking, great heat and weight in the womb and vagina, dragging, aching pain in the back, also from the abdomen down into the thighs. During the menses, abdominal spasms and headache, disposition to miscarriage, menses too early and too profuse, leucorrheal discharge of fetid, yellow mucus.

Sepia, irregular menstruation, too early, too feeble or suppressed, heat in the womb, pains in the back and abdomen, aggravated by walking, frequent desire to urinate, contractive, pressive pain in the abdomen, as if everything would be pressed out, colic before the menses, itching, excoriating leucorrhea, with a discharge of a yellowish or reddish water or a mattery fetid fluid.

The treatment, in most cases, may commence by administering one dose of *Nux Vomica* every four hours, and be continued for one week, during the next week no medicine should be given, but the week following, the patient may take one dose of *Sepia,* night and morning. If the symptoms indicate *Belladonna,* that remedy should be preferred to *Nux Vomica,* at the beginning and followed by *Sepia,* or *Calcarea Carb.*

Calcarea Carb., this is an excellent remedy for persons of a weak or lax muscular system, or of a scrofulous habit, and especially when menstruation is exhaustive, too profuse, and too frequent.

Secale Cor., is occasionally called for, especially when there is prolonged bearing-down, forcing pains, profuse menstruation, depression, lowness of spirits, deficient contraction after miscarriage. Other remedies as *Mercurius Sol., Thuja, Kresote, Nux Mosch., Stannum Met.* are at times called for.

Cold water when properly used in this disease, will be highly beneficial. The most convenient and advantageous mode of application is the wet bandage, renewed two or threee times a day. Frequent sitting-baths, of short duration, will be of great benefit.

At the commencement of the treatment, it is often necessary for the patient to maintain a recumbent position for a greater part of each day, and in all cases it is absolutely necessary to refrain from all active work or exercise, and running up and down stairs is especially objectionable. The patient should strictly avoid taking purgative medicines, as well as coffee and tea.

9. LEUCORRHEA–WHITES

Definition: This term is applied to light, colorless discharge from the female genitals, varying in hue from a whitish or a colorless to a yellowish, light green, or to a slightly red or brownish, varying in consistency from a thin, watery, to a thick, tenacious, ropy substance, and in quantity from a slight increase of the healthy secretion, to several ounces, in the twenty-four hours.

Leucorrhea may occur at any period of life, from early infancy to old age, but it is most frequent between the ages of fifteen and forty-five. It seldom continues beyond this period, except when the discharge has is origin in some organic disease of the womb. It may occur even before the first menses have made their appearance, especially in scrofulous subjects, and materially interfere with the full and free development of this important function. As a general rule, the leucorrheal discharge is more copious at the time of the menses than at any other time.

The disease may be acute and chronic. A large majority of the mild cases consist simply of a catarrhal inflammation, occasioned by taking cold. The chronic form is merely a continuation of the acute, the inflammatory stage, if neglected or improperly treated, passes in the chronic form, with ulceration of the neck of the womb.

Causes

As is generally supposed, 'general debility' is not the cause of the disease, nor is the discharge. They are simply the outward manifestation, or the result of morbid action going on in some portion of the uterine organism. What that disease is, or has been, which has given rise to these symptoms, can generally be ascertained by the nature of the discharge, and the peculiarities which each particular case presents. For instance, the discharge from the vagina are of three kinds, namely mucus, purulent or mattery and watery, and the morbid conditions capable of producing each of these discharges. It is very necessary to ascertain definitely the cause of the various forms of the malady in order to treat the disease intelligently.

Leucorrhea is a hereditary disease depending upon the nature of the constitution, for instance, those possessing a lymphatic, nervous constitution, with soft flesh and pale skin are *hereditarily predisposed* to uterine affections. In the case of such people, a cold, errors in diet, or wrong habits of living would result in leucorrhea, or some kindred disease, while other women differently constituted may be quite free even though they may commit any imprudent acts sometimes.

The exciting causes are generally—exposure to cold, sitting upon very cold ground, stones, irritation from stimulating injections, inflammation of the rectum, miscarriages, uterine displacements,

DISEASES OF WOMEN

ulceration of the womb, purgatives, improper diet, excessive use of tea and coffee, sudden emotions, etc.

Treatment

To obtain satisfactory results from remedies, it is necessary that all those conditions and irregular habits which are responsible for the disease should be avoided.

The following remedies will be found efficient in arresting the disorder in a large majority of cases.

Calcarea carbonica, particularly suited to women of lymphatic constitution, light complexion, and who have copious menstruation which is liable to return too soon, when the discharge is *milky,* often passes with the urine, and on lifting, and usually comes on, or is *worse immeditely before menstruation,* often attended by itching and burning, shooting pains through the parts, and falling of the womb. It suits leucorrhea in infants and young girls often recurring before puberty, leucorrhea before menses, or in *recurring attacks between the menses.*

Pulsatilla, when the discharge takes place during pregnancy, or immediately before, during and after menstruation, when produced by fright, and when occurring in young girls who have not yet menstruated, the discharge is thin and acrid, excoriating the parts, or the discharge is thick, like cream, sometimes corrosive and attended by itching of the parts, and attended with crampy or cutting pains in the abdomen.

Sepia, leucorrhea of a yellowish green colour, somewhat offensive and often excoriating, milky, worse before menses, with bearing-down, the patient has a sallow, pimply face. Most suitable in leucorrhea of little girls.

Sulphur, for inveterate cases of leucorrhea, the discharge sometimes yellowish, burning and corrosive, and preceded by colic, also when it results from suppressed eruptions or ulcers.

Cocculus, watery, bloody leucorrheal discharge during pregnancy, scanty menses, with leucorrhea between the periods, leucorrhea instead of the menses.

Alumina, leucorrhea after the menses, profuse, discharge of *transparent mucus* during the day, corrosive leucorrhea, producing heat, soreness and itching of the vulva, between and after the menses, *discharge of bloody water, profuse leucorrhea just before and after menstruation.*

Kreosotum, whitish, acrid leucorrhea, attended with great weakness, discharge of blood and mucus from the vagina on rising in the mornings, excessive pains in the small of the back, falling of the womb, smarting and itching of the external parts.

Natrium Muriaticum, when the discharge is copious and consists of transparent, whitish and thick mucus, or is acrid, with yellow colour of the face, also when accompanied by headache, disposition to diarrhea, with slimy evacuations and colic.

Silicea, leucorrhea like milk, acrid, excoriating leucorrhea, with itching of the parts.

Administration of the remedy : Give one dose morning and evening for 3 days. If there is no improvement, give a dose of *Sulphur,* and omit for four days, when the remedy may be repeated. If this gives no relief, or if the symptoms change, select a new remedy.

Injections of cold water, or cold hip baths are beneficial. In severe and obstinate cases, injections of the solution of *Hamamelis* tincture have been helpful, after the parts are washed with warm water. They may be used three or four times a day.

CHAPTER – XVIII

DERANGEMENTS DURING PREGNANCY

1. GENERAL REMARKS

The women whose privilege it is to bear within herself a human being occupies a high position in the scale of humanity.

It is true, in the highest possible degree, that the habits of mind, the impulses and emotions of the mother during pregnancy, do have a direct and powerful influence upon her offspring, and to such an extent too, that it is in the power of the mother to determine, at least in a great measure, what class of passions shall have predominance, in the souls of her children. It is, therefore, very important that she should maintain a proper state of the mind and feelings during this period. All sorts of mental excitement should be avoided as it causes in most cases abortion. She should also pay all possible attention to her diet and mode of life.

Diet, should be well regulated. Whatever tendes to disturb the general health should be strictly avoided. Many females, during this period, have a morbid desire for things which, if indulged in, would prove highly injurious, producing dyspeptic and other troublesome symptoms, which, besides being a source of much suffering to the mother, may seriously affect the future health of her offspring. Each one, by using a little discrimination, can best regulate her own diet. The diet should be simple, purely nutritious, liberal, but not excessive, and everything medicinal or stimulating, such as all highly seasoned foods, strong tea, coffee, etc., should for the most part be avoided.

Exercise, she should keep herself sufficiently active and may attend to her normal household duties without causing fatigue. She should spend a greater part of her time in open air. She should avoid quick and violent action, such as lifting heavy articles, or exert herself in moving them.

2. DERANGEMENTS DURING PREGNANCY

Although pregnancy is a perfectly natural and perfectly healthy condition, yet owing to the increased activity going on in the constitution, we very often meet with disorders peculiar to this condition. As there are constitutions which are differently affected during this period, it is better to take note of these and take the best means for removing them.

The following are some of the most common of the deviations from health which are met with during this period.

(a) Continued Menstruation

This is comparatively rare, yet when it occurs it should receive attention. The following remedies will arrest the discharge.

Cocculus Ind., when there is severe spasmodic pain low down in the abdomen.

Crocus Ind., when the discharge is dark and copious.

Phosphorus, Platina and Sulphur are also useful. For their indication, and also for other remedies, see under 'Painful menstruation' and 'Profuse menstruation.'

(b) Headache and Vertigo During Pregnancy

Very often, pregnant women are seriously affected with giddiness and pain in the head. With these headaches there is almost always a sense of dulness, and disinclination for active employment, sometimes there are nausea, dimness of sight, sparks before the eyes, palpitation and nervous tremblings. These symptoms are generally caused by nervous irritability, and whatever tends to

DERANGEMENTS DURING PREGNANCY

derange the general health of course predisposes the patient to their frequent occurrence. To prevent these, it is necessary that the patient should observe the rules of diet and exercise rigidly, and avoid all mental and physical excitement. These symptoms are generally worse in the morning.

Aconitum Nap., for persons of a full habit, with a florid complexion, and nervous temperament, and especially if there is giddiness, as if intoxicated, on rising from a seat, frequently causing one to fall, faintness and dimness of vision on rising rom a recumbent posture, determination of blood to the head, and pressure in the forehead, stupefying pains in the head, eyes red and sparkling, with intolerance of light, black spots before the eyes.

Belladonna, for congestion to the head, with vertigo, staggering and trembling, buzzing in the ears, intolerance of noise, heaviness and pressive pain on top of the head or in the forehead, over the eyes, pain, with a sense of expansion of the head, and violent throbbing of the large arteries of the neck, redness of the face, soreness and redness of the eyes, sparks before the eyes, objects appear double. The symptoms are mostly *worse in the morning.*

Glonoine, for symptoms see under 'Headache'.

Nux Vomica, most suitable for women of a hasty temper, and those who are of sedentary habits, or addicted to coffee. The symptoms are generally *aggravated* in the *morning* and *better* in the *open air.* It is valuable for giddiness with a feeling of confusion in the head, with cloudiness of sight and buzzing in the ears, pains in the head of a tearing, drawing or jerking character, or periodical pains, constipation, insipid or acid, bitter and putrid taste.

Opium, for giddiness on rising from a stooping or sitting posture, vertigo, with stupidity as if from a debauch, *great drowsiness,* and imperfect sleep, with puffed face, *thick, heavy breathing,* and illusions of the imagination.

Platina, if there is headache, which increase gradually until it becomes violent and then diminishes in the same way and also for headache produced by vexation or passion, constant disposition to spit, the saliva being tasteless or sweetish. It is particularly valuable in suffering of *nervous* and *hysterical women.* The symptoms are *worse* during repose and relieved by motion.

Pulsatilla, for giddiness, which is worse after stooping with momentary blindness and staggering, throbbing and shooting pains in the head, one-sided headache, headache every other day. The sufferings are sometimes attended with numbness of the limbs, are *worse* in the *afternoon* and *evening* and better in the *morning.* It is most suitable for women of a mild disposition.

Sulphur, if there is congestion of blood to the head, with pulsative pains and sensation of heat in the head, vertigo and staggering, principally when seated, or after a meal, attended sometimes by nausea, fainting, weakness and bleeding from the nose, confusion of the head, with difficulty in meditating, *worse* in the *morning* or *evening,* one-sided headaches, or headaches on top of the head, the back part, or intermittent headaches, *worse* in the *morning* or *evening,* or at night. The pains in the head are mostly *aggravated* by movement, walking in the open air and meditation.

(c) Morning Sickness

Nausea, vomiting, heartburn, etc. are at the same time the most common and the most distressing accompaniments of pregnancy. They usually begin five or six weeks after conception and continue until the sixteenth week. After which time they generally abate or cease entirely, in some cases, however, they continue with but slight modification to the end of pregnancy.

These troublesome symptoms commonly arise immediately on rising from bed in the morning and are often exceedingly harassing for two or three hours. Sometimes they return again in the evening.

Attention to the diet must be particularly observed in this affection. The food may be taken at more frequent intervals and in smaller quantities and when the vomiting is very persistent, liquid food alone should be used.

Ipecac., when there is nausea and vomiting, with great uneasiness in the stomach, vomiting of drink and undigested food, bilious vomiting and tendency to looseness of the bowels. Two globules of *Ipecac. 30,* in one oz. of water, one tea-spoonful twice a day for some days.

Nux. Vom., when there is nausea and vomiting, especially in the morning, while eating, or immediately after eating or drinking, violent hiccough, water-brash, pain and sensation of weight in the pit of the stomach, constipation and irritable temper. Two globules of *Nux. Vom. 30* in one oz. of water, one tea-spoonful *thrice* a day for a number of days.

Sepia, in obstinate cases and if there is the vomiting of milky mucus and the woman is of a melancholy temperament and is subject to sick headache or any derangement of the uterus. Two globules of *Sepia 30* in one oz. of water, one tea-spoonful every morning for eight days.

Natrium Mur. in obstinate cases accompanied by loss of appetite and taste, constant flow of water from the mouth, acid stomach, pain and soreness at the pit of the stomach. Two globules of *Nat. Mur. 30* in one ounce of water, one tea-spoonful, morning and evening, for *three* days and repeated after three days' interval.

Arsenicum Alb., if there is excessive vomiting, especially after eating or drinking, with attacks of fainting, great weakness and emaciation. Two globules, No. 10, of *Arsenicum Alb. 30* in one ounce of water and one tea-spoonful, morning and evening for some days, or in severe cases every three hours.

Pulsatilla, nausea after eating, vomiting of food, heartburn, eructations, acid, bitter, or with the taste of food, depraved appetite, or craving for acids, etc., whitish coated tongue.

Two globules, No. 10, of *Pulsatilla 30,* in one ounce of water and tea-spoonful doses, morning and evening for three days and after three days' interval repeat in the same way.

(d) Constipation During Pregnancy

Pregnancy is frequently accompanied by a sluggish condition of the bowels and especially in persons of a naturally constive habit. When it is not due to a mechanical cause, a change in diet, a little more of vegetables or fruits, more exercise in the open air and a good drink of fresh cold water on rising in the morning will be beneficial. Indigestible foods and coffee and tea should be avoided to remove the difficulty.

One dose of *Nux Vom. 30,* morning and evening, may be taken for three or four days, when there is dull headache, heat in the abdomen, frequent but ineffectual desire for stool. If *Nux Vom. 30* alone is insufficient, it may be taken in alternation with *Opium 30.* If both these remedies fail and when constipation has continued for a long time, *Lycopodium Clav. 30* or *Sulphur 30* may be taken. *Bryonia Alba, Alumina* and *Sepia* are often of service.

(e) Diarrhea

Diarrhea in a pregnant female is an untoward symptom and should be checked as soon as possible, otherwise the health of the patient may suffer severely.

The medicines called for are-*Chamomilla, Pulsatilla, Dulcamara, Lycopodium Clav., Sulphur, Antim Crud.* and *Calcarea Carb.*

Chamomilla, should be given when there is violent colic, with yellow, greenish stools, or resembling stirred eggs.

DERANGEMENTS DURING PREGNANCY 331

Pulsatilla, when the stools are watery, or greenish, preceded by colic, with slimy, bitter taste in the mouth.

Dulcamara, when the diarrhea results from a cold or after getting wet.

For further indications regarding the other remedies see under 'Diarrhea'.

(f) Itching–Pruritis

Itching of the private parts is a very annoying trouble. Sometimes the trouble arises from a vitiated condition of the mucus secretion of the parts and in others it depends upon an aphthous eruption when it is accompanied by a burning heat with dryness, redness and perhaps some swelling. This affection is not confined to the pregnant state alone, but may occur at any time.

Bryonia Alba, Arsenicum Alb., Rhus Tox., Pulsatilla, Silicea, Sulphur, Lycopodium Clav. and *Graphites* are the chief remedies for this disease. Give each remedy for three or four days before selecting another and use the remedies in the order given.

A very efficacious external application is a solution of one ounce of *Borax* in a pint of rose-water or distilled water. The parts affected may be washed several times a day with this solution. As an alternative, water in which lemon juice is mixed may also be used.

(g) Hysterical Fits–Fainting

Females of a nervous, hysterical or delicate constitution are frequently, especially during the early months of pregnancy, attacked with fainting, hysterical spells. They are occasioned by want of sleep, excessive fatigue or a disordered digestion. The attack is usually preceded by a constriction about the throat, by sobbing, or repeated attempts at swallowing. Then the patient rolls about from side to side, or sometimes lies perfectly still and motionless for some little time, then the sobbing become violent, or the patient bursts out into tears and the paroxysm then terminates.

Generally the attack passes over in a short time, without any bad consequences. When the attacks are light, attention to proper diet and plenty of fresh air, will generally prevent their recurrence. But should the attacks be more severe, it will be necessary to treat the cause, and, if possible, remove it.

The speediest means of reviving a patient from fainting is to sprinkle cold water upon the face and admit plenty of fresh air into the room. When the paroxysm is over, a single dose of two globules of *Chamomilla* or *Coffea* should be given and the patient permitted to go to sleep. On waking, she will feel quite restored.

Where these derangements arise from a disordered stomach, the diet should be changed and *Nux vom.* or *Pulsatilla* should be given. *Nux Vom.* is suitable for nervous and peevish patients and *Pulsatilla* for mild and easy ones and when the attacks are attended by great excitability with disposition to low spirits, etc.

Chamomilla, when the disorder arises from excitement or fit of anger.

Belladonna and Aconitum Nap., may be useful in preventing a return of the attacks in individuals of full habit and *Belladonna* may follow after *Aconitum Nap.* when there is congestion to blood to the head.

Ignatia, is one of the most valuable remedies when the patient complains of a severe headache, *as if a nail were driven into the head,* melancholy, frequent sighing and concealed sorrow.

Administration of Remedies : The medicines may be given dry or in a solution. When given dry, two globules dry on the tongue, or in a solution, two globules in one ounce of water, one teaspoonful for a dose every two, three or four hours according to the severity of the case.

(h) Palpitation of the Heat

Palpitation of the heart not unfrequently causes pregnant women a great deal of annoyance and sometimes serious alarm. If it occurs for the first time, there is no fear of it being connected with organic disease of the heart and it should cause no uneasiness.

The principal remedies are-*Coffea, Ignatia, Chamomilla, Nux Vom., Pulsatilla, Belladonna.* When caused by anger, *Chamomilla,* by fear, *Veratrum Alb.,* by joy, *Coffea,* by sudden fright, *Opium,* for nervous persons, *Ignatia, Coffea, Chamomilla,* for plethoric persons, *Aconitum Nap., Belladonna.*

The medicine may be given in water solution, teaspoonful doses every hour, or oftener in severe cases.

(i) Toothache

This is a very common affection in pregnancy and frequently it is of exceedingly severe character. It generally commence in a decayed tooth and extends to others, but sometimes even a sound tooth may have it. The pains are of a neuralgic character and may be removed by suitable remedies.

WHEN THE PAIN IS ERRATIC, FLYING FROM ONE TOOTH TO ANOTHER–*Pulsatilla.*

FOR TOOTHACHE IN CARIOUS TEETH–*Antim Crud., Chamomilla, Nux Vom., Staphy sagria, Mercurius Sol., Sulphur.*

FOR VIOLENT PAINS, WHICH COME IN PAROXYSMS – *Coffea, Chamomilla, Belladonna.*

FOR NERVOUS TOOTHACHE–*Ignatia, Coffea, Chamomilla, Belladonna, Sepia.*

The medicine may be given dry on the tongue, from one to six hours according to the severity of the pain.

(j) Neuralgia

On account of the increased irritability of the nervous system during pregnancy, the neuralgic pains may appear in any part of the body.

The following remedies are useful–

Belladonna, Aconitum, Coffea, Chamomilla, Bryonia Alba.

The medicine may be given from one to four hours according to the severity of the pain

(k) Pains in the Back and Sides

Women often suffer very much from pain in the lower part of the back during pregnancy. Sometimes the pain is seated deep in the right side under the ribs. The patient also feels a sensation of heat in the affected part. It is usually most troublesome from the fifth to the eight month. The sensation experienced is that of an almost indescribable aching, or of a dull heavy pressure, as if caused by a dead weight resting on the part affected.

FOR THE PAIN IN THE BACK–*Bryonia Alba, Rhus Tox., Belladonna, Pulsatilla, Nux vomica, Causticum* or *Sulphur.*

FOR THE PAIN IN THE SIDE–*Aconite Nap., Chamomilla, Pulsatilla* or *Phosphorus.*

WHEN THE PAINS ARE OF A DULL, HEAVY CHARACTER–*Chamomilla.*

IF THE PAIN IS ATTENDED WITH MUCH HEAT– *Mercurius Sol., Aconitum Nap.*

(l) Cramps

Cramps in the calves of the legs, hips, feet, back or abdomen are common accompaniments of pregnancy and are exceedingly painful and annoying.

The best remedies for CRAMPS IN THE LIMBS ARE–
Veratrum Alb., Colocynth, Nux Vomica, or *Sulphur.*

THOSE OF THE BACK–*Ignatia, Rhus Tox.* or *Opium.*

THOSE OF THE ABDOMEN–*Nux Vomica, Pulsatilla, Belladonna, Hyocyamus Nig.,* or *Colocynth.*

(m) Varicose Veins or Swelling of the Veins

Some women suffer a great deal during pregnancy from distension of the superficial veins of the lower extremities. This distension is caused by the pressure of the enlarged uterus upon the veins within the abdomen and pelivs, thus preventing a free return of the blood upward. Usually the swelling commences at the ankles and gradually extends upwards towards the thigh. Very often the swelling is confined to the leg below the knee, the veins of the calf of the leg alone presenting any unnatural appearance. Both limbs may be involved, or the disease may be confined to one.

When the disease first commences, the veins beneath the surface assume a reddish hue, but as the distension increases and the vessels become knotted and swollen, they change to a dark blue or leaden color. The swelling decreases when the patient is lying down or when the limb is kept in an elevated position, as lying upon a chair when the patient is sitting, but when the patient is compelled to be constantly or for a large part of the time upon her feet, or when the limb is allowed to hang down, the disposition is very much increased and the disease aggravated.

This condition of the veins, at first, is not painful and becomes so only from actual distension of the vessels. Sometimes the swelling is so great, that the veins actually burst and large quantities of blood is discharged, either externally or effused beneath the skin.

After delivery, the pressure of the pregnant uterus on the

large veins of the abdomen and pelvis being removed, the swelling disappears and the veins resume their natural size.

Treatment : At the commencement of the difficulty and in case where the swelling is not extensive, nor the pain so severe, frequent bathing with cold water, or diluted alcohol, will give relief. But when the veins are large and painful, or when they are knotted, the leg requires the careful application of a bandage and rest in the recumbent posture.

Persons who are constantly on their feet, should constantly wear the bandage, or a laced stocking. The stocking or bandage should be applied in the morning on rising, at which time there is the least swelling, beginning at the toes and progressing upwards, with a moderate and equal pressure. At night, on retiring, the bandage should be removed and the whole limb freely bathed and rubbed *upward* with cold water or water and alcohol or a weak solution of *Arnica Tincture.*

Varicose veins, though occurring more frequently during pregnancy, are not by any means confined to this state, they may take place at any time in the females and are often met with in the male sex. When occurring under any other circumstances than those which we have been considering, they are indicative of constitutional debility.

The remedies which will be required in this affections are– *Arnica Mont., Hamamelis, Pulsatilla, Nux vomica, Arsenicum Alb., Lachesis, Lycopodium Clav., Carbo Veg.*

Nux Vomica, when the disease is attended with hemorrhoids, constipation, frequent bearing-down pains, enlargement of the abdomen and irritable temper.

Pulsatilla is the principal remedy for varices, especially when there is much swelling of the veins and of the whole limb, with severe pain and more or less inflammation, or when they are of a bluish or livid colour, which is imparted to the whole limb. Should

'Pulsatilla' give some relief, while the swelling and discoloration continue the same, *Lachesis* may be substituted. In some cases, especially where the occupation of the patient compels her to be constantly upon her feet, *Arnica Mont.* given in alternation with *Pulsatilla* proves very efficacious.

Arsenicum Alb., when the swelling is of a livid colour and attended with a good deal of burning pain, when the burning continues after the administration of *Arsenicum Alb.*, give *Carbo Veg.*

Lycopodium Clav., in inveterate cases, after the failure of other remedies.

Administration of the Remedies : Give the indicated remedy in water solution, one teaspoonful every four hours for two days, if there is no relief, select another remedy.

(n) Hemorrhoids or Piles

Pregnant women are very often subject to piles. This is chiefly owing to the pressure of the enlarged uterus on the contents of the abdomen causing more or less inactivity of the bowels and obstruction to the circulation Those who are subject to habitual constipation are more liable to this affection. It is, therefore very important that a pregnant woman, especially if it is her first pregnancy, should pay particular attention to the state of her bowels and avoid constipation or diarrhea to continue for any length of time by taking suitable precautions or appropriate remedies in time

Treatment : The appropriate remedies for this disease are:

Pulsatilla, Nux Vomica, Ignatia, Opium, Sulphur also *Arsenicum Alb., Carbo Veg., Belladonna, Hepar Sulph., Natrium Mur., Hamamelis.*

Pulsatilla, when blood and mucus are discharged with the stools, with painful pressure on the tumours, pains in the back, pale countenance. When this remedy proves insufficient, follow it with *Sulphur.*

Nux Vomica and *Sulphur,* are the principal remedies for this trouble, *Nux Vomica,* especially, when there is burning, pricking pains in the tumours, also when there is a discharge of light blood after each evacuation of the bowels and a frequent tendency to evacuate. This remedy may be given at night and *Sulphur* in the morning. *Sulphur* is well suited for all forms of piles and like *Nux Vomica,* is especially called for when there is that constant, ineffectual inclination to stool. It is also useful when there is considerable protrusion of the tumours, so much so that it is difficult to place them back. Also when there are violent shooting pains in the back.

When these two remedies, after two or three days' trial, fail to afford relief, they should be followed by *Ignatia,* especially if the pains, like violent stitches shoot upward, or where after the evacuation, there is painful contraction and soreness, or the rectum protrudes after each evacuation.

As regards other remedies, see the chapter under the heading of 'Hemorrhoids'

***Administration of Remedies* :** The remedy may be given dry on the tongue, night and morning, or in severe cases, in watery solution, in tea-spoons every hour until relief is obtained.

In addition to the administration of remedies, much benefit may be obtained by a proper use of cold water. When the piles do not bleed, cold applications, either as sitz baths, compresses or injections are of great benefit. As evil results sometimes follow the sudden suppression of the discharge, it is not advisable to use cold water when there is much bleeding. When however, the bleeding is profuse, so as to cause alarm, cold applications are best. Warm water or steam is preferable when the tumours do not bleed, or when, from any cause, the bleeding is caused and there is considerable pain.

DERANGEMENTS DURING PREGNANCY

The use of condiments and stimulants of every description, such as coffee, tea, etc., which are responsible for this complaint should be strictly avoided. The diet should be simple and nourishing.

(o) Jaundice

This disease occurs sometimes towards the end of pregnancy and is caused partially, perhaps, by the mechanical pressure of the distended uterus upon the bile-duct and partially by the sympathetic action going on in the liver, in common with the other digestive organs.

The symptoms of this disorder are constipation with whitish, almost colourless stools, urine of an orange color and dry skin, with slight remittent or intermittent fever.

To commence with, take *Mercurius Sol.* at intervals of four hours (3 doses per day) for three days and follow with *Hepar Sulph. 6* or *Lachesis,* night and morning, for a few days.

When the disorder arises from a fit of pain, take *Chamomilla* and *Nux Vomica,* in alternation (3 doses per day) as in the case of *Mercurius Sol.* for 3 days.

(p) Incontinence of Urine

This disorder consists of a partial or total inability to retain the urine. There is a frequent desire to urinate which is sometimes so violent, that a few drops of urine will escape before the patient is able to reach her place for the purpose.

The principal remedies are : *Pulsatilla, Sepia, Belladonna, Causticum, Hyoscyamus Nig.*

Commence with *Pulsatilla* and if this is insufficient, next try *Sepia.*

(q) Dysuris and Strangury

These two affections are equally frequent among pregnant females. *Dysury* means, simply, difficulty in passing urine, while *Strangury* refers to the frequent painful urgings to discharge urine and it passes only by drops, or in very small quantities.

The causes which give rise to these troubles are the pressure of the extended uterus upon the bladder and urethra, the irritation of the mucous membrane excited by this pressure, spasms at the neck of the bladder, excesses in eating or drinking, exposure to cold, etc.

The best remedy for this trouble is *Pulsatilla.* One dose every two hours and, if this is not sufficient, *Nux Vomica will be of service.*

Aconitum Nap., Belladonna, Cocculus Ind., Cantharis, Phosphoric acid and *Sulphur* are also valuable remedies and may be taken in the same way.

In addition to the internal remedy, barley water or thin parboiled rice water may be taken freely, mixed with butter milk.

(r) Depression of Spirits

Aconitum Nap., if depression results from fright and fear of death is the most important symptom.

Belladonna, if there is great agitation and restlessness at night, fear of ghosts, fear and disposition to run away and hide, involuntary laughter, disposition to laugh or sing, or to fall into a passion and rave, frightful visions, indisposition for exertion, etc.

Pulsatilla, for depression, with sadness and weeping, uneasiness in the pit of the stomach, sleeplessness, she imagines herself to be oppressed with a multitude of cares, dislike to conversation, headache and heartburn.

Sulphur, lowness of spirits with great anxiety on the subject of religion, despair of salvation, forgetfulness of proper names and of words when about to speak them, disposition to get angry.

Administration of Remeies : Give the indicated remedy morning and evening for three days and after an interval of three days, repeat again in the same way and if there is no relief choose another remedy.

3. INFLUENCE OF EXISTING DISEASES UPON PREGNANCY–PROPHYLACTIS APPLIED TO CHRONIC AND HEREDITARY DISEASES

The various acute disease which are likely to occur during the pregnant period and the manner in which they have to be treated have been dealt with so far. The question which next arises is what influence pregnancy has over the chronic or constitutional diseases of the patient and how they should be treated during this period.

Chronic diseases do not modify the course of pregnancy in anyway, but pregnancy sometimes slackens the course of chronic maladies and even suspends the development of th symptoms. The period of pregnancy is, therefore, exceedingly favourable to their treatment, as the female organism is never more sensitive to the action of the drugs than during pregnancy. It is at this time that the germs of disease are most easily extinguished in the human body. Both the mother and the child which she bears in her womb are benefited by a wisely directed treatment.

It is, therefore, advisable to give the mother at different periods of pregnancy, two globules of *Sulphur 30* which should be allowed to act for six weeks, after which a dose of *Calcarea Carb. 30* may be given and allowed to act for a similar period. This is applicable to all cases and has the effect of purifying the fetus from the psoric taint which it may have inherited from the parents and bringing forth healthy children. Similarly, if either of the parents had been suffering from chronic skin troubles, it is desirable to give two doses of *Sulpur 200* at intervals of two months and after the same interval, one dose of 1 M potency during this period and if the father had suffered from venereal diseases and the mother had been infected thereby, two doses of *Mercurius Sol. 200* and one dose of the same in 1M potency, allowing the same intervals, will be useful. If the mother had one or two children who were subject to epileptic fits, or who were puny and had defective bone development, it will be necessary for the mother to take *Sulphur 200* and *Calcarea Phos. 200* in the latter, at intervals of two months between the doses. If either of the parents had tuberculosis, *Tuberculinum* in the higher potencies will be necessary for the mother during pregnancy allowing the same intervals.

4. MISCARRIAGE OR ABORTION

Definition

By miscarriage, or abortion, is understood the expulsion of the fetus from the womb before the sixth month, subsequent to this period, it is called premature labour. Women are liable to miscarriage at any period of pregnancy, but most frequently about the third or the beginning of the fourth month. When it takes place before or about this period it is not very dangerous, though repeated miscarriages, from the profuse discharge with which they are usually accompanied, impair the constitution and very often lead to some chronic trouble. Miscarriages occurring at a later period are much more serious and very often highly dangerous.

Females who have miscarried once, are exceedingly liable to its recurrence, which liability is greatly increased, if it has occurred two or three times.

The most common causes of miscarriage are-mechanical injuries, as a fall or blow, etc., sudden and powerful mental emotions, the abuse of purgative drugs, great physical exertion, too free use of stimulating foods and drinks, neglect to take air and exercise, late hours, etc.

DERANGEMENTS DURING PREGNANCY

The following symptoms generally precede and attend this affection, chilliness followed by more or less fever and bearing-down pains, severe pains in the abdomen, cutting pains in the loins, or pains resembling labour pains, discharge of mucus and blood, sometimes of a bright red color, at others dark and clotted, followed by a flow of thin fluid. The miscarriage generally occurs along with this discharge, which, if not stopped by appropriate means, may continue for hours and endanger the life of the patient.

In case of threatened miscarriage, the patient should immediately lie down and remain in that position until the danger is passed, or, in case the miscarriage has taken place, she should still remain in this position for a few days to guard against a fresh discharge, which is more likely to occur in the upright posture.

Arnica Mont. if the attack has been brought on by a fall, blow, violent concussion, over-lifting, misstep, or walking, or great physical exertion of any kind.

If Arnica Mont. fail, you may try cinnamon next.

Chamomilla, when there is excessive restlessness, severe pain in the back and loins, also periodical pains, resembling those of labour and each pain is followed by a discharge of dark-colored blood.

Secale Corn. is very valuable, after miscarriage has occurred and particularly in females who have miscarried more than once, or in those who have a weak and debilitated constitution, or when the discharge consists of dark liquid blood and the pains are but slight.

China off., for weak and exhausted persons, also when there is spasmodic pain in the uterus, or a bearing-down sensation, with a considerable discharge of blood at intervals. This is a *most valuable remedy in restoring the exhausted energies* of the patient, after the hemorrhage has ceased.

Hyoscyamus Nig., for miscarriages, attended with spasms or convulsions of the whole body.

Ipecac., in alternation with *Secale Corn.,* if, with flooding, there is nausea and cramps profuse and continuous discharge of bright, red blood, disposition to faint, whenever the head if raised, chills and heat, cutting pain in the umbilical region. If *Ipecac.* does not help, *Platina* may follow.

Platina, when there is a discharge of dark, thick, or clotted blood, attended with pressing or bearing-down pains.

Belladonna is a valuable remedy at the commencement, especially when there are great pains in the loins and the entire abdomen, severe bearing-down as though the intestines would be pressed out, pain in the back, as though it was dislocated or broken, profuse discharge of blood.

Crocus Sat., is especially indicated when there is discharge of dark, clotted blood, with a sensation of fluttering or moving about in the umbilical region, an *increased discharge of blood on the slightest movement.* If other remedies fail, this sometimes will help.

Nux Vomica and *Bryonia Alba,* may be given alone or in alternation, for the following symptoms; severe burning or wrenching pain in the loins, painful pressure downward, with a mucous discharge. Also in cases attended with obstinate constipation.

In cases where there is a disposition to miscarriage, or if the patient had previously miscarried, as she approaches again the same period, she should lie on the bed the greater part of the day, taking an occasional dose of *Sabina,* until the period is passed.

As preventives of this disorder, the main remedies are- *Sabina, Secale Cor., Lycopodium Clav., Calcarea Carb., Sepia.*

Administration of the Remedy : Give the selected remedy in watery solution (2 globules in one ounce of water)-one tea-spoon every fifteen to twenty minutes in severe cases, in milder ones every two hours and in the early stages when no danger is apprehended, every six or twelve hours. If relief is not obtained in five or six hours, select another remedy.

5. FLOODING DURING PREGNANCY OR AT DELIVERY

When this accident occurs, the woman should lie down quietly, should move as little as possible, her mind should be kept free from tensions and the greatest quietness preserved in the whole house.

Internally, the *Tincture of Cinnamon* should be administered, two or three drops in half a tumbler of water, well stirred and a teaspoon every half hour or oftener according to the urgency of the case. If the *tincture of Cinnamon* is not at hand, a piece of *cinnamon* may be chewed. If this does not produce a salutary effect, give sugar and when the burning sensation has passed, *Arnica Mont.*

Arnica Mont., in all cases, arising from mechanical injuries, such as a fall, blow, lifting or carrying weights, etc.

Ipecac., very copious continued flooding, particularly when occurring during pregnancy, the blood flowing regularly, without interruption, with cutting pains around the navel, much nausea, great pressure and bearing-down, chills and coldness of the body, feeling of heat rising into the head, great weakness and inclincation to lie down. This is also a *most important remedy in flooding after delivery.*

Chamomilla, after *Ipecac.*, if there is no improvement, or when the flooding is accompanied by pains resembling labour-pains.

Bryonia Alba, when dark red blood is discharged in great quantities, with violent pressive pain in the small of the back and headache, particularly in the temples, as if the head would burst and constipation.

China off is very important in the *most dangerous cases*, when the heaviness of the head, giddiness, loss of consciousness and drowsiness appear, for sudden weakness, fainting, coldness of the extremities, paleness of the face, convulsions, contortions of the eyes, or when the face and hands turn blue, or single jerks pass through the whole body. While giving this remedy the abdomen may be rubbed gently, or cloths dipped into vinegar or water applied to it. Also when accompanied by colic, frequent urging to make water and sore tension of the abdomen. It is *always* serviceable for the *debility or other troublesome symptoms* which frequently remain after the flooding has ceased.

Hyoscyamus Nig., for flooding attended by labour-like pains, with drawing in the thighs and small of back, or in the limbs, heat over the whole body with a quick or full pulse, great uneasiness, excessive liveliness, trembling over the whole body or numbness of the limbs, loss of consciousness, darkness before the eyes, delirium, twitching in the muscles of the extremities, jerking in one or the other limbs alternating with stiffness of the joints.

Belladonna, when the blood discharged is neither particularly dark, nor light colored, with pressure in the privates, as if everything would fall out, pale or flushed face, heat about the head, palpitation of the heart and thirst.

Platina, when the discharge is *dark and thick,* but *not clotted,* the pain in the back drawing towards the groins, with pressing-down internally towards the *genitals,* which are *excessively sensitive.* This remedy is *particularly applicable to cases of flooding produced by any violent mental emotion.*

Ferrum Met., when the blood is *sometimes black and clotted,* at others, liquid, with labour-like pains, the *face usually red, China off.* follows *Ferrum Met.* very well.

6. PREPARATION OF THE BREASTS

By paying proper attention to the breasts before confinement, mothers will in many instances save themselves much suffering after delivery from sore nipples, gathered breasts, etc. The most common affections to which the nipples are subject are excoriation, cracks, inflammation and scaly eruptions.

For several weeks previous to delivery the entire breast and chest should be bathed with cold water daily and afterwards well-dried and rubbed with coarse towels. If there is tenderness or slight excoriation, it is better to bathe the parts with diluted *tincture of Arnica Mont.* and administer internally *Aconitum Nap.* or *Chamomilla*. In some cases, *Silicea* or *Sulphur* may be required.

The swelling, burning, itching, cracks and eruptions will be removed by *Lycopodium Clav., Mercurius Sol., Hepar Sulph.* or *Sulphur.*

7. EASY DELIVERY

To facilitate easy labour and delivery, it is advisable to give *Caulophyllum 30,* one dose every fourth day for a fortnight during the last month of pregnancy. One globule No. 10 may be given dry on the tongue in the morning on empty stomach for a fortnight.

8. FALSE PAINS

Previous to delivery, sometimes but a few days or a week, women are very much troubled with what is termed *spurious* or *false pains*. They differ from labour pains in the irregularity of their recurrence in being unconnected with uterine contractions and principally confined to the abdomen, which is tender to pressure and movement and in not increasing in intensity as they return. In some instances it is exceedingly difficult to discriminate between them and genuine labour pains. In such cases, the period of pregnancy will be the chief guide and when they come on a week or two before labour is expected, they should be checked by the administration of a suitable remedy.

The exciting causes of these pains are congestion of blood to the uterus, a chill affecting the abdomen, mental emotions, errors in diet, clothing etc.

Bryonia Alba is most suitable when the symptoms have arisen in consequence of a fit of passion and consist of pains in the abdomen, followed by dragging pains in the back and loins, constipation and irritable temper. They are aggravated by motion.

Nux Vomica, for pains in the abdomen and back like those under *Bryonia Alba,* also when there are pains as if from a bruise in the region of the pubes, constipation. The pains occur chiefly at night. Applicable to *passionate persons a*nd when the exciting cause appears to be *indulgence in stimulants,* such as *highly seasoned foods, coffee, tea etc.*

Pulsatilla, pains in the abdomen, pains in the loins, as if from continued stooping, with a feeling of stiffness and painful dragging and aching in the thighs, constipation or diarrhea, most applicable to *mild tempered persons a*nd when *due to eating rich or fat, indigestible food.*

Dulcamara, when the pains are sharp and violent in character, or when they arise from taking cold, the effect of a chill or dampness. The pains are mostly confined to the small of the back coming on or aggravated at night.

Aconitum Nap., is most suitable for young persons of a full habit, when the pains are attended with a full, strong and frequent pulse, with congestion to the head, flushed face and hot skin. *Belladonna* may be given after *Aconitum Nap.,* when the head is

DERANGEMENTS DURING PREGNANCY 349

hot and the feet are cold and also when the pains are spasmodic in their character.

Administration of Remedies :

The selected remedy may be given in watery solution in teaspoon doses, in severe cases every half hour, in other cases, every three or four hours, until relief is obtained, or another remedy may be selected.

CHAPTER – XIX

TREATMENT AFTER DELIVERY

1. LABOUR– CHILD-BIRTH

Natural labour generally takes place at the end of the ninth month-after two hundred and eighty days from the last menstruation. It not unfrequently happens. However, that pregnancy is protracted to the two hundred and ninetieth day or even later.

The commencement of actual labour is usually preceded by some of the following premonitory symptoms-agitation, nervous trembling, lowness of spirits, irritability of the bladder with frequent inclination to urinate, nausea and vomiting, flying pains through the abdomen, followed by the increased mucous discharge or flow sometimes streaked with blood.

The true labour pains usually commence in the back, sometimes they are first felt at the lower and interior part of abdomen and extend to the loins and lower part of the back. They are at first slight and of a short duration, lasting but a few moments and with intervals of rest lasting from half-an-hour to an hour or more. By degrees they become more and more frequent, gradually increasing in intensity, until labour is completed, which usually takes from four to six hours.

Cases frequently occur in which labour is prolonged much beyond the usual period, or is attended with a great deal of suffering, such labours are more likely to take place with women in their first confinement, who are already somewhat advanced in life and those of a slender form and highly nervous and sensitive habits.

The sufferings in these cases may be greatly alleviated by using the following medicines :

TREATMENT AFTER DELIVERY

Coffea, will prove generally serviceable when the pains are ineffectual and extremely violent, following each other in quick succession and attended by great agitation, restlessness and tossing about.

Aconitum Nap., when the above remedy is insufficient, or when the patient has been in the habit of drinking coffee frequently as a beverage.

Chamomilla, after the above, if required, especially if there is a great mental excitement, excessive sensitivity to pain, anguish and discouragement.

Pulsatilla, in the absence of any exciting symptoms as above, as soon as labour pains commence, one dose of *Pulsatilla 200* may be given in watery solution (one globule in one ounce of water). If delivery does not take place normally within 3 or 4 hours, a second dose may be repeated.

Nux Vom., when the labour is protracted from the irregularity and insufficiency of the pains and there is *constant inclination to evacuate the bladder and rectum.*

Secale Corn. 200, will be useful when the labour pains are attended by spasms of the stomach and vomiting, or with acute pains in the back and loins and painful drawing sensation in the thighs, when *Pulsatilla* is not sufficient in increasing the activity of the uterine contractions, also for women who are very feeble, with a disposition to cramps in the legs and feet and if she has had already a number of previous labours. The medicine should be given in watery solution, *tea-spoon doses every half hour* until the pains are developed.

Spasmodic pains, cramps and convulsions.

Chamomilla, if there are very acute pains, mostly of a cutting description, extending from the region of the loins to the abdomen and attended with spasmodic convulsions, redness of the face, with great sensitiveness of the nervous system and excitement.

Belladonna when there are excessively violent bearing-down pains, attended with convulsive movement of the limbs, great agitation and constant tossing, congestion to the head, with throbbing and distension of the blood vessels, red and bloated face and profuse sweating.

Hyoscyamus Nig, for severe convulsions *with loss of consciousness,* great anguish and cries, with oppression of the chest.

Stramonium, for trembling of the limbs and convulsions *without loss of consciousness.*

Ignatia, when there is a confused feeling in the head, spasmodic and compressive pains, with sensation of suffocation, convulsions.

Ipecac., spasmodic convulsions, paleness or bloatedness of the face, nausea or vomiting.

Cocculus Ind., cramps or convulsions of the limbs or whole body, cramps in the lower part of the abdomen with heat, redness and puffiness of the face.

2. TREATMENT AFTER DELIVERY

Two globules of *Arnica Mont. 30* may be dislocated in one ounce of water and given as four doses, one dose immediately after delivery, the second twelve hours later, the third on the third day and the fourth on the fourth day. If the local pains and soreness continue, at the same time, 20 drops of *Arnica Mont. Tincture* (external) may be dissolved in half a tumbler of water and the solution applied externally by wetting a cloth and using it as a compress over the part for some days. After the delivery, if the patient is unable to get sleep and is excited, a few doses of *Coffea 30* will be enough.

TREATMENT AFTER DELIVERY

(a) Flooding After Delivery

The directions for the appropriate treatment of this trouble will be found under the heading of 'Flooding' in the previous chapter.

The medicines which are useful are *China, Chamomilla, Corus, Platina, Belladonna* and *Tincture of Cinnamon*.

(b) After Pains

Arnica Mont., when the pains are not violent and are accompanied with a feeling of soreness, with pressure on the bladder and retention or urine.

Chamomilla, if *Arnica Mont.* proves insufficient and the patient is nervous and excitable with great restlessness, tossing about, etc.

Nux Vom., after *Chamomilla*, will often be serviceable, especially when the pains are of an aching or a violent colicky description and press towards the rectum with desire to go to stool.

Pulsatilla, is indicated in persons of a mild and feeble disposition, when the pains do not return very frequently, but are protracted and continue for several days.

Secale Corn., for very weak women, who have borne many children, great exhaustion, complains of burning heat and cannot bear warmth.

(c) Duration of Confinement

The mother should remain in bed for six or eight days after delivery, the length of time depending on circumstances. After the first nine or ten days, the mother may be seated in an easy chair for a short time every day, after this period, she may walk about the room if she feels strong enough. It is not safe for any woman to resume her normal activities until the end of the sixth week after delivery.

The diet should be light but nutritious and everything stimulating, both food and drinks and all strong odours should be strictly avoided.

If the patient is in normal health, three weeks after delivery, a dose, or two three week's interval, of *Psorinum 200* may be given for quick convalescence.

(d) Diseases Following Parturition–The Lochia

The discharge which take place after confinement are called *Lochia* and very considerably in different individuals, sometimes it is thin and scanty and cease in a few days and in others it continue for several weeks and is so profuse as almost to amount to a hemorrhage. In the majority of the cases it cease about the tenth day. In color and consistence, it at first resemble menstruation, but gradually grow lighter colored, lose the redness entirely and become successively, yellowish and whitish before it cease finally.

When this discharge continues too long, or is too profuse and also when it is checked suddenly or suppressed from exposure to cold, errors of diet, or other causes, it is necessary to take suitable medicines.

Crocus Sat., is indicated when the discharge is too long continued, in too great quantity and consists of dark colored or black blood of viscid consistency.

Pulsatilla, is the principal remedy for sudden suppression, either from mental emotions, exposure to dampness, or any accidental causes, particularly if it is followed by fever and headache, coldness of the feet and frequent desire to pass water.

Bryonia Alba, if the suppression is accompanied by headache, fullness and heaviness in the head with pressure in the forehead and temples, throbbing in the head, aching in the small of the back and scanty discharge or urine. It is also useful when the lochia is too profuse in quantity and of a deep red colour, with internal burning pains in the region of the uterus.

TREATMENT AFTER DELIVERY

Aconitum Nap. is also valuable in too profuse lochial discharge of a deep red color and may be found sufficient to check it in two or three days. If *Aconitum Nap.* is insufficient, *Calcarea Carb.* may follow with advantage, especially if the discharge is attended with itching in the uterus.

Belladonna, if the discharge continues too long and becomes thin and offensive, producing excoriation of parts.

Nux Vom., if the pulse is hard, with paleness of the face, pains in the back and weight in the anus, chills alternating with heat.

Dulcamara, after *Pulsatilla,* when suppression arises from exposure to cold or dampness. It may also precede *Pulsatilla.*

Chamomilla, if the suppression is followed by diarrhea and colic.

Platina, for suppression consequent on some mental emotion.

China off. and Ipecac. In alternation, if the discharge takes place in paroxysms, with nausea, vertigo, fainting, coldness of the extremities, paleness of the face and debility.

Rhus Tox., in case where the lochia return after they once had ceased.

Administration of Remedies, the selected remedy may be taken-2 globules No.10, dry on the tongue, once in four hours until better.

(e) Milk Fever

Arnica Mont., given internally and the diluted tincture applied externally to the breast as a lotion, once or twice a day, will be beneficial, when there is much distension, with soreness or hardness.

Aconitum Nap., if there is much fever, with hot, dry skin, breasts hard, restlessness and anxiety.

Bryonia Alba, after *Aconitum Nap.,* when there is oppression in the chest, violent pains in the head and constipation.

Belladonna may be given after *Bryonia Alba,* to remove the symptoms completely.

Chamomilla, will have the preference when there is much nervous excitement, with restlessnes, tenderness of the breasts and inflamed nipples.

Pulsatilla, in severe cases, when there is great distension of the breasts, with soreness and rheumatic pains, extending to the muscles of the chest, shoulders, under the arms, etc. A timely administration of this remedy with prevent a threatened attack of child bed fever.

Rhus Tox., in cases similar to *Pulsatilla,* with rheumatic pains throughout the system, swelling, heat and hardness of the breasts, headache, stiffness of the joints and general constitutional disturbance.

(f) Suppressed Secretion of Milk

The evil effects of a suppression of this secretion are frequently of so serious a nature that the slightest diminution in the quantity of milk should receive immediate attention. In the majority of cases, the administration of *Pulsatilla* will be sufficient to check this disorder at the outset and restore the flow of milk. If any unpleasant symptoms still remain, after the use of *Pulsatilla,* then *Calcarea Carb.* will be helpful. If symptoms of fever set in, with hot, dry skin, thirst, etc., give *Aconitum Nap.* at short intervals, until amelioration of the symptoms takes place. If there is great restlessness and nervous excitement, *Coffea* may be given in alternation with *Aconitum Nap. Belladonna* and *Bryonia Alba* will be found serviceable when there is congestion of the head or lungs, with fever, pain and aching in the limbs and especially if these symptoms were preceded by a chill.

TREATMENT AFTER DELIVERY

(g) Excessive or Involuntary Secretion of Milk

China off., when it is caused by debility from loss of fluids.

Rhus Tox., from over-distension in consequence of excessive secretion of milk.

Calcarea Carb., or *Pulsatilla* in other cases.

(h) Diarrhea after Confinement

Pulsatilla, if the diarrhea occurs mostly in the night, or early in the morning, if accompanied by much ineffectual straining, if it makes the parts sore, or if there is only a discharge of mucus with pain in the anus, chilliness.

Secale Corn., for offensive, very weakening diarrhea.

Phosphoric acid, in *obstinate, protracted* cases, when the discharge is watery, or painless and almost involuntary.

Dulcamara, when arising from checked perspiration, produced by chills, from exposure to cold or dampness.

Rheum or *Antimonium Crud.*, for watery and offensive evacuations, *Rheum*, if the stools smell sour and fetid, with much pain and straining after each evacuation, *Antimonium Crud.*, when the tongue is coated white and there are frequent, bitter eructations, diarrhea worse during the night and early in the morning.

For diarrhea with clay-whitish, curdled, or sour-smelling, mustly evacuations, accompanied with nursing sore-mouth, give *Nux Vomica* and *Hepar Sulph.*, in alternation every three hours.

Administration of Remedies : The selected remedy may be taken dry upon the tongue (2 globules) or in watery solution, teaspoon doses, from two to four hours, till there is relief.

(i) Constipation after Confinement

It is natural for the bowels to remain inactive for a few days after delivery and nothing should be given to disturb this state, as it is always a good symptom and serves to promote the strength of the patient. Purgative medicines should in no case be given at this time, as they can do no good whatever and are often highly injurious to the patient. If, after the lapse of five or six days, the patient complains of fullness of the head, or pain in the bowels, a dose or two of *Bryonia Alba* will gradually bring about an evacuation and give relief. If this should be insufficient, a dose of *Nux Vomica* may be given in the evening and followed by a dose of *Sulphur* next morning. If after waiting for a day or two no evacuation takes place, an injection of lukewarm water may be given.

(j) Retention of Urine or Painful Urination

It not unfrequently happens, especially after severe labour, particularly with first children, there is retention of urine or painful urination. The following medicines will give relief.

Arnica Mont., should be the first remedy, as it is especially indicated in cases like the present, where the difficulty arises from mechanical injuries. Should *Arnica Mont.* fail and there be much fever, with burning heat in the region of the bladder, give *Aconitum Nap.*

Belladonna, when there are darting and pricking pains, extending from the lower part of the back to the bladder and there is great agitation and colicky pain.

Camphor, when the retention arises from spasmodic contraction of the neck of the bladder.

Nux Vomica and *Pulsatilla,* the former especially, if there is also constipation.

The application of warm fomentations to the parts, or sitting over a pan containing warm water will often have the desired effect.

Administration of Remedies : Give tea-spoon doses of the selected remedy in watery solution every two hours till there is

TREATMENT AFTER DELIVERY

relief and if no relief is obtained after eight or ten hours, select another remedy.

(k) Sore Nipples

The chief difficulty in the way of healing sore nipples, arises from their being constantly torn open afresh by the efforts of the child in sucking. In the majority of cases, if proper attention is paid to the preparation of the breasts before confinement, this could be avoided. When, however, there is a tendency to tenderness and excoriation, the internal administration of *Arnica Mont.* and bathing the nipples with a solution of *tincture of Arnica Mont.*, consisting of ten drops in half a tumbler of water, several times a day will give relief. If this should be insufficient, *Sulphur*, when the nipples are sore and chapped, with deep fissures around the base, which bleed and burn like fire, *Calcarea Carb.* in cases similar to *Sulphur* when it fails to relieve, *Nux Vomica* for soreness of the nipples with painful excoriation of the adjacent parts.

In obstinate cases, *Lycopodium Clav., Mercurius Sol.* and *Silicea* will be found valuable.

Washing the nipples with cold water every time the child has taken the breast and then sprinkling them with finely powdered white sugar will be helpful.

(l) Gathered Breasts

Inflammation and suppuration of the breasts are likely to occur during the whole period of nursing and may arise from several causes, such as cold, passion, fright, bruise etc., or putting the child too late to the breast, or the sudden stoppage of suckling on account of the death of the child. The most effectual means of preventing suppuration is to take out the milk.

Bryonia Alba is the principal remedy in the beginning, when the breasts become swollen, hard and feel heavy, with shooting pains, dry skin, thirst and other feverish symptoms.

Belladonna, after *Bryonia Alba,* when there is much swelling and hardness of the breasts, shooting and tearing pains and redness of the skin, sometimes like erysipelas. These two remedies will generally be sufficient. If, however, some hardness remains, *Mercurius Sol.* should be given every six hours.

Hepar Sulp., when suppuration has already commenced and frequently preceded by a chill.

Silicea, in cases in which the discharge becomes fetid, thin and watery and comes from several openings, which are not disposed to heal.

Sulphur, in inveterate cases when there is profuse discharge of matter, with emaciation, fever, etc.

Arnica Mont., in all cases when the disease arises from external injuries.

Should the above remedies fail to effect a cure, try *Graphites* or *Calcarea Carb.*

ADMINSITRATION OF REMEDIES: When at the commencement, *Bryonia Alba* or *Belladonna* is given, it is better to give them in watery solution, tea-spoon doses every hour. The other remedies may be given at intervals of three to six hours. Towards the end when *Sulphur* or *Calcarea Carb.* is used, one dose dry, on the tongue, will be enough morning and evening.

(m) Child-bed Fever or Puerperal Peritonitis

Child-bed fever or Puerperal Peritonitis is an inflammation of the peritoneum or serous membrane lining the abdomen and covering the bowels. It is not unfrequently complicated with inflammation of the womb and its appendages.

TREATMENT AFTER DELIVERY

Among the exciting causes of this disease are, violence during delivery, taking cold, diarrhea, irritation of the bowels, induced by purgative medicines, severe mental emotions, suppressed secretion of milk, etc.

Child-bed fever is generally preceded or attended by shivering and sickness or vomiting and is marked by pain in the belly, which is sometimes very extended, though in other cases it is at first confined to one spot. The abdomen very soon becomes swelled and tense and the tension rapidly increases. The pulse is frequent, small and sharp, the skin hot, the tongue either clean or white and dry, the patient thirsty, she vomits frequently and the milk and lochia usually are obstructed. The belly becomes as large as before delivery and is often so tender that the weight of the bed-clothes can scarcely be endured, the patient also feels much pain when she turns, the respiration becomes difficult and sometimes a cough comes on, which aggravates the distress, or it appears from the first to be attended with pain in the side, as a prominent symptom. Sometimes the patient has a great inclination to belch which always gives pain. The bowels are either constipated, or the patient purges bilious or dark coloured stools.

Aconitum Nap. is the first remedy called for in a majority of cases, especially if the disease commences with a chill and is succeeded by a dry, hot skin, thirst, clean tongue when tachycordio and attended with anxiety, forebroodings of evil, etc.

Belladonna, especially, when there is deep-seated pains in the abdomen, with dragging downwards, throbbing pains in the head, face at times flushed and full, glassy appearance of the eyes, delirium, spasmodic eructations, mostly bitter, retention of urine, distension or excessive tenderness of the abdomen, sometimes with shooting and digging pains, painful pressure on the genital organs.

Bryonia Alba, sensitiveness of the abdomen, constipation, with shooting pain in the abdomen, high fever, with great thirst. This remedy may be given in alternation with *Aconitum Nap.*

Pulsatilla, in patients of gentle disposition, where the attack is mild in the beginning, great pressure downwards, with frequent inclination to pass water, suppression of the lochia, tendency to diarrhea. Other remedies applicable to this disease are -*Apis Mell., Arnica Mont., Arsenicum Alb., Chamomilla, Hyoscyamus Nig., Nux Vomica, Rhus Tox.* and *Sulphur.*

Administration and Dose : In the beginning of childbed fever, it is safest to give *Aconitum Nap.* and *Belladonna* in alternation, every one, two, three, or four hours, according to the urgency of the symptoms. Two globules for a dose, dry on the tongue.

(n) Milk Leg or Crural Phlebitis

It is an inflammation of the veins of the leg, due to the effusion of lymph and serum from the blood into the cellular tissue.

The exciting cause is generally due to exposure to cold.

In the beginning, there is uneasiness or pain in the lower part of the abdomen, extending along the brim of the pelvis through the hips. The patient is irritable, depressed and complaints of great weakness. As soon as the inflammation is fairly set in, the region about the groin becomes swollen and in a short time, twenty-four to forty-eight hours, the thigh becomes swollen, tense, white and shiny. The swelling, which sometimes increases the limb to the size of a man's body, or an elephant's leg, may be confined to the thigh, or it may extend down to the foot. Along the course of the inflamed vein, although there is great tenderness, there is neither redness nor other discoloration. In most cases, the vein may be traced from the groin down the thighs, feeling hard and folding under the finger like a cord.

Either leg may be affected, though the left appears to be more frequently attacked and it happens that the sound leg participates in the disease before the disease is perfectly removed and then the disease runs a similar course a second time.

Treatment : The treatment of this disease should be undertaken only by an experienced physician. The following remedies may be employed at the commencement of an attack.

Aconitum Nap., if the disease has an acute character, with high fever, heat all over and violent pains.

Arnica Mont., if phlebitis sets in after tedious labour, or after an injury.

Belladonna, this seems to be the better remedy in the commencement of most cases, especially when there are sharp, stitching pains, as with knives, heaviness in the thighs and lower part of the abdomen, creeping in the limbs, violent fever, with burning thirst, great sensitiveness to touch or motion.

Bryonia Alba, when there are drawing or lancinating pains from the hip to the foot, with copious sweat and excessive tenderness to touch or motion.

Pulsatilla, if *Belladonna* or *Bryonia Alba* effected no improvement. Other remedies recommended for this disease are :-

Rhus Tox., Sulphur, Nux Vomica, Arsenicum Alb.

Administration of Remedies : Of the selected remedy, give two globules, dry on the tongue, once in two hours.

(o) Nursing Sore Mouth

In this disease, the soft part and sometimes the whole interior of the mouth becomes very red and so sensitive and tender, as to render it almost impossible for the patient to partake any solid food whatever. This is quite different from what is generally called canker sore mouth. In some females, it appears to be constitutional. This form of sore mouth arises from the peculiar irritation which the act of nursing produces upon the digestive organs.

If not properly treated, it sometimes becomes so severe and is attended with so much suffering and debility, that the weaning of the child becomes necessary. The weaning of the child has a magical effect upon this disease, the whole of it vanishing as soon as nursing is discontinued.

In the majority of cases, this disease, can be readily controlled by one of the following remedies.

Mercurius Sol., this is a prominent remedy and may be given in alternation with *Nux Vomica* or *China off.* With *China off.,* especially, when there is great debility and exhaustion.

Should this fail, *Borax* may be used and in severe and obstinate cases, *Nitricum acid* or *Sulphur* will be necessary.

Sometimes an exhausting diarrhea accompanies this disease. When such is the case. and evacuations are sour, curdled or musty, *Nux Vomica* and then *Hepar Sulphur* are useful.

Administration of Remedies : The selected remedy may be taken in tea-spoon doses, every four to six hours, or dry upon the tongue (two globules), once from six to eight hours, the repetition of the dose being regulated according to the severity of the case.

When *Nux Vomica* and *China off.* are used in alternation, the dose may be repeated once in four hours. When taking *Sulphur*, a dose, night and morning, will be enough.

(p) Perspiration after Delivery

The increased perspiration, which takes place immediately after delivery and continues for several days, acts as a substitute for the suspended mucous secretion and consequent inactivity of the alimentary canal. Therefore its sudden suppression from exposure to cold, or a sudden chill, is unavoidably followed by some injurious result, such as, gathered breasts, diarrhea or child-bed fever.

When sudden exposure to cold, especially dampness, has caused the suppressed action of the skin, *Dulcamara* will be found the most efficient remedy to bring about a renewed action. A dose of *two globules* may be taken every four hours, until four doses have been taken, when the interval between the does may be prolonged. If this remedy does not help and there is great excitability and restlessness, with colic and looseness of the bowels, give *Chamomilla* and *Mercurius Sol.* in alternation.

Belladonna, should lateral headache occur, with pain in the back of the neck.

Bryonia Alba, will be found serviceable when the suppression is followed by chills, or severe pain in the head and limbs. If there is much fever, *Aconitum Nap.* may be given in alternation with *Bryonia Alba.* In some cases, *Sulphur* or *Nux Vomica* may be required.

Administration of Remedies : The remedy may be taken dry, or in tea-spoon doses and repeated every three or four hours, according to the urgency of the case.

(q) Excessive Perspiration after Delivery

Excessive perspiration, besides causing great debility, predisposes to other disorders, by the high susceptibility of catching cold which it causes. A few doses of *China off.* will remove this condition.

Sulphuric acid is called for especially, when the perspiration is *profuse while lying still,* but diminishes by moving about.

The medicine may be taken dry on the tongue once in three hours.

(r) Weakness from Nursing

If the mother cannot sleep well, feels bad in the morning, has no appetite, or perspires much, commences to cough and is very sensitive to the least breath of air, give *China off.,* dry on the tongue, 3 doses per day, for a few days.

(s) Falling Off of the Hair

Some females, while nursing, suffer from falling off the hair of the head.

Sulphur, Lycopodium Clav. or *Calcarea Carb.* will be useful.

CHAPTER – XX

TREATMENT OF INFANTS

NOTE– As regards the doses suitable for infants, *single drop* doses of the solution made up, by dissolving one globule, No.10 in one ounce of distilled water, have been found most suitable and are recommended. (For details see 'Introduction'). As the ailments of infants are of acute character, single drop doses have to be repeated at intervals of one to four hours, according to the urgency of the complaining. Doses must be stopped as soon as improvement commences.

1. ANTIPSORIC PROPHYLACTIS

In order to protect the child from the development of the psoric taint which it may have inherited from its parents, it is advisable, as soon as possible after birth, to put in the mouth of child a dose of *Sulphur 200*. As the child is very sensitive to the action of the homeopathic remedy, this may given by dissolving *one globule, No.*10 in an ounce of water and touching the tongue of the child with just *one drop* of this solution. If no morbid symptoms demand another medicine meanwhile, after 4 or 5 weeks, another dose of *Sulphur 200* may be repeated in the same way. Towards the third month, a dose of *Calcarea Carb. 200* may be given in the same way.

2. ECCHYMOSIS ON THE SURFACE OF THE SKULL
(COLLECTION OF BLOOD IN ONE PLACE)

If this appears at the time of labour, or some time after, one account of the sojourn of the head in the pelvis, or due to the use of forceps during the delivery, one or two applications of the solution of *Arnica Mont. tincture* will remove it.

3. DEFORMITIES, MONSTROSITIES

Deformities are the effect of a deviation in the action of the vital forces in the formation of the organs and in bringing back this force to its normal state we may obtain a resolution of the vicious forms which they have produced by the use of suitable homeopathic remedies. Many deformities may be corrected in this way. In all deformities, a few doses of *Sulphur 30* and *Calcarea Carb. 30* may be given, in alternation at fortnightly intervals. If the deformity involves the bones, after these medicines are given, *Silicea 200* may be given monthly.

4. MARKS

The different marks which appear on the surface of the body of the new-born child are the products of a defect of the organic tissues of the skin and ordinarily of the excessive development of the capillary vessels. To correct these, *Sulphur 30* followed by a few doses of *Calcarea Carb. 30* will be useful.

5. CYANOSIS–BLUE DISCOLORATION

Children remain blue, because the arterial duct remains open and the venous blood is not consequently forced to pass through the lungs and get orggenated. In this condition, a dose or a drop of the solution of *Sulphur 30* should be administered immediately and after an interval of three hours, a dose or more of *Calcarea Carb. 30*. After an interval of two months, a dose of *Digitalis 30* may be followed, after a fortnight, by a dose of *Calcarea Carb. 200*.

6. SWELLING AND ELONGATION OF THE HEAD

In the case of difficult and protracted labour, it is common for the head of the infant to be swollen and elongated immediately after birth and occasionally a tumour may appear on the back or top of the head. These may disappear in a few days. If they continue, repeated washings with cold water, or a weak solution of *Arnica Mont. Tincture (3* drops in half a tumbler of water) will correct it. If not better in two or three days, give *Rhus Tox.*

7. THE MECONIUM OR FIRST DISCHARGE FROM THE BOWELS

If the first discharge is delayed too long and the child becomes uneasy and restless, a few tea-spoonfuls of warm water mixed with sugar will have the desired effect. If this is not sufficient and the child's bowels are not moved freely during the first few days, a dose or two of *Nux Vomica, Bryonia Alba* or *Sulphur* may be administered to both mother and child. *Laxative medicines should never be given to the infants for the purpose of purging out the meconium, as this will bring about many chronic diseases in after-life.*

8. SORE EYES

Aconitum Nap., should be given first, especially if the inflammation arises from exposure of the eyes to too much light and the entire eye becomes red and discharges a good deal.

Belladonna, after *Aconitum Nap.,* when the whites of the eyes are very red, with bleeding from the eyelids, intolerance of light.

Chamomilla, when the eyelids are swollen, bleed and are glued together in the morning with a yellowish secretion.

Mercurius Sol., when there is redness of the eyes and eyelids, small yellowish ulcers along the margins of the eyelids with discharge of yellowish matter, etc.

Pulsatila, when there is profuse discharge of purulent matter from the eyes, with redness of the whole eye and interior of the lids.

Argentum Nitricum, is very important when there is profuse discharge of creamy pus, the eyelids are very much swollen.

Calcarea Carb. and *Rhus Tox.* are also useful.

(For particular see 'Affections of Eyes'.)

9. CONGENITAL HERNIA

Whether inguinal or umbilical, a dose of *Sulphur 30* may be given first and if the tumour still protrudes in a fortnight, a dose of *Nux vom.* 30 and eight days after, another dose of *Sulphur 30.* If the trouble continues, *Cocculus Ind.* or *Veratrum Alb.* may be given daily till there is relief.

10. HARDENING OF THE CELLULAR TISSUE

A few dose of *Aconitum Nap. 30,* followed by *Bryonia Alba 30* will correct this. If the disease still persists, give *Sulphur 30* and then repeat *Aconitum Nap. 30* as before.

11. SWELLING OF THE INFANT'S BREASTS

It is generally the effect of improper pressure upon the parts. If there is no redness, give *Arnica Mont.* 30, otherwise, *Chamomilla 30.* If there is inflammkation, *Aconitum Nap. 30,* followed by *Belladonna 30* or *Bryonia Alba 30.* If an abscess has formed, *Hepar Sulph.* 6, three doses per day and then *Silicea 30* to complete the cure.

12. HICCOUGH

The child should be warmed against the breast of the mother or nurse and sweetened water should be given in drops. If this does not help, the child should be given a dose of *Nux Vomica*.

13. OBSTRUCTION OF THE NOSE— "SNUFFLES"

The disorder which consists of an inflammation and consequent thickening of the mucous membrane which lines the nasal passages, prevents infants from breathing while sucking.

Nux Vomica, given at night will mostly afford relief, it should be given when there is obstruction with no running from the nose, or if there is running, it is in the morning, with dryness at night. If the *30th* potency does not help, the *200th* acts better.

Chamomilla, if the obstruction is attended with much running of water from the nose.

Carbo Veg., when the complaint is worse every evening.

Dulcamara, when worse in the open air.

Mercurius Sol., when there is much swelling and a thickish discharge from the nose.

Antimonium Tart, if there is rattling of mucus in the chest, which is worse at night, along with the running of the nose.

Lycopodium Clav., is often useful.

Arsenicum Alb, obstruction of the nose with, at the same time, a discharge of watery, acrid mucus and burning heat in the nose, the discharge from the nose producing excoriation and swelling of the adjacent parts. Also, when there is redness and watering of they eyes. If the *30th* potency does not give relief, the 200*th* acts better. When this remedy gives partial relief, it may be followed by *Ipecac., Sulphur,* in obstinte cases, when there is profuse discharge of thick mucus.

14. SORE MOUTH –THRUSH

Mercurius Sol., should be given when the disease first appears and also in cases where there is much salivation and the thrush shows a tendency to ulcerate.

Sulphur, should follow *Mercurius Sol.,* when the latter does not give relief in a few days.

Arsenicum Alb., when the thrush assumes a livid or bluish appearance, attended with great weakness and diarrhea.

Bryonia Alba and Nux Vomica are also useful in some cases.

15. SORE THROAT

Aconitum Nap., if they are restless, cry before passing water and have red cheeks.

Belladonna, if the whole face is red, also *Rhus Tox.*

Rhus Tox., if the throat is dark red, if they do not perspire, but become very hot during night and remain dry. If *Rhus Tox.* is not sufficient, give *Bryonia Alba.*

Belladonna, if they perspire much, the throat looks bright red, if the eyes are congested. If *Belladonna* is not sufficient, give *Mercurius Sol.*

16. JAUNDICE

Chamomilla may be given first and will be sufficient in many cases.

Mercurius Sol., may follow *Chamomilla* when the symptoms have only been partially removed, or when that remedy has not given relief.

China off. may follow for the remaining symptoms.

TREATMENT OF INFANTS

Nux Vomica, if the child is very irritable and has constipation also.

17. Excoriation or Raw Surface

Chamomilla, will be sufficient in most cases.

Mercurius Sol., when the excoriation is extensive and there is yellowness of the skin, which *Chamomilla* has not removed.

Rhus Tox. will cure, if red pimples appear on the head.

Sulphur or *Carbo Veg.* in obstinate cases.

18. THE "GUM" OR "RED GUM"

This term applies to an eruption of red pimples which appears in early infancy and chiefly on the face, neck and arms and sometimes over the whole body. A few doses of *Rhus Tox.* or *Sulphur* are enough.

19. RETENTION OF URINE

A few doses of *Aconitum Nap.* will afford relief. If this does not help, *Pulsatilla* will generally suffice. If constipation is present, *Nux Vomica* will be useful.

20. CONSTIPATION

Bryonia Alba or *Nux Vomica* will ordinarily be sufficient. If they don't help, *Opium,* if the constipation returns often, a dose of *Sulphur.* In chronic cases, *Alumina.* The same medicines may be given to the mother also. Injections of warm water may also be given.

But never use soap, as bad consequences develop by using soap for a long time.

21. DIARRHEA

Ipecac., when caused by overloading the stomach and especially if accompanied by nausea and vomiting, paleness of the face, frequent crying, stools of a bilious, slimy or greenish-yellow color, sometimes blackish, or streaked with blood and of a putrid odour.

Rheum, due to acidity and with flatulent distension of the abdomen, colic, crying and straining both before and after the evacuations, *which smell sour, the whole body also emits a sour smell.*

Chamomilla, in diarrhea of a bilious, watery, frothy or slimy character and of a whitish, greenish or yellowish color and of an offensive odour, with colic, crying, restlessness and drawing up of the legs toward the abdomen and redness of the face or of one cheek.

China off., in watery, painless diarrhea with more wind in the stomach and undigested appearance of the milk in the stools.

Belladonna, in the commencement, when the child is disposed to sleep a good deal, but is restless and starts up suddenly, the evacuations are greenish, small and frequent.

Aconitum Nap., in diarrhea attended with much fever.

Opium or *Aconitum Nap.*, when produced by fright.

22. COLIC

Chamomilla, will be sufficient in most cases, especially if the pain is attended by distension of the abdomen, crying, writhing and twisting, drawing up the legs towards the abdomen and coldness of the feet. If this remedy does not cure, give *Colocynth.*

Ipecac., when the colic is attended by sickness and diarrhea, the stools of a putrid odour.

China off., for colic with distension and hardness of the abdomen, the attack generally *appearing in the evening.*

Nux vomica, when caused by constipation.

Pulsatilla, in flatulent colic, with rumbling of wind in the abdomen, shivering and paleness of the face and tender abdomen.

23. CONTINUAL CRYING OF INFANTS WITHOUT APPARENT CAUSE

Belladonna, will be serviceable in most cases and also when the infant starts suddenly from sleep and begins to cry violently.

Aconitum Nap. or *Coffea,* if *Belladonna* fails, especially when there is much uneasiness and heat.

Chamomilla, if there is reason to think that the crying is due to some pain, such as earache or headache.

24. RESTLESSNESS AND WAKEFULNESS

Coffea, will often be sufficient for restlessness, hot skin, etc.

Opium, when *Coffea* is not sufficient and *there is red face.*

Chamomilla, if the restlessness is attended by flatulence and griping, with startlings and jerking of the limbs, or feverishness with one cheek red.

Belladonna, when the child is drowsy but cannot sleep or starts from sleep suddenly and cries.

Pulsatilla or *Ipecac.,* when due to overloaded stomach.

Nux Vomica, if caused by the child or mother taking coffee.

25. SCURF ON THE HEAD

Sulphur, administered night and morning for some days will remove the trouble.

26. MILK-CRUST

This is an eruption of numerous small white pustules appearing in clusters upon a red surface. They appear first on the face, the cheeks and forehead, from where they spread over the whole body. In a short time, they become yellow or dark coloured, burst and form thin yellow crusts. The eruption is often attended with considerable redness and swelling of the surrounding parts and with troublesome itching, which renders the child exceedingly restless and fretful and causes it to rub the affected parts constantly, by which the scabs are torn off and the disease is aggravated.

Aconitum Nap., should be given first, when the eruption is surrounded by redness and inflammation of the skin and the patient is very restless and uneasy.

Rhus Tox. may follow *Aconitum Nap.,* of after the lapse of a few days the eruption is not improved.

Sulphur, will be useful after *Rhus Tox.,* when the improvement is slow.

Viola tricolor is probably the remedy that cures more cases than any other.

Hepar Sulp., Arsenicum Alb and *Lycopodium Clav.* may be serviceable in tedious cases.

27. SCALD HEAD–RINGWORM OF THE SCALP

This disease is characterised by circular, red-colored patches, covered with numerous small yellowish points or pustules, which do not rise above the level of the skin. These pustules soon break and form thin scabs. The patches frequently unite with adjacent patches and assume an irregular and extensive appearance and sometimes cover the whole head. These incrustations, by accumulating, become thick and hard and when removed, the surface beneath is left red and glossy, but studded with slightly elevated pimples. If these eruptions continue long, the hair is frequently destroyed. It is commonly found in children from the age of two years to the age of puberty. It is not confined to the scalp, but appears on the face, neck and other parts of the body and in such cases, they are less difficult to cure than when located in the scalp.

This disease is often extremely obstinate and especially so, when it has been treated with local washes and external ointments, the effect of which is generating aggravation of the complaint and render the cure much more difficult than when proper remedies are used from the beginning.

Rhus Tox. will generally be the most appropriate remedy to start with and under its action the disease will change favourably.

Sulphur may follow *Rhus Tox.*, when the eruption becomes dry and begins to scale off.

Staphysagria, if it becomes most and offensive, attended with violent itching, to be followed by *Rhus Tox.* again.

Arsenicum Alb. must be given if, not withstanding the use of the above remedies, the disease becomes worse, with corrosive discharge or formation of ulcers, after this, *Rhus Tox.* will have a better effect. If the above remedies are insufficient, then the following will be required.

Hepar Sulp., especially when the disease extends to the forehead, face and neck, or when the eyes and eyelids become red and inflamed.

Bryonia Alba, when the glands of the neck and throat become *swollen, red and painful,* or if they are swollen and hard but not painful, *Dulcamara.*

Antimonium Crud. will be useful when a *thick scab* is formed on the head and the eruption extends over the entire face, with itching of the whole body.

In protracted cases, *Calcarea Carb., Lycopodium Clav.* and *Sulphur* will often prove useful.

28. SPASMS OR CONVULSIONS

(See the chapter on this subject)

29. TEETHING–DENTITION

The period of dentition in children is generally attended with a general derangement of health, greater restlessness than usual, especially at night, flushes of heat and alternate paleness of the face, the gums become swollen and hot, difficulty in sucking, the child frequently takes hold of the nipple and bites, disposition to bite at everything, inclination to loose bowels.

Aconitum Nap., when there is fever with much restlessness, sleeplessness and pain, as indicated by the child's crying and starting.

Belladonna, in convulsions caused by teething, the convulsion is followed by sound sleep, which continues for a long time, or until another fit comes again. The child starts from sleep as if frightened and looks around as if terrified, with a changed expression of the face, the pupils of the eyes are dilated and the eyes fixed, the whole body becomes stiff with burning heat in the palms of the hands and in the temples.

Calcarea Carb., when the teething is too slow in children of light complexion and who are inclined to be fat.

Chamomilla is *particularly* adapted to the *various diseases* of children *during* the period of *dentition* and especially when a child is *very spasmodic jerks and twitching of the limbs during sleep,* starts at the slightest noise, general heat, redness of one cheek and of the eyes, moaning, groaning, agitation, short, quick, noisy respiration and oppression of the chest, hacking cough, mouth

TREATMENT OF INFANTS

dry and hot, *diarrhea,* with watery, *slimy and greenish evacuations,* worse at night.

China off. may be given to children who wet the bed at night and grind their teeth during sleep and at other times, have hardness and distension of the abdomen, rub the nose and have a dry cough, resembling whooping cough.

Coffea, when the child is very excitable, does not sleep, is sometimes fretful and at other times too lively, with some fever.

Ignatia, when there are convulsive jerking of single limbs, frequent flushes of heat, sometimes followed by perspiration, the child wakes up form a light sleep with piercing cries and trembles all over.

Ipecac. is very useful in nausea and vomiting with diarrhea, the stools are mixed, of different colors.

Mercurius Sol. is useful for cases of *excessive flow of saliva from the month,* redness of the gums and *green evacuations* from the bowels with *straining.*

Sulphur, when the stools are whitish or hot and sour and excoriate the parts.

30. SUMMER COMPLAINTS

This disease is most prevalent during the summer and usually commences with nausea and vomiting, followed by diarrhea. The evacuations from the bowels are very frequent and may assume various forms, sometimes greenish, thin and watery, or yellowish, at others whitish or slimy and mixed with blood. Often the food is passed undigested and the odour is very offensive.

The most common exciting causes are improper diet, great changes of temperature, want of fresh air and teething. The latter is possibly the most frequent cause in children at this time.

Antimonium Crudum, when the tongue is coated white or yellow, dryness of the mouth, with thirst, nausea with vomiting or retching and cough, distension of the abdomen with flatulence, offensive, slimy stools and frequent passages of water.

Arsenicum Alb., if the child is very weak, pale and emaciated, inflammation of the abdomen, cold extremities, loss of appetite, nausea and vomiting, intense thirst, yellow and watery, white or brownish offensive diarrhea which is worse after midnight, towards morning and after eating or drinking.

Bryonia Alba, when the *diarrhea* comes on *in hot weather* and is *accompanied by much thirst,* vomiting of food, nausea and vomiting after eating, diarrhea with colic, the stools have a putrid smell, are white or brownish and lumpy.

Carbo Veg., if *Bryonia Alba* gives only temporary relief, especially if the evacuations are *very thin* and *offensive a*nd are *attended* with *burning* and *much pain.*

Dulcamara, if the complaint returns *every time the weather gets cool,* or *occur after drinking cold water,* while in a heat, violent thirst for cold water, *diarrhea of a greenish or brownish mucus, worse at night.*

Ipecac., if given at the *commencement* of the disease *will arrest its progress at once.* The symptoms for this remedy are- nausea and vomiting of food and drink, or of mucus and bile, with diarrhea of fermented stools, with white flocculent particles or tinged with blood, coated tongue, dislike for all food and extreme thirst. May be followed by *Nux Vomica, if Ipecac.* is not sufficient to arrest the disease.

Mercurius Sol., when the *diarrhea* is *worse before midnight* and is attended with *colic, straining at stool a*nd *perspiration,* evacuations scanty, greenish, sour, with nausea and eructations, if the children have a *great desire for butter.*

Calcarea Carb., for diarrhea with *thin, light colored stools, smelling like bad eggs,* vomiting, *much sweat on head, belly enlarged.*

China off., when there is *diarrhea after every meal*, the stools are very fetid and contain undigested portions of the food and there is *much wind in* the bowels.

Veratrum Alb, weakness from the *nausea* and vomiting is *so great as almost to cause fainting*, great exhaustion, vomiting and diarrhea, vomiting after swallowing the least liquid, *slightest movement excites vomiting*, great thirst for *cold water*, sensitiveness over the pit of the stomach, colic with burning and cutting pains in the abdomen, loose, brownish and blackish stools and small unnoticed evacuations of liquid stools.

Sulphur, useful in *protracted cases*, especially when the evacuations are *frequent and greenish*, thin and watery, or whitish and slimy.

31. HEAT SPOTS–PRICKLY HEAT

During the heat of the summer, infants and young children are troubled with an eruption consisting of small vesicles, generally, about the size of a pin's head, they are red, inflamed at the base and filled with watery fluid. After breaking, they sometimes form into thin scabs and sometimes ulcerate. There is more or less fever along with the eruption. *Aconitum Nap.* or *Chamomilla*, when there is much fever and restlessness. *Rhus Tox.*, if the eruption is extensive and if this is insufficient, *Arsenicum Alb.* or *Sulphur.*

Sulphur 200, at fortnightly intervals, to correct the tendency to the complaing.

32. DISCHARGE FROM THE EARS

Belladonna, Mercurius Sol., Chamomilla and *Pulsatilla* are the best remedies for the pain.

Mercurius Sol., Pulsatilla, Calcarea Carb., Rhus Tox. and *Sulphur* for the discharge.

33. LEUCORRHEA OR WHITES OF CHILDREN

Calcarea Carb., followed by *Pulsatilla* will be enough.

34. WEANING

Children may be weaned at about the age of ten months, or when the teeth have come out to enable them to chew solid food and the mother's milk may be dispensed with. At the same time *Pulsatilla* may be taken by the mother to stop the secretion of milk and relieve any discomfort caused by the continued secretion.

35. STUTTERING

This should be arrested in the beginning. It is cured by the use of *Belladonna*, followed later by *Mercurius Sol.* or *Platina* or *Euphrasia off.*, followed later by *Sulphur.*

36. BEDWETTING

Pulsatilla, for tender, gentle children inclined to weep, particularly if fat food does not agree with them, if little girls have the *whites,* if they put *the hands upon the abdomen, or both arms above the head.*

Nux Vomica, for children who become easily angry or are obstinate, if they put the arms *above or under the head.*

Rhus Tox., if the urine is acrid and passes *too quickly* even by *Bryonia Alba,* if the children are very peevish.

Sulphur, for pale, thin children with large bellies who are frequently unwell and eat much sugar. It is the *chief remedy in all cases* when you cannot decide upon the proper remedy.

Calcarea Carb., for stout fat children who drink much and perspire easily, if they pass urine more than once at night and have

TREATMENT OF INFANTS

frequent desire to pass urine during the day and passing little at a time, if they sleep lying on the belly, or put the arms over their head, follows *Sulphur* if it is not sufficient. *Belladonna*, if the urine passes involuntarily also during the day, especially when standing, or if the water passes *often* and in *large quantities*, if they *easily perspire* and *catch cold easily*.

Mercurius Sol., for easily perspiring children, who sometimes become suddenly weak, who have *great desire for butter*, if the urine is hot and smells sour.

Silicea, for children with swelled neck or boils, if wounds heal slowly, if the complaint came *after vaccination*.

Causticum, if they wet the bed during the first sleep, the urine *passes while coughing, sneezing, walking*, for children who can pass the stool or urine *only when standing*, but *not when sitting*.

Carbo Veg., if the urine is offensive.

37. OLDISH APPEARANCE OF A SUCKLING

If a suckling, three or four weeks old, had not grown and its face was like that of an old man, limbs lax, skin wrinkled, the bones of the skull had lapped over during birth, the parietals over each other and over the occiput. *Opium* 30, one dose *daily* till there is a change and may be repeated after a short interval, till there is relief.

CHAPTER XXI

DISEASES OF CHILDREN

Children are in the acute stage of life, rapidly growing and developing. The cell-life that clothes and binds them to earth is in a marvellous stage of activity. They are hypersensitive to influences that normally exercise less power later on. They are subject to disease that seldom attack adults. Besides this, with them, labelled diseases do not always run the same course as with their elders. For instance, what we call rheumatism-acute rheumatism is very different with widely different symptoms in the case of children, from that of adults.

First, we have to settle whether the ailment is acute or chronic and if it be the former, whether it occurs in a healthy or diseases child. A healthy child getting sick may present a few prominent symptoms due to some causes, which can be easily met by suitable remedies and the child will get cured more rapidly. A diseased child on the other hand, has been born with a family history and will require careful treatment even for acute troubles as these are based on the constitutional make-up and are brought about by various causes.

In Homeopathy the essentials, i.e., the symptoms so easy to get in the child and so all-important, if marked for a successful prescription, are briefly–

(a) *Disposition,* or more important still, change of disposition due to illness.

(b) *Fears,* habitual or, more important, new to child.

(c) *Sensitiveness,* even to the least noise or any outside impression.

DISEASES OF CHILDREN

(d) *Food cravings and loathings.*

(e) Any *rare* and *peculiar pathological symptoms,* which may be noticed.

    (i) Disposition : There may be extreme of this type. There may be obstinate *Natrium Mur.* and *Sepia* children who are not amenable to sympathy and there may be *Pulsatilla* children who are weepy, there are the heavy, lethargic and rather dull *Calcarea Carb.* type and the restless, suspicious and anxious *Arsenicum Alb. type a*nd there are the defiant, obstinate, passionate, sensitive and irritable *Nux Vom.* type and *Chamomilla* one which is not easily satisfied. Whatever the disease, these things must be taken into consideration in selecting the suitable medicine.

    (ii) *Fears:* One type of child will wander about alone, while another will want some one near. In some there may be fears of the dark, of wind of thunder, of strangers, of falling down, or of a bath.

    (iii) *Cravings and Loathings:* These are very strong in children and are very important in the selection of the remedy, as over-eating of any such article may be responsbile for the illness. Some are found of salt, some of sweets and some of earth, chalk or slate pencils, while others may dislike milk, salt or sweets.

    (iv) There are the dirty-nosed *Sulphur* children, the sweaty *Calcarea Carb.* children and the shy *Baryta Carb.* ones and the diseased children with glands and poor resistance to tubercle-all these points should be taken into consideration in the selection of the suitable remedies.

Some of the more common diseases to which children are subject, which come under the term 'scrofulosis' (see chapter XXII) and which may be treated more effectively by homeopathy during this period of life, are now dealt with. If these are attended to at an early stage, the children will be free from disease and will grow into healthy adult life, as they advance in age.

1. RICKETS-RACHITIS

Definition : This is a constitutional disease of childhood marked by increased cell growth of the bones, deficiency of earthy matter and deformities and changes in the liver and spleen, said to be due to lack of Vitamin D.

Causes : They are hereditary influences-chronic tuberculosis in the father and constitutional syphillis in the parents and cold, damp and ill-ventilated buildings.

Symptoms : Its premonitory symptoms are:-intestinal and bronchial catarrh, feverishness and restlessness towards evening and through the night, perspiration about the head, slow, irregular teething after a while, changes in the bony structure become apparent and the particular ends of the long bones swell.

Remedies

Calcarea Carb., for the fat, fair and lethargic type of child, with profusely sweating head, especially in sleep (*Silicea, Sanicula*), with soft, fat, flabby inadequate limbs that bend under its weight, with big abdomen.

Calcarera Phos., like *Calcarea Carb.*, head large, fontanelles long, open, but less sweating, bones of skull thin, even emaciated, sunk, flabby abdomen (reverse of *Calacarea Carb.*), spine too weak to support body, thin neck, too weak to support head, child pale and cold, seems stupid.

DISEASES OF CHILDREN

Silicea, pale, waxen, earthy face, head large (*Calcarea, Sulphur*) fontanelles open, body small and emaciated, except the plump abdomen, bones and muscles poorly developed, i.e., slow in learning to walk, worse from milk, infant unable to take any kind of milk (aethusa); diarrhea from milk; offensive sweat on head, neck, face and feet.

Sanicula, invaluable remedy for unflourishing, ill-developing children. Defective nutrition, thin and old-looking, dirty brownish skin, stubborn and touchy, cold, clammy hands and feet, profuse sweat about occiput and neck.

Sulphur, large head (like *Calcarea Carb.*), tendency to rickets (*Calc Carb.*), voracious appetite, defective assimilation, hungry, yet emaciated (*Iodum*), shrivelled and dried up, like a little old man, skin hangs in folds, yellowish wrinkled and flabby.

Chamomilla, intensely sensitive, intensely irritable, changeable, never satisfied, wants to be carried, can't keep still, painful gums, pain-colic, doubles and screams, kicks, diarrhea, grass-green stool, one cheek red, the other pale, coughing or ailments from anger, sleepy but can't sleep.

Arnica Mont. tender to touch, does not want to be disturbed, or irritated, or handled, worse from heat, especially if there has been any injury at birth or otherwise.

Alumina, abnormal cravings, liquid stools, with much straining, absence of sweat, dry, lustreless hair, persistent squint in the eye, slow in walking, speaking, cutting teeth, large head, open fontanelles, bathed in cold sweat, voracious appetite, distended abdomen, progressive wasting, persistent watery diarrhea.

Natrium Mur. particularly useful when the thighs are notably emaciated and the disese is in its very early stages, with slight pliability of the bones.

2. SCURVY

Arnica Mont., as detailed above a *great remedy here*.

Phosphorus, bruising, effusion of fluid into the tissue.

Kreosotum, gums bleed and ulcerate, offensive odours, mouth etc.,

As a constitutional treatment is required in all the cases referred to in this chapter, the instructions given in the *'Introduction'* for the treatment of chronic diseases of children, regarding the potencies to be employed from time to time and intervals to be allowed between doses, should be followed.

As all these diseases are deficiency diseases, due to lack of vitamins and essential salts. It is necessary to attend the proper dieting of the children, in addition to the administration of appropriate remedies. The general use of the sunbaths and the addition to the daily diet of plenty of green vegetables, fruit juices, wheat oats or other whole-grain preparations and whole milk, in place of white bread, meat, coffee, tea and white sugar and the use of egg-yolk and codliver oil are essential, for the improvement of the constitution.

3. MALNUTRITION, WASTING, MARASMUS

The principal remedies with diagnostic symptoms are:

Calcarea Carb., coldness, profuse sweats, head (*silicea*), at night (*silicea*), cold, damp feet, cold legs with night sweats, milk disagree (*Calcarea Phos, Natrium Carb., Magnesium Carb., Aethusa Sil*), big head, with large hard abdomen *(Sil)*, stomach swollen, distended, even with the rest of body emaciated, malnutrition, glands, bones and skin, faulty bone development, late teething and deficient teeth, sourness of sweat, of sweating head, sour stool, sour vomit, constipation with white stools, pass and vomit worms, chew and swallow, or grit teeth in sleep *(Cina)*, cross and fretful, easily frightened.

DISEASES OF CHILDREN

Calcarea Phos, vomits milk *(Calcarea Carb., Natrium Carb., Magnesium Carb.),* stools green slimy with foetied flatus, face pale, white, sallow, neck cannot support head, marasmus, shrunken, emaciated and very anemic, tall scrawing children with dirty, brownish skin, peevish, restless, fretful, flabby, sunken abdomen (opposite of *Calc. Carb.*).

Phosphorus, tall, slender, delicate, grows too rapidly, delicate, waxy anemic, hectic blush, bleed easily, bruise easily, sensitive to cold, love to be touched and rubbed, fear that something will happen, of thunder, of the dark, of being alone, indifferent, desire for cold water, ices, salt, savouries, may complain of a hot spine, chilly patient, yet stomach and head better from cold, chest and limbs better from heat, *better from sleep-* from short sleep *(Sepia).*

Tuberculinum, deep-acting, long acting, affects constitutions more deeply than most remedies *(Sulph., Sil. Dros.),* Tubercular family history, debilitated and anemic, hopelessness, desire to travel, to go somewhere, sensitive, dissatisfied, fear of dogs, aversion to meat, craves cold milk, excessive sweat in chronic diarrhea, driven out of bed with diarrhea, air hunger, suffocated in a warm room, better riding in a cold wind worse damp cold, old dingy look, very red lips *(Sulph.)* and very blue outer skin of the eye-balls.

Sulphur, ravenous hunger, especially at 11 a.m. *Heat vertex, with cold feet,* wakes screaming, great voracity, puts everything into its mouth, drinks much and eats little, craves much fat, slow, lazy, hungry and always tired, red lips, nostrils, eye-lids, anus, stool offensive, excoriating, frequent, slimy diarrhea or obstinate constipation, hates bath, worse after bath, limbs emaciate with distended abdomen, emaciates even with good appetite *(Iodum),* eruptions, itching, worse at night, boils.

Psorinum, pale, sickly, delicate children look unwasted, *(Sulph.)* have a filthy smell even after a bathin, dread of the bath *(Sulph.),* very chilly, worse open air, also worse warm bed, stools fluid, fetid.

Sepia, indifference, absence of joy, comprehension difficult, progressive emaciation, skin wrinkles, child looks like a shrivelled, dried-up old man, freckled, across nose and cheeks, child wets the bed in first sleep, damp cold legs and feet *(Calc).*

Silicea, child weak, puny, from defective assimilation, large head, body small, emaciated, except abdomen which is round and plump, face pale, waxy, earthy or yellowish, pinched and old looking, limbs shrunken, bones and muscles poorly developed, for the reason late walking, coldness, chilliness, head sweats profusely, in sleep *(Calcarea Carb.),* offensive sweat, head and face, offensive foot sweat, little injuries fester, poor healing, boils and pustules and sepsis, want of self-confidence.

Natrium Mur., nutrition impaired, eats and emaciates all the time *(Iodum),* emaciation, weakness, nervous prostration, nervous irritability, skin shiny, pale, waxy, as if greased, or skin dry, withered, shrunken, an infant looks like a little old man *(Iodum, Abrotanum, Sanicula),* collar bones become prominent and neck scrawny, but hips and lower limbs remain plump and round (opp. of *Abrot, Lycopodium* also emaciates downwards). Children with *voracious appetite, yet emaciates (Iod., Sulph.).* One of the few mapped-tongue remedies, gets herpes about lips, terrible headaches, craving for salt, hates bread and fats, weeps easily, but not amenable to sympathy.

Abrotanum, emaciation mostly of legs; Ascending type (rev. of *Natrium Mur., Lycopodium),* bloated abdomen, cross, irritable children, pale, hollow-eyed, old face *(Iodum, Natrium Mur., Sulph.),* wrinkled, appetite very great, *ravenous opposite while emaciating (Iodum),* in marasmus, skin flabby and hangs loose.

Iodum, general emaciation, wants to eat all the time, While the body withers, the glands enlarge, *(Abrotanum, Natrium Mur.),* always hungry, eats between meals and is yet hungry, better eating, emaciates with an enormous appetite, excitement, anxiety, impulses,

DISEASES OF CHILDREN

worse trying to keep still, worse heat, better cold *(Lyc.)* (Opp. of *Sil.*), *always too hot.*

Sanicula, child looks old *(Argentum Nit.),* dirty, greasy and brownish, progressive emaciation, kicks off clothing in coldest weather *(Sulph.),* sweats on falling asleep, mostly neck, wets clothing through *(Calcarea Carb., Sil.),* cold, clammy sweat, occiput and neck, child craves meat, fat, salt. *(Natrium Mur.), child wants to nurse all the time, yet loses flesh.* After intense straining, the stool nearly evacuated, recedes *(Sil.),* foul foot-sweat, chafes toes *(Sil.).*

Lycopodium, emaciates from above downwards *(Sanicula, Natrium Mur.),* lower limbs fairly nourished, flatulent, distended like a drum *(Argentum Nit.).* Can hardly breathe, so full, he cannot eat, wakes 'ugly', worse 4 to 8 p.m., no self-confidence *(Sil.)* miseries of anticipation *(Argentum Nit., Sil.),* cries when thanked, when receiving a gift, withered lads, with dy cough, headache, better from cold, worse warm room *(Iod.),* red sand in urine, craves sweets *(Argentum Nit.),* hot drinks, *one foot hot, one cold (characteristic).* Sickly, wrinkled face with contracted eye-brows.

Argentum Nit., child looks dried up like a mummy, old looking, pale, bluish face, progressive emaciation, craves sweets *(Lycopodium Clav.)* which disagree, wants cold air *(Lycopodium Clav.),* cold drinks (opp. of *Lycopodium Clav.),* craves salt *(Phos., Natrium Mur.).* A most flatulent remedy *(Lycopodium Clav.)* distended to bursting *(Lycopodium Clav.).* Emotional diarrhea, from anticipation *(Gels.),* examination funk, fear of high places.

Arsenicum, atrophy of infants, marasmus, face pale, anxious, distored, skin harsh, dry, tawny, rapid emaciation, sinking of strength. Least effort exhausting, chilliness, diarrhea as soon as begins to eat or drink, stools undigested, offensive, *anxiety, restlessness, prostration, burning* and *cadaveric odours,*

Hepar Sulph., sour smell *(Calcarea Carb.)*, white *(Calcarea Carb.)*, fetid evacuations, undigested stools, seems better after feeding *(Natrium Mur.)*, chilly, over-sensitive to cold, to dry cold, to draughts *(Nux Vom., Sulph.)*, to touch, mild, also over-sensitive every little thing makes him angry, abusive impulsive *(Nux Vom.)*. Quarrelsome *(Nux Vom.)*, little injuries fester *(Sil.)*, are very sensitive, ears discharge, lax, chilly, sweats all night, *worse* cold, *better* warm, wrapped up *(Sil.)* Nux Vom., over-sensitive, irritable, touchy, never satisfied, violent temper uncontrollable, very chilly cannot uncover (rev. of *Sulph.*), always selecting his food and digesting almost none, yellow, sallow, bloated face, constipation, alternately diarrhea and constipation, irregular peristalsis, i.e., contents of intestines driven both ways, i.e., fitful or fruitless urging to stool.

Natrium Carb., nervous, withered infants, cannot stand milk, diarrhea from milk, aversion to milk, abdomen hard and bloated, much flatus, loud rumbling, worse and especially hungry at 11 p.m. and 5 a.m., headache from any mental exertion, 'ankles turn'-weak.

Baryta Carb., 'dwarfishness of mind and body and of organs', enlarged glands, enlarged abdomen, emaciation of tissues, emaciated limbs and dwarfishness of mind shy, bashful, easily frightened.

In cases that make no progress, on account of syphilitic or sycotic taint, the following remedies will be useful:

Leuticum. Dwarfish *(Baryta Carb.)*, marasmic, *worse at night*, impulse to wash hands, where the syphilitic taint is far to progress.

Medorrhinum, sycotic taint blocks progress, poor reaction, lies on abdomen, sleeps in knee-elbow position, fiery-red, moist, itching anus *(Sulph.)*, worse by day (opp. of *Leut.*).

4. TUBERCULOSIS

Diseases of Glands and Bones

The treatment of 'T.B.' glands and bones in children is a

DISEASES OF CHILDREN

great triumph for homeopathy. There have been numerous cases of children of 6 or 8 years of age, 'eaten up' with tubercle, who, from babyhood have been 'never without a bandage' and subject to repeated operations, where homeopathic treatment has not only promptly stopped further progress of the disease, but has closed the wounds, while long suffering and feeble existence were replaced by new energy and health. There were others also of children with tubercle who had hideous scars round the neck, on chest, arm and leg and who were successfully treated and brought to health in 2 or 3 years. These cures have been possible only with the constitutional treatment followed with the use of several remedies proved and worked out by Hahnemann and his fellow workers.

Therapeutic Hints

Drosera, excels all other remedies in T. B. gland and bone and is indicated in all tubercular manifestations, or a strong family history of tuberculosis. Under its influence, glands of neck, if they have to 'break', produce only very small opening, old suppurating glands soon diminish in size and close old cicatrical tissues yield and soften, deep tied down scars relax and come up so that deformity is greatly lessened. While the improvement in health, in appearance in nutrition, is rapid and striking, *Drosera* has also great use in the diseases of joints and bones (in persons with a T.B. history), even when these are not tuberculous, quickly taking every pain and improving health and well-being. Hahnemann urged that *Drosera* should be given in frequent doses and in the 30th potency. It is advisable to give *Drosera* 30 at fortnightly intervals to start with.

Silicea, hardened glands, especially about the neck, "Scrofulous glands", a deep remedy for eradicating the tuberculous tendency, when symptoms agree, *worse,* in wet, cold weather, *better* in dry, cold weather, but very chilly, tendency to swelling of glands, which suppurate, the *Silicea* child is timid, lacks confidence, 'grit, head sweats in sleep *(Calcarea Carb.)*; for nearly all diseases of bone, fistulous openings, discharge offensive, swollen, pouting, bluish-red; sweat of feet, often, offensive feet.

Symphytum, in a case of necrosis of lower jaw after an accident where *Sil.* and *Tub.* failed to improve, *Symphytum* healed, the *left, lower jaw* being an *important location* for the remedy. It is an out-standing remedy for bone *(Dros. Phos.).*

Sepia, a case of T. B. bone with a sinus on each side of the right middle finger, one above and one below the first joint, was cured, *because the individual symptoms demanded Sepia* and this is an important point to remember that *it is the remedy called for by the individual symptoms of the patient, that will stimulate him to put his house in order and get well.* The typical *Sepia* patient is indifferent, over-burdened, dull, has auxiliary sweats, offensive *(Sil.),* hates noise and smells, only wants to get away, alone and be quiet.

Sulphur, princes of remedies in scrofula-in caries in early childhood, voracious appetite, greedily clutches at all that is offered, edible or not, as if starved, shrivelled and dried up, like a little old man.

Tuberculinum, patients with a T. B. family history, or with T. B. manifestations, glands etc., a deep acting, long acting remedy, closely related to *Calcarea Carb.,* the one may be indicated, then the other *(Sil., Dros.),* always wanting to go somewhere-to travel, feeble vitality, tired, debilitated, losing flesh, emaciation, with hunger *(Iodum),* worse, in a close room, in damp weather, *better,* cold wind open air, desire for alcohol, bacon, fat, ham, smoked meat, cold milk, refreshing things, sweets.

Calcarea Carb., affects the glands of the neck and all the glands, glands of abdomen become hard, sore, inflamed, useful in T. B. formations, calcareous degenerations, necrosis of bone in

DISEASES OF CHILDREN

such children, very useful in T. B. abdomen when symptoms agree *(Psorinum,* when odour of child is very offensive)

Phosphorus, like *Drosera* appears to break down resistance to tubercle, since workers in match factories have been especially liable to consumption and have suffered from caries and necrosis of bone. It helps to cure not only bone troubles, but also 'scrofulous glands', but always in the typical slender *Phos.* children, who grow too rapidly, delicate, waxy, anemic, bruise easily, easy bleeders with thirst for *cold water,* hunger for salt, love of ices, are nervous alone-fear the dark, rather apathetic and indifferent.

Iodum, scrofulous swellings and induration of glands, large, hard, usually painless, torpidity and sluggishness, cross and *restless,* impulses, anxiety, the more he keeps still, the more anxious, always too hot, eats ravenously, yet emaciates, dark hair and complexion *(Bromium,* fair and blue eyes). Enlargement of all the glands, except the mammae, these waste and atrophy, compelled to keep on doing something to drive away his impulses and anxiety *(Arsenicum Alb.),* but *Iodum* is warmblooded and wants cold, while *Arsenicum Alb.* is cold and wants heat, warm room, warm clothing etc.

Bromium, very useful in enlarged glands with great hardness without any tendency to suppurate, glands that take on tuberculosis, tissues take on tuberculosis, glands that inflame for a while, begin to take a lower from of degeneration swelling and induration of the gland is a strong feature of the remedy; the needing *Bromium* for chronic glands, will have a grey earthy color of face, oldish appearance, or plethoric children with red face easily over-heated, left-sided remedy, *worse* dampness, weak and easily overheated, then sweaty and sensitive to draughts, glands in persons of light complexion, fair skin and light blue eyes (distinguishes from *Iodum),* tonsils deep-red, swollen, with network of dilated vessels.

Baryta Carb., glands swell, infiltrate, hypertrophy, sometimes suppurate, dwarfish children, late to develop, with dwarfish minds, slow, inept, mistrustful of strangers, shy, affected by every cold;

cold, foul foot-sweat *(Sil.)*, tearing and tension in long bones, boring in bones.

Mercurius Sol., a curious but useful symptom, "sensation of shivering in an abscess", or in a sinus from diseased bone.

Calcarea Iod., for cases of suppurating glands, sometimes causing them to reabsorb and disappear without discharging, when there would be only a little thickening of tissue, like a tiny scar, left, cases which are typical *Calcarea Carb.* patients, except that they were *hot and hungry*.

5. EPIDEMIC DIARRHEA OF CHILDREN

Baptisia Tinct., taken *suddenly* and frightfully ill. Sudden attack of diarrhea and vomiting, with a typhoid condition. Foetid, exhausting diarrhea, with excoriation. Odour of stool putrid, penetrating. Tongue swollen, dark, dry, yellow or brown centre, cracked, ulcerated (comp. *Arsenicum Alb.*). Drowsy, as if *drugged* or intoxicated. If a roused, begins to speak, then fades back into stupor. *Dark, red, besotted countenance.* Hot-flushed-dusky. Influenza cases.

Veratrum Alb., diarrhea *with violent vomiting, vomit- stools, sweat very profuse.* Thirst for much cold water, for acid drinks. Exhaustion after each spell. *Cold sweat* on forehead from least movement.

Carbo Veg., putrid or bloody, offensive stools. Acrid. Face pale or greenish, abdomen distended, in lumps. Emission of large quantities of flatus. *Skin damp, cold, tongue and breath cold.* (The Homeopathic veritable corpse-revivor).

Bryonia Alba, diarrhea *from hot weather* and the return of hot weather. Vomits food immediately. Colic, with thirst for big drinks and lumpy diarrhea. Dry, parched lips.

DISEASES OF CHILDREN

Dulcamara, every change of weather to cold, brings diarrhea (rev. of *Bry.*). Exposure to cold or damp. Nausea with desire for stool. Colic, before and during stool. Prostration, changeable stools.

Croton Tig., yellow, watery stools, *come out like a shot,* while nursing and immediately after. Any food or drink starts this stool. A hand pressing on umbilicus produced protrusion of rectum.

Aloes Soct., hurry to stool after eating or drinking. *Inability to retain-or to evacuate stool.* (Straining may fail to produce stool, which presently slips out unnoticed).

Kreosote, cholera infantum in teething infants, *with very painful dentition,* seems painful, spongy. Severe cases with incessant vomiting and stools cadaverously smelling. Intensely irritable *(Cham.).*

Chamomilla, watery, greenish stools, excoriating, smell like rotten eggs, very cross *(Kreos.),* must be carried. Especially in teething babies.

Belladonna, drowsiness *(Baptisia),* with dry, burning heat. Pupils dilated. Stools green, small, frequent. Colic before stool, straining. Child starts with every noise, twitches.

Colocynth, paroxysms of severe colicky pain precede stools. Immediately after eating. *Relief from doubling up and pressure.* Frothy stools. Stools watery, then bilious, then bloody, excoriating, frquent, not profuse.

Magnisium Phos., very like *Colocynth,* but *urgently demands heat as well as pressure.*

6. SEVERE URGENT CASES WITH COLLAPSE

Aethusa, intolerance of milk. Face expresses anxiety and pain. Pearly whiteness on upper lip, bounded by a distinct line to anges of mouth. Violent vomiting of milk, after milk. Stool undigested, thin, green bilious. Violent straining before and after stool. *Collapse,* almost as bad as *Arsenicum Alb.,* except restless. A remedy of violence, violent vomiting, violent convulsions, violent pains, violent diarrhea.

Arsenicum Alb., worse at night, 1 to 3 A.M. Rapid emaciation, *exhaustion and collapse, intense restlessness (Pyrog.),* (opp. of *Aethusa).* Painless, offensive, watery stools. There may be simultaneous vomiting and diarrhea *(Ipec.).* After cold drinks, when heated, in older persons, after ices. Thirst for cold water, immediately vomited, coldness of extremities. Pale, cadaverous face. Skin dry, wrinkled, toneless.

Camphor, skin cold as marble (Carbo Veg.), but child will not remain covered. Great prostration and diarrhea. Dosage, give a drop of strong tincture on sugar. Repeat it within 5 to 15 mts., if case urgent. Keep *Camphor* away from homeopathic medicines.

Pyrogen, extreme restlessness, has to keep on moving. Only momentary relief from moving, but has to move for that relief (comp. *Rhus Tox.).* Diarrhea with frightfully offensive stools *(Bapt Tinct.).* Profuse, watery, painless stools, sometimes with vomiting.

CHAPTER –XXII

GENERAL DYSCRASIAS AND CONSTITUTIONAL TREATMENT

1. SCROFULOSIS

This terms is applied to a deprived condition of nutrition which appears among children and young people upto the age of pubescence in the form of glandular swellings, skin eruptions, affections of the bone of every description, marasmus, malnutrition, and tubercular tendency. The scrofulous diathesis (constitutional and predisposition to disease), can be inherited from scrofulous or tuberculous parents, although children from such parents may be entirely free from any scrofulous taint. It has also been attributed to parental tentiary syphilis, carcinoma, advanced age, or when parents have been near-relatives. *Acquired,* it may be, by poor or faulty diet, or by the want of exercise and fresh air, frequently, by the joint action of different, unhealthy influences.

It is possible to confine the scrofulous disease to this early period, by suitable constitutional treatment with Homeopathic remedies. The remedies required for this purpose are detailed in Chapter XXI. If, however, this disease is not treated in the early stage, it develops in adult life in the form of tubercles in the lungs, brain, liver, bowels and other organs, and later on, as chronic skin affections, polypi, cataract and other analogous forms of disease which in their complex, furnish a striking parallel to what Hahnemann has grouped together under the name of *'psora'* in his "chronic diseases". Even the scrofulous diathesis in adults can be treated by Hahnemann and his followers, on the basis of the totality of the most prominent, characteristic symptoms observed in each individual case, before they develop into the fully formed disease. Even modern medicine is slowly beginning to realise the fundamental teachings of Hahnemann over a hundred years ago. Tuberculin, 'Diphtheria Serum', the various organ preparations, and vaccines, and their mode of employment, the attention given to mental symptoms, to special bodily constitutions and tendency to disease (vitamin and mineral salt deficiencies, glandular deficiencies, allergy etc.) show, how for this change has been accomplished. The vaccines and serum therapy is closely similar to homeopathy in the use of similar remedy, and small dose. In fact, the vaccine of today is the nosode of yesterday.

There are, however, fundamental differences between homeopathy and modern allopathy in the matter of diagnosis and administration of medicines.

(*a*)   Hahnemann showed that 'homeopathy is absolutely inconceivable without the most precise individualisation.' The name of diseases should never influence the physician who has to judge, and cure diseases, not by names, but by the signs and symptoms of each individual patient. That, since diseases can only express their need for relief by symptoms, the totality of the symptoms observed in each individual case of disease, can be the only indication to guide in the choice of the remedy. He taught also that all parts of the body are intimately connected to form an invisible whole in feelings and functions, that all curative measures should be planned with reference to the whole system, in order to cure the general disease by means of internal remedies.

(*b*)   The allopathic doctor makes a physical examination of the patient, in order to give a name to the disease, and prescribe therefore, but does not take into consideration the general constitution of the patient, and the symptoms he feels, and also the cause of the trouble. He has to prescribe a remedy which will give the patient immediate relief.

The homeopathic physician, however, prescribes appropriate constitutional remedy, based on the symptoms, small in dose, and of a suitable potency, so as to fit in with the condition of the patient, without reference to the name of the disease. It is intended to give him relief as quickly as possible, and at the same time to tone up the constitution so as to give him a cure of the present trouble, and prevent a recurrence of the trouble, or leave any after-effects.

(c) As the allopaths are of the opinion, that the dose should be the largest tolerated, and that its repetition is a matter of opinion or individual practice, they prescribe their doses as strong as may be required for giving quick relief to the patient. The strong doses may give relief to the patient for time being, but by their strong action suppress the trouble, and do not effect a cure. So long as the root cause of the trouble is not eliminated, the chances are, that the patient may get the trouble again in some other form, and is never free. It is unfortunate that the allopaths don't realise the idea, which was propagated by Hahnemann that there is a law of nature governing all these matters. The Arndt law, which was arrived at, after numerous experiments, states that the same poison given to the same cell, may be legal, inhibitive or stimulating, according to the largeness and smallness of the dose. Professor Bier of Germany, also endorse Hahnemann's idea as regards the infinite sensitiveness of diseased parts to the vital stimulus. The small homeopathic dose which is dynamized, as taught by Hahnemann, has a distinct, curative action, and leaves no bad effects.

(d) *Vaccine and Serum Therapy*

(i) Vaccines and sera have been used in allopathy on the basis of their bacterial relationship alone, without taking into account, reactions and idiosyncrasies of the patients treated with them.

Homeopathic remedies, on the other hand, have been proved on healthy human beings, who could express their feelings and reactions to the remedies taken by them, and all the symptoms produced have been verified and recorded in the Materia Medica. So, medicines, prescribed according to the law of similar, have their specific action on the patient.

(*ii*) The doses of vaccines and sera are far too large, and, therefore, the sections caused by their use are, for the most part, strong and injurious.

(*iii*) The vaccines and sera are administered by hypodermic injections. It is well-known that foreign proteins, when introduced into healthy organisms direct, without the intervention of the natural channel of absorption, may produce many complicated reactions, and thus prove deleterious. Homeopathic remedies taken orally are quickly absorbed in a few minutes, and leave no after-effects.

(e) *Vitamins and hormone therapy*

In the case of deficiency diseases, the lack or deficiency of the mineral salts, in spite of our taking plenty of foods rich in vitamins and mineral salts, was due to the inability of the system to appropriate the same from the foods, and this defect cannot be remedied by administering the same vitamins and salts in a *concentrated form* in the form of tablets, or with the idea, that it will be much more readily absorbed in the system, but, as in that condition of the body, it can appropriate only a small fraction, and repeated doses of the same concentrated product will be necessary to produce any appreciable change. So, the more rational way of improving the constitution will be, to give the deficient mineral salt in an extremely attenuated preparation, to stimulate the system to better action. Homeopathic remedies in suitable potencies, if administered to the patient, will stimulate the digestive system sufficiently to enable it to absorb the natural vitamins and mineral salts from the cereal foods and vegetables we ordinarily take, and will have a better effect on the whole.

(f) Allergy and Allergens

Allergy is a condition of unusual or exaggerated specific susceptibility to a substance in some persons, which is harmless to a majority of persons, given in like amounts, and under the same conditions.

Certain food products produce urticaria, nausea, vomiting, diarrhea, etc., in some persons, which are harmless to others. Similarly certain drugs and medicines would be borne by the majority, while the same would produce allergic symptoms, and even toxic manifestation in those specifically sensitive. This food and drug allergy is, probably, more extensively present than is ordinarily known, and may first show itself in childhood, and continue throughout life, unless corrected in time.

Over one hundred years ago, Hahnemann recognised this fact, and called this *'Idiosyncrasies'*. In para. 117 of the *Organon,* he defines this as "peculiar constitutions which, though otherwise healthy, possess a disposition to be brought into a more or less morbid state by certain things which *seem* to produce no impressions or changes in many other individuals".

To this he adds a note as follows– "Some persons are apt to faint from smell of roses and to fall into many other morbid and, sometimes, dangerous states from partaking of mussels, crabs, and fish roe, or from touching the leaves of some kinds of sumach *(Rhus Tox.)*."

Dr. Kent notes that certain subjects cannot take opium, because of dangerous congestions arising, even from the smallest doses. He also cites that quinine made some alarmingly sick, while, one would take 15 grains and have no symptoms, that lavender flowers produce coryza in one, the eating of peaches always produce diarrhea in another. He regarded craving for salt as a distinctive symptom of the psoric or tubercular diathesis.

This idiosyncrasy, or hypersensitivity is called 'Allergy' in modern medicine, and is purely constitutional. It can be corrected at a very early stage in children, by suitable homeopathic remedies prepared according to the law of *'Similia Similibus Curantar'*. Thus, we have for cases of chronic poisoning by cane sugar- *'Saccharum Officinalis'*,

For Quininism–*Cinchona Sulphuricum'* high,

For susceptibility to parsley–*'Petroselinum 30'*,

For Hypersensitiveness to *Rhus* Poisoning–*'Rhus Tox.30'*,

For Rabies–*'Hydrophobinum'*,

For Anthrax–*'Anthracinum'*,

For Tuberculosis–*'Tuberculinum'*, in potency, etc.

For adults of a scrofulous diathesis who have not been treated in their early years, it will be helpful to give constitutional treatment for some of the more common diseases, before they reach the *incipient* stage, and so avert a development into full-fledged diseases. The course of treatment is given in outline for all such cases, in general, and, if it is pursued vigorously for some time, it will be possible to prevent further development.

2. TUBERCULOSIS

The earliest indications for this trouble are:
(*a*) Chronic, periodical headache at a circumscribed spot, where a dull pressure is experienced, which is, now and then accompanied by paroxysms of vertigo, or
(*b*) Painful pressure at a circumscribed spot in the vertebral column, from which very violent, burning and lancinating

GENERAL DYSCRASIAS AND CONSTITUTIONAL TREATMENT

pains sometimes emanate, with occasional twitching in more remote localities, or

(c) A variety of gastric and digestive complaints, when accompanying a seated pain in the region of the liver, with periodical lancinating pains flashing from below upwards.

In all these cases, it is better to commence with *Sulphur 30*, and after *four weeks*, a dose of *Calcarea Carb. 30*, and after *eight weeks*, a dose of *Lycopodium Clav. 30*. These three remedies if allowed to work for long periods, will have cleared the system sufficiently in most cases, and the patient will feel better. If, after *four weeks*, the improvement is not *sfuficient*, the same medicines may be given, in the 200th potency, with an interval of *six weeks* between each.

If, however, after the first three doses are given there is no *real improvement*, on account of particular organs being specifically affected, it will be necessary to give other remedies to supplement the action of the three remedies.

Four weeks after the dose of *Lycopodium Clav. 30*, the following medicines may be given:

If the brain is principally affected, *Phos. 30*, if the spinal cord, *Caust. 30, Baryta Carb. 30* or *Phos. 30*, according to characteristic symptoms.

If the liver, *Silicea 30*. These medicines may be given after intervals of *four weeks* between each. If, however, pulmonary tubercles are distinctly present, eight weeks after the dose of *Calcarea Carb. 30, Phos. 30* may be given, and if, after four weeks, this is not enough, *Hep Sulp. 30* and then, after *four weeks, Spong 30*.

Each dose consisting of two globules No.10 (or one globule No.20), may be dissolved in one ounce of distilled water, and given as one dose. If there is only slight improvement, after the doses are given as above, and if further doses may be necessary, the same medicines may be given in the *200th* potency with an interval of *six weeks* between each.

The idea of giving *Sulphur, Calcarea Carb.* and *Lycopodium Clav.* to start with, in this order in all cases, is that they will regulate all kinds of constitutions, and improve them sufficiently, but if they are not enough, on account of particular organs being affected, they will, at least, have prepared the ground for the speedier action of the indicated remedy, which may be given after these. Longer intervals between doses are specifically mentioned in these cases, as scrofulosis being a chronic and slowly progressing disease, there should be no objection to allow an anti-scrofulous medicine to act for a long time, since by this means, all other *voluntary* manifestations of the scrofulous disease are prevented, rather than promoted, and, if any should take place, are very generally wiped out by the power of the progressively acting drug.

3. GLANDULAR AFFECTIONS

Although in the majority of cases, these affection of a scrofulous nature, yet, they may likewise arise from other causes, and may require a more immediate, somewhat palliative treatment. If scrofulous persons are afflicted with simple glandular swellings on the neck, inguinal region, or in the axilla, *Sulphur 30, Calcarea Carb. 30, Lycopodium Clav. 30, Silicea 30,* with intervals of *four weeks* between each. If they fail to disappear within *four weeks,* after the last medicine, *Dulc. 30, Hep. S. 30, Bell. 30,* or *Merc Sol. 30,* according to indications, may be given at intervals of *four weeks.* If the glands are very much inflamed, and threaten to break, *Merc Sol. 30* may be given first. If the glands have begun to suppurate, *Hep. Sulph. 30* and *Silicea 30,* or *Mercurius Sol. 30,* according to indications, may be given at intervals of *four* weeks. or, in chronic cases, *Bell. 30, Sulph 30* and *Calcarea Carb. 30* may be given in this order at *weekly* intervals. If the glands have hardened, *Baryta Carb. 30* and then *Carbo An 30,* may be given at intervals of *four weeks.*

4. DISEASES OF THE BONES

The treatment may be commenced with *Sulphur 30, Calcarea Carb. 30, Lycopodium Clav. 30.* and *Silicea 30*. If these are not enough, the following remedies, indicated by the nature of the affection, will be required, and may be given *four weeks* after the dose of *Silicea 30.*

In syphilitic bone diseases:
> *Mercurius Sol., Aurum Met., Phos., Phos. Ac.*

In mercurial bone diseases:
> *Aurum Met., Asaf., Fluor Ac., Mez.*

In inflammations:
> *Mez., Phos., Mercurius Sol., Phos. Ac.*

In swelling of the bones:
> *Asaf., Aurum Met., Mercurius Sol., Fluor Ac.*

In curvatures:
> *Bell., Puls., Asaf.*

In Necrosis:
> *Silicea, Calcarea Carb., Sulph.*

In Caries:
> *Silicea, Sulph., Calcarea Carb., Aurum Met., Fluor Ac.*

One dose of the indicated remedy, in one ounce of water, as *one* dose. In chronic diseases of the bone where the nature of the affection is known, it is best to commence with one dose of the *indicated* remedy, in one ounce of water, one dose in the *first week*, and then, after an interval of *four weeks*, *Sulph. 30, Calcarea Carb. 30, Lycopodium Clav. 30, Silicea 30* with intervals of four weeks, and then after an interval of four weeks, one dose of the indicated remedy again. That is one dose of the indicated remedy during the first week, followed by *Sulph. 30, Calarea Carb. 30, Lycopodium Clav. 30* and *Silicea 30* and last of all another dose of the indicated remedy. If the improvement is not distinct, another more suitable indicated remedy should be chosen and given in the same way as indicated above. If, however, there is some improvement, but not enough, the same order of medicines in the *200th* potency may be taken as before, the indicated remedy in the *200th* potency, to be followed by *Sulphur, Calcarea Carb., Lycopodium Clav.* and *Silicea* in the *200th* potency, and last of all, another dose of the indicated remedy in the *200th* potency.

5. ADVANTAGES OF CONSTITUTIONAL TREATMENT

Summary

Preventive treatment is far better than the treatment of a disease, after it is fully developed, while allopathy can treat patients only after a disease is fully developed and diagnosed, and a name given to it, as medicines are prescribed only for removing the pathological symptoms which appear as the effect of the disease. So, numerous medicines are prescribed, either in the form of mixtures or as sub-cutaneous injections, which are *strong* and *powerful* in action, and on account of the strength and massiveness of the doses, although they remove the symptoms of the patient, and give him relief, they have not a *mild curative* action, but merely *suppress* the trouble for the time being, 'Dr. William Howard Hay, M.D., an eminent surgeon of U.S.A. in his book, "A New Health Era", has said that all the powders, pills, mixtures tonics, etc., which the allopathic physicians prescribe, contain minerals and acids, which are not eliminated from the system, in spite of several purgatives, etc., but are embedded in the tissues and joints of the body, and are the causes of further ill health and disease, and that this fact is not generally recognised, and there are no medicines to counter-act these effects, or eliminate them from the system.

If the patients who have had allopathic treatment, fall sick again, it may be the return of the old trouble, due to the same original cause, but, in a new form, or may be a drug disease. With further treatment along the old lines for all the diseases that may crop up from time to time, the body becomes a repository of the remnants of the drugs. The patient always has the elements of disease in his body, threatening to break out, for any reason and at any time, such as, either exposure to any sudden change of weather, or due to wrong, or improper diet. Such patients cannot claim to be healthy, in the real sense, though they may appear to be healthy, and may be able to carry on their ordinary avocations normally. These conditions apply to both acute and chronic diseases. So, there is no constitutional treatment, and no preventive treatment, except in the vaccine and serum injections, given during epidemics, which leave their own effects. The efficacy of B. C. G. injections, which are now given on a large scale, can be judged only after some years.

Homeopathic treatment is both preventive and curative. In the case of fevers, for example, though there may be violent symptoms which may indicate influenza, malaria or typhoid, yet by the administration of suitable remedies, according to the symptoms, in the early stages, it is possible to prevent it from developing into the full form of the disease, whatever it may have been. Similarly, other acute diseases may also be treated suitably and prevented from becoming chronic. Persons of a scrofulous diathesis can also be treated, and helped from developing serious chronic diseases.

The small doses of potentized homeopathic remedies have no material substance in them, and act *dynamically* on the patient, and help to remove the cause of the trouble, and relieve the patient of the pathological symptoms. The patient is cured, and there are no after-effects. Hahnemann's doctrine of 'Psora' has helped to diagnose the deeper underlying root causes of chronic diseases of the human body, which are a source if intense suffering, and to prove suitable antipsoric remedies, which could effectively cure them. Thus, homeopathic remedies, cure patients of their diseases as and when they appear, and, if they are given suitable constitutional treatment, according to their symptoms, from time to time, they need not fall ill again, except in the case of accidents, or due to any epidemics, or any special causes. Even these latter can be treated successfully, if they are taken in hand in time. People who are under homeopathic treatment can keep fairly normal health, and live up to a good old age, provided they observe correct eating habits, use their judgement in the selection of simple, wholesome and non-irritating foods and in balancing them in accordance with the needs of the body, their age and their state of health and lead a well ordered life.

CHAPTER –XXIII

DISEASES OF THE AGED

The case of the ageing, as well as those already aged, is equally important. Senescence (the state of growing old) commences from the age of 40, and more can be accomplished for the group of sensescents, than for those fully senile. Care between the two decades of 40 and 60 determines the future health of the aged, and so, to be fully effective, the treatment, during this period must be largely preventive.

Ageing represents a series of complex mechanisms and degenerative processes which may begin at any age, but which most commonly start in the individual, past forty. These processes are gradual, but definite in character, and are manifested in readily discriminable, anatomic, physiologic, chemical and psychologic changes.

Appetite failure frequently is due to decrease in production of digestive enzymes and hormone secretions, not only those of sexual implication, but those involving nutritional balance, are slowly lost. Impairment of mineral metabolism results in the imbalance of the calcium-Phosphorus ratio, frequently resulting in the development of fragile bones. Low back pain, with muscle atrophy and weakness, particularly of the erector muscles of the spine, is a common feature, resulting in the characteristic stooped position of the aged. Many other evidences of reduced homeostatic efficiency are found, such as, chronic rheumatoid arthritis and fibrous tissue disorders.

Treated early, most of these may be halted or delayed, but, if ignored, will inevitably lead to the development of those progressive, chronic, disabling conditions which afflict our ageing population.

Before considering specific therapy, a few generalities may be enumerated. From the age of forty, and onward, the need for building material, as protein foods and concentrated starches, has been reduced to the barest minimum, as compared with earlier needs. The major mistake made by most elderly persons is, eating too heavily of concentrated starch and protein foods with the idea that they can be digested easily. Such foods should be eaten sparingly.

As the years advance, the food practices must definitely revert to those foods which were best suited to the earlier years of life. Milk or butter milk, and alkali-ash-forming fruits and vegetables well cooked, a small amount of well-prepared cereal and finely ground nuts are the easiest to digest, and therefore best suited for aged persons. All concentrated heavy foods and complicated made-up articles of food, should be avoided.

For further particulars, see 'Introduction'. Some of the more common ailments, and the indicated remedies are given.

Ambra Grisea, great remedy for the aged, with impairment of all functions, weakness, coldness and *numbness*, usually of single parts, fingers, arms, etc. One sided complaints call for it.

Ammonium Carb., fat patients, with weak heart, wheezing, face suffocated. Erysipelas of old people, when cerebral symptoms are developed, while the eruption is still out, debility and soreness of the whole body, tendency to gangrenous destruction.

Aurum Muriaticum, for arteriosclerosis, with hypertrophy of the heart, congestion to the chest and head, strong palpitation, of old age. Paraesthesias, stitches and heaviness about the heart.

Baryta Carb., diseases of old men, when degenerative changes begin cardiac, vascular and cerebral, who have hypertrophied prostate, or indurated testes, very sensitive to cold, offensive foot-sweats, very weak and weary, must sit or lie down, or lean on something. Very averse to meeting strangers. Blood vessels soften and degenerate, become distended, and aneurisms,

DISEASES OF THE AGED

ruptures, and apoplexies result. Loss of memory, mental weakness. Irresolute, vertigo, stitches, when standing in the sun, extending through head.

Baryta Mur., for arteriosclerosis of the large blood vessels and aorta. Dizziness of old people. Apoplexy or threatened apoplexy, with buzzing in the ears. In bronchial affections of old people, with cardiac dilation. In arteriosclerosis of the lung, in senile asthma. also, in all sclerotic degenerations, especially of the spinal cord, liver and heart.

Calcarea Carb., impaired nutrition, changes in the glands, skin, and bones. Tickling cough, fleeting chest pains, nausea, acidity and dislike for fats. Gets out of breath easily. Persons of scrofulous type, who take cold easily, with increased mucous secretions. They are fat, fair, flabby and perspiring, and cold, damp and sour. Apprehensive, worse towards evening, fears loss of *reason, misfortune,* contagious diseases. *Forgetful, confused, low spirited, Vertigo* when walking in open air, as if he would reel, especially when turning the head quickly, on going upstairs, *worse* in the morning, with nausea and vomiting. Rush of blood to head with heat, redness and puffiness of the face.

Calcarea Phos., vertigo and constipation of old people. Vertigo., on motion, when walking in open air, worse in windy weather, with costiveness. Hard stool, with depression of mind, causing headache.

Calcarea Fluor., in arthritis and hypertension, causes absorption of abnormal out-growth of bone on the fingers.

Carbo Vegetablis., in old people, with venous congestions, states of collapse in cholera, typhoid, with a lowered vital power from loss of fluids, after drugging, after other diseases. Asthma of old people, weakness, trembling, looks as if dying, full of wind, but cannot raise it, better in cold air, *worse* in morning. Desires to be fanned, must have more air. Breathing short, with cold hands and feet. Patient seems to be too weak to hold out.

Conium Mac., is suitable for old age, difficult gait, trembling, sudden loss of strength while walking, painful stiffness of legs, etc., debility, hypochondriasis, urinary troubles, weakened memory, sexual debility, vertigo, like turning in a circle, on rising from a seat, worse when lying down, as though the bed was turning in a circle, when turning in bed, or when looking around, from downward motion , when walking, venous abdominal hyperemia. Arterio sclerosis, chronic hypertrophy of the prostate, with difficulty in voiding urine, it stops and starts with sharp, lancinating pain in neck of bladder. Dribbling in old men.

Crataegus, in arterio-sclerosis. Said to have a solvent power upon crustacious and *calcareous deposits in arteries.* Chronic heart disease with extreme weakness. Will often prolong life for several years, if taken in small doses daily. (See under Chapter VII).

Fluoric Acid, complaints of old age, also premature old age, in consequence of syphilitic, mercurial dyscrasia. Acts especially upon lower tissues, and indicated in deep, destructive processes, bed-sores, ulcerations, varicose veins and ulcers. Patient is compelled to move about energetically. He is worse from warmth, and cannot remain in a heated room, is relieved by cold. It often lowers blood pressure and causes an improved circulation of the feet.

Thus, we see than in homeopathic treatment, senescence, though inevitable, may be delayed, and the ills, commonly associated with later life, be made less incapacitating.

Kalium Bich., is indicated in obese, light complexioned people, subject to catarrhs, or with a scrofulous or syphilitic history, in diseases of the kidneys, heart and liver, in aged persons, a general weakness, bordering on paralysis, dilation of heart and stomach.

Kalium Carb., for fleshy, aged people, with dropsical and paretic tendencies, *weakness is characteristic,* with soft pulse,

DISEASES OF THE AGED

coldness, general depression, and very characteristic *stitches,* which may be felt in any part of the body, or in connection with any affection, all pains are *sharp* and *cutting,* nearly all, better by motion, sensitive to every atmospheric change, and *intolerance of cold weather. Early morning aggravation very characteristic.*

Nux Vomica, digestive disturbances, portal congestion and hypochondrial states, due to excessive indulgence in stimulating articles like coffee, tea and liquors. *Irritable,* nervous system, hypersensitive, and over-impressionable, *zealous, fiery temperament.* Easily chilled, avoid open lair, etc.

Opium, especially suitable for old people, insensibility of the nervous system, depression, drowsy stupor, painlessness and torpor, the general sluggishness and lack of vital reaction constitute the main indications. *Vertigo, lightness* of head in old people. Obstinate constipation, no desire to go to stool, *round, hard, black balls.* Lessens voluntary movement, contracts pupils, depresses higher intellectual powers, lessens self control and power of concentration, judgment, stimulates the imagination, checks all secretions, except that of the skin.

Phosphorus, produces a picture of destructive metabolism. *Tall, slender, narrow-chested individuals, with great nervous debility are characteristic.* Yellow atrophy of the liver, and sub-acute hepatitis, faulty degeneration of the blood vessels, hemorrhage and hematogenous jaundice, usually respond to this remedy. One of the outstanding indications in senescence, is a burning sensation in the brain, and sensation of heat and congestion coming up the spine to the head. In the gastro-intestinal sphere, we find hunger, even soon after a meal, often must eat at night as well. *Similar* to *Pulsatilla,* thirst for cold drinks, but with *Phosphorus,* they are vomited as soon as they warm up in the stomach. For those hypersensitives who crave salt, *Phosphorus* will counter-act the bad effects. There are numerous stool symptoms, ranging from profuse, watery, gushing movements, with lumps of white mucus, or bloody, with small white particles, to constipation with long, dry, tough, doglike stools. In both sexes, the sexual appetite is affected, the excitement frequently causing the patient to expose himself or herself. This phase is frequently succeeded by impotence, though the desire remains. In fact, *Phosphorus* is a remedy frequently called for in older people in disorders of appetite, brain, heart, lungs, stomach and liver. A good rule to follow is, when any two systems are involved, such as heart and lungs, or brain and kidneys, think of and study *Phosphorus*.

Plumbum Met., hypertension and arterio-sclerosis associated with chronic nephritis. Patient feels the pulse in the fingers. Slight motion causes fainting. It suits the anemic, pale, emaciated patients with extreme weakness.

Sulphur, inertia and relaxation of fiber, hence feebleness of tone characteristic. *Ebullitions of heat, dislike of water, dry and hard hair and skin, sinking feeling of stomach about 11 a.m., and cat-nap sleep. Standing is the worst position, it is always uncomfortable.* Very forgetful. Difficult thinking. Childish peevishness in aged people. Affections vitiated, *very selfish,* no regard for others. They are nearly always irritable, depressed, thin and weak, even with good appetite.

CHAPTER- XXIV

DISEASE OF THE BRAIN AND NERVOUS SYSTEM

1. Inflammation of the Brain

Definition

Inflammation of the brain itself is called *encephalitis*, inflammation of the membranes which invest the brain is called *meningitis*.

Symptoms and Causes

The most common and striking phenomenon of the inflammation of the brain and of its investing membranes is a sudden and long-continued attack of general convulsions. Stills, convulsions, especially in children, frequently arise from various other causes, for instance, from teething, from overloading the stomach, or from worms.

More commonly the attack may come with severe pains over the entire head, throbbing of the arteries of the neck and temples, fits of shivering, vertigo, sleeplessness, or restless sleep, disturbed dreams, unsteady gait, quick pulse.

The *predisposing* cause of acute attacks of *Tubercular Meningitis* or *Acute Hydrocephalus* is a hereditary scrofulous or consumptive taint, which forms a constitutional tendency toward tubercular diseases. The *exciting cause* may be a fall, difficult denition, or gastric irritation. These, in children otherwise constituted, would produce scarcely any trouble.

In its *earliest* stages, the precursory symptoms are :

The child loses his appetite, he sometimes appears to dislike his food and sometimes devours it voraciously, his tongue is foul, his breath offensive, his belly enlarges, and is sometimes tender, his bowels are constipated, the stools are pale, or are dark, fetid, sour-smelling, slimy, or hard and lumpy, and the child loses his former healthy appearance. There are also some indications of unusual behaviour, the child is dull and dejected, he gets excited, and is uneasy and sometimes shows a little unsteadiness in walking. A frequent, sudden cry or scream, a clenching of the fists, and a turning in of the thumb toward the palm of the hand, given warning also of the approaching malady.

At the beginning of an attack, there is often pain and stiffness at the back of the neck, sometimes extreme tenderness of the scalp, the child cries and shrieks when taken up. Vomiting is nearly a constant symptom, and is often excited by raising the child to an erect position, the headache and vomiting are both aggravated by motion, there is a total loss of appetite, the tongue is coated white, the breath is offensive. Constipation is almost always a prominent symptom. Occasionally, there may be diarrhea, but this is rare. The constipation is generally obstinate for the first week or ten days of the disease, and then toward the termination of the case, gives way to a diarrhea with involuntary stools.

The head is usually hot, the pulse is variable, the senses of sight and hearing become painfully acute, the patient shuts his eyes and contracts his brows, whenever the light is thrown upon his face, the slightest noise or jar, even walking across the room, irritates and distresses him.

When the disease passes to the next stage, which it does sometimes with great rapidity, there is marked change in the symptoms. Noises do not disturb the child, who lies on his back, with his eyes half closed, in a state of drowsiness, which is occasionally interrupted by some cry or exclamation expressive of pain. Convulsions frequently occur, but not uniformly, slight and partial spasmodic twitchings, or general and long-continued convulsions, sometimes paralysis. The urine and stool are passed unconsciously. Sometimes the child, with feeble and tremulous hands, incessantly picks his lips or bores his finger into his ears or nostrils. This stage may last a week or two, and sometimes there may be a remission of these symptoms.

During the last stage, the child rolls his head prepetually from side to side, waves his hands in the air, or one hand, the other frequently being palsied, sometimes there is paralysis of one side, and convulsive twitchings of the other. The circulation is very unequal, one part of the body will be found hot and dry, and another covered with a cold sweat, the cheeks are alternately pale and flushed, the child is raving or insensible, the rapid pulse gets more and more weak, and, at length, the patient expires. In many, instant death takes place in the midst of a strong convulsion.

Treatment for Acute Meningitis

Belladonna 30, is one of the most important remedies in the beginning, and should be given, in watery solution, one tea-spoon every three hours, and continued. In most cases, a decided improvement will be noticed after even twenty-four hours. If this does not help sufficiently, it may be followed by *Bryonia Alba 30*, one globule dry on the tongue, every three hours, and then *Sulphur 30* also in the same manner.

Bryonia Alba, constant inclination to sleep, sudden starting from sleep, with delirium, starts, cries, burning and shooting pains through the head, cold sweat on the forehead. *Bryonia Alba* is very often indispensable after *Belladonna* if pains remain which it was not able to subdue, likewise at the beginning, if *violent lancinating pains shoot through the head from one side to the other*, whereas *Belladonna,* corresponds more to *throbbing and hard, aching, pressing pains.*

Glonoine, the most distinguished remedy for *cerebral irritation from sunstroke.*

Apis Met., useful in cerebral affections occasioned by suppressed exanthemas, especially *urticaria.*

Helleborus Nig., painful heaviness of the head, with heat in the head, and cold extremities. The pain is less violent when the patient lies still and quiet. The pain in the head is of a stupefying nature, as if the brain were bruised. There is a predisposition to bury the head in the pillow. The child sleeps with its eyes half-open. The child shrieks and cries when roused up, or taken from its cradle. *Helleborus Nig.* may be given alone, or in alternation with *Bryonia Alba.*

In all cases where head symptoms supervene upon any other derangement, as teething, or intestinal irritations, or where, from suppression of eruptive diseases, or from suppression of discharges from the ear, the head becomes affected, *Helleborus Nig.* and *Bryonia Alba* should be given without delay, in alternation, from one to two hours apart, according to the urgency of the symptoms. Should these remedies prove insufficient, and the case grow worse, with the addition of the following symptoms, loss of consciousness, eyes motionless, with insensible pupil, skin of a bluish color, coldness of the surface, and pulse imperceptible, give *Belladonna* and *Zincum Met.,* in place of *Helleborus Nig.* and *Bryonia Alba.*

Hyoscyamus Nig., drowsiness, loss of consciousness, delirium, sudden starting, red face, constant muttering, desire to escape, picking at the bed clothes, low muttering,-to be given either alone, or in alternation with *Belladonna.*

Stramonium, when there is starting or jerking in the limbs, staring look, red face, sleep almost natural, but followed by absence of mind after waking. Sometimes the patient has frightful dreams or visions, moans and tosses about during sleep.

DISEASES OF THE BRAIN AND NERVOUS SYSTEM

Pulsatilla, if the brain has become irritated by a metastatic suppression of *coryza,* otorrhea or any other discharges, this remedy will, in *such cases only,* restore the original discharges, and bring about a change in the condition of the patient. If it does not do so in 24 to 48 hours, other remedies should be tried.

Sulphur, very useful not only in desperate cases of acute hydrocephalus, but more particularly in cerebral irritaitons from suppressed measles, or other exanthemas, and is often indispensable even while these exanthemas are on the point of braking out. In these cases, the remedy should be given in the form of watery solution of three to six tea-spoons a day.

Zincum Met., eminently useful in *paralytical* and *dropsical* conditions of the brain, especially when consequent upon *exanthematic* fevers, not only in the 30th but also in the 200th potency.

Cuprum Met., one of the best brain remedies, *if there are spasms in the fingers* or *toes,* oppression on the chest, lockjaw, or if the cerebral disease develops itself after *suppression of erysipelas* or some other eruption, or even after suppressed catarrh or during the process of dentition. It acts very well in the 30th as well as in the 200th potency, *especially if it is indicated by convulsions of the extremities.*

In *Tubercular Meningitis,* which is almost always certain to exist if, in the case of young people who are affected with tubercles in the chest and abdomen, a violent fever with headache and delirium sets in, the only remedies which are useful are *Calcarea Carb.,* and *Phos.* In these cases *Calcarea Carb. 30* should be given in watery solution, a tea-spoon every three hours till there is a change in the condition, and should be followed with *Phos. 30,* in the same way for the remaining pains.

2. CONVULSIONS, SPASMS OR FITS

Definition

By the term fits, spasms, or convulsions, is meant a violent and involuntary agitation of a part or of the whole body. These agitations consist in alternate contractions and relaxations of the muscles of the part affected. Convulsions may be either general or partial. When general, or universal, the muscles of the face and body, as well as those of the extremities, are affected. When partial, the spasmodic action is confined to a particular part. All convulsive diseases consist in affections of the spinal system of nerves.

Causes

Among the *predisposing* causes of the disease, may be mentioned a highly susceptible irritable or nervous temperament.

Convulsions occur most frequently in children under seven years of age, particularly during first denition.

The *exciting* causes of convulsions are-the most common being irritation of the bowels, difficult dentition and worms. Among others are overloading the stomach, very large use of drugs and patent remedies, excessive crying from anger or pain, excessive joy and fear, exposure with the head uncovered, to a hot sun, severe pains, as earache or colic, and suppressed eruptions as after measles, small-pox, etc.

Symptoms

In mild cases, the muscular twitchings may be confined to the face, or rapid shocks may affect a few parts, the face, neck and arms, or half the body. But in severe cases, when the spasm becomes general, the whole body is violently convulsed, the head is drawn backward, or to either side, the body may become stiff and rigid, or variously contorted, the fingers are drawn into the palms of the hands, the arms are thrown backward and forward, or jerked and drawn into all conceivable positions, the lower extremities are likewise affected, but not generally in so violent a manner.

The duration and recurrence of an attack depends upon the *cause* of the disorder. As long as this continues in action, we can expect no permanent improvement. Our first effort is, therefore, to remove it, but this is not easily done, because in many cases it cannot be detected.

Treatment

In the treatment of convulsions, our first and chief attention should be given, *first,* to the *cause* of the disorder, and *second,* to the *disordered condition* of the nervous system, which this cause has produced.

In *all cases,* whatever the nature of cause of the attack, it is better to start the treatment of a child with a *warm bath* by keeping the child in the water from ten to twenty minutes, or until the convulsion ceases, while at the same time cold water would be applied to the head. The child should then be wrapped up in a warm flannel or woolen blanket. In mild cases, a warm foot-bath may be enough, but cold water pack should be applied to the head at the same time.

Special Treatment

(a) **Indigestion:** If the convulsion has been caused by the child eating some indigestible substance, the feet and legs up to the knees, should be immediately placed in hot water, as hot as it can be borne.

Give internally, *Nux Vom., Ipecac., Pulsatilla* or *Veratrum Alb.*

Nux Vomica, should be preferred when there is *constipation,* colic, eructations, violent spasms attended by shrieks, bending of the body backward, jerking backward of the head, eyes set in the head, trembling of the limbs.

Pulsatilla, when the trouble can be traced directly to an overloaded stomach, may be given in alternation with *Nux Vom.*

Veratrum Alb., especially if the patient is cold and pale, with *cold perspiration on the forehead.*

Ipecac., if the vomiting continues after the convulsion has ceased.

If the medicines don't break the fit, place the child again in the warm bath, applying cold water to the head.

For the symptoms, which remain after the spasm is broken, give *Nux Vomica, Chamomilla* or *Aconitum Nap.*

Nux Vomica, for griping and distension of the abdomen.

Chamomilla, if the child is cross or fretful, and especially, if it is teeting.

Aconitum Nap., if there is fever.

(b) **Teething:** When the spasms arise from difficult dentition, as they very frequently do, and when the gums are red and swollen, a warm bath may be given, and the following remedies may be given.

Belladonna, in the case of fat children especially, the child starts suddenly from sleep, stares about wildly, the pupils of the eyes are dilated, the body is rigid, the forehead and hands hot and dry, clinching of the hands, great nervousness, the least touch being sufficient to excite an attack, convulsions attended by smiles and laughter. Should *Belladonna* afford to relief, or but partial relief, it may be followed by *Chamomilla,* or *Belladonna* and *Chamomilla* may be given in alternation.

Chamomilla, is especially applicable to nervous children, those who are extremely sensitive, cross and fretful. It may be given when there are convulsive jerkings of the limbs, twitching of the muscles of the face and eyelids, eyes drawn up beneath the upper lids, constant rolling of the head from side to side, clinched thumbs, great restlessness, disposition to drowsiness between the fits, jerks and convulsions of the arms and legs, one cheek red and the other pale. When *Chamomilla* fails to suppress the fit, *Belladonna* may be given again, or the two may be given in alternation.

Aconitum Nap., when there is high fever, congestion of blood to the head, with red face, great restlessness, crying and starting.

Ignatia, convulsive starts, tremors of the whole body, attended with violent crying and shrieks. Convulsive movements of single limbs, or of single muscles, in different parts of the body, the fits returning at regular hours each day, and followed by fever and perspiration.

When *Belladonna* and *Chamomilla* fail, try *Ignatia.*

(c) **Worms:** When convulsions are caused by worms, give *Cina 200, Mercurius Sol., Cicuta, Ignatia* or *Hyocyamus.*

Ignatia, when there are sudden and violent startings from sleep, with the symptoms detailed above.

Cicuta Virosa, when there are violent griping in the abdomen sudden shocks and jerkings of the limbs.

Cina, when there are spasms of the chest, with stiffness of the entire body, especially suitable for scrofulous children, for those who are troubled with cough, and for convulsions during an attack of whooping cough, may follow *Mercurius Sol.,* or may be given in alternation with it, or with *Hyoscyamus Nig.*

Mercurius Sol., tossing and stiffness of the limbs, distension and hardness of the abdomen, painful eructations, dropping of water from the month, fever and moist skin. After a paroxysm there is great weakness, the child lying a long while in an exhausted condition. This remedy may precede or follow *Cina*.

Hyoscyamus Nig., for sudden attacks after eating, the child gives a shriek, and becomes insensible, nausea and vomiting, convulsive movements of the limbs and whole body, especially twitching of the muscles of the face, pale-blue ring around the eyes and mouth, foaming at the mouth, and great wildness.

(*d*) **Repelled Eruptions:** If the eruption has been a chronic one upon the head, and its suppression has caused spasms, give *Antimonium Tart*. If this does not help, give *Sulphur*, if not better in a couple of hours, give *Stramonium*, and especially if the following symptoms are present-sudden flushes of heat, trembling of the limbs, the eyes fixed, pupils dilated, rigid stiffness of the body, respiration laboured, tossing of extremities, and involuntary passing of urine and faeces.

If the spasms arise from suppressed measles, give *Bryonia Alba*. If it does not gve relief, give *Cuprum Met.*, either alone or in alternation with *Belladonna*. If not better within three hours give *Stramonium* or *Opium*.

(*e*) **Suppressed Catarrh:** Cold on the chest is occasionally the cause of convulsions, the disease is transmitted to the head or spinal nerves, and produces spasms which are very obstinate. Should the head be hot, apply cold water and persevere in its use till the trouble leaves the brain. Also put the child in a warm bath, and give immmediately *Belladonna* and *Cuprum Met.*, afterwards Opium *and Camphor.*

(*f*) **Fright:** Convulsions from fright require *Opium*, especially if there is trembling over the whole body, or when the child

DISEASES OF THE BRAIN AND NERVOUS SYSTEM

lies as if half-stunned, breathes like snoring, with blue face, loud screaming during the fits.

Ignatia is also useful. *Stramonium,* if *Opium* should fail.

Hyoscyamus Nig., when there is foaming at the mouth, twitching of the muscles of the face. Where the child is over excited, and presents symptoms bordering on convulsions, caused by fright, fear, or joy, give *Aconitum Nap.,* if no better within an hour, give *Coffea.*

(g) **Mechanical Injuries:** When convulsions arise from blows or falls upon the head, give *Arnica Mont.* In such cases, it may be necessary to have surgical assisgtance.

(h) **Unknown Causes:** There are many cases for which we can find no adequate cause. In all such cases, use the warm bath, and apply cold water to the head, and give internal *Ignatia,* if this should fail, give eiher if the preceding remedies, whose symptoms. whose symptoms coincide with convulsive phenomena.

Administration of Remedies : Give the selected remedy in watery solution, one teaspoon for a dose every ten, fifteen or twenty minutes, according to the urgency of the case. As the child improves, prolong the interval between the doses, or stop the doses altogether, when the child becomes normal.

After the child has, to all appearances, recovered from the attack, it is desirable to give two or three doses of *Sulphur* at intervals of six hours.

DIET: After a convulsive attack, it is best to keep the child on a low, non-stimulating diet for a few days, especially if the attack was due to indigestion.

3. HYSTERIA

Definition

Hysteria is purely a nervous disorder occasioned by some morbid modification of the reproductive apparatus. It manifests itself mostly in unmarried ladies, between the ages of fifteen and thirty-five, and occurs oftener at, or about the period of menstruation, than at any other time. Females, possessing great susceptibility of the nervous system and of mental emotion are more liable to the disease than those otherwise constituted.

Causes

The predisposing causes are a highly, nervous, irritable and sanguine temperament, and a delicate or a full habit of body with deficient tone. Children of weak and exhausted or aged parents, whether this delicate state of body may be due to heredity or mismangement during early education or development, are most likely to be subject to this disorder. These propensities are further accelerated by wrong mode of living and highly stimulating foods or drinks.

The immediate exciting causes of an attack may be sudden mental emotions, anger, jealousy, fright, sudden intelligence of exciting nature, or unsightly objects.

Treatment

Ignatia is one of the most effective remedies. During the attack, cold water is the best remedy. Frequent bathing and washing of the head are the principal modes of application.

If *Ignatia* is not sufficient, *Silicea* is the next best remedy. *Cocculus Ind.*, *Cuprum Met.*, *Causticum*, *Chamomilla*, *Natrium Mur.*, *Pulsatilla*, *Sepia*, *Sulphur* and *Veratrum Alb.* are also useful remedies.

4. EPILEPSY

This complaint is also due to the several causes already mentioned under nervous troubles, and these fits are more recurrent and of a chornic nature. In the dealing with this kind of spasms also, it is important to take into account (*a*) the *causes* which excite the spasms, (*b*) the accompanying symptoms, (*c*) the time or period when they usually occur, and (*d*)the parts of the body affected.

As patients treated by allopathic doctors for the affection are invariably given preparations of *Opium* or *Potassium Bromide*, it is always best to commence the treatment of these patients iwth a dose of *Sulphur* 200, dry on the tongue, or repeated in watery solution, for 3 days in succession, in order to neutralise the effects of the previous medication.

Special indications for the selection of the remedies.

(a) Causes and Period

DUE TO FRIGHT OR FEAR– *Ignatia, Caust., Cuprum Met., Hyoscyamus Niger.*

DUE TO SUPPRESSED ERUPTIONS–*Arsenicum, Causticum, Cuprum Met., Sulphur, Calcarea Carb.*

DUE TO EMOTION–*Bell., Hyosyamus Nig., Ignatia, Nux Vom., Puls.*

EXCITED BY THE LEAST CONTACT-*Bell., Cocculus Ind., Stram.*

BROUGHT ON BY WASHING–*Sulphur.*

IF THEY OCCUR EARLY IN THE MORNING– *Calcarea Carb., Lycopodium.*

IF THEY OCCUR AT NIGHT–*Calcarea Carb., Caust., Silicea.*

IF AT NEW MOON–*Silicea, Sulph., Caust.*

IF AT FULL MOON–*Calcarea Carb.*

IF BY DRINKING WATER–*Calcarea Carb., Rhus T.*
IF DRINKING WATER ARRESTS THE SPASM–*Caust.*
IF DURING SLEEP–*Silicea, Kalium Carb.*

(b) Accompanying Symtoms

HEADACHE BEFORE AND AFTER THE SPASM–*Bell., Caust., Calcarea Carb., Cham.*
LOSS OF CONSCIOUSNESS–Stupor–*Hyosyamus Nig., Bell., Stram., Opium.*
FLUSHED FACE–*Bell., Stram., Cuprum Met.*
IF ACCOMPANIED BY GREAT ANXIETY–*Cuprum Met., Bell., Verat Alb.*
PALPITATION OF·THE HEART, especially–*Arsenicum Alb., Aconitum Nap., Laches, Hyosyamus Nig.*
FROTH AT THE MOUTH–*Calcarea Carb., Caust., Silicea, Bell., Cupr Met., Ign., Lachesis, Hyosyamus Nig.*
PERSPIRATION AFTER THE SPASM–*Silicea, Bell., Secale Corn.*
VERTIGO, BEFORE OR AFTER–*Bell., Lachesis, Calcarea Carb., Silicea, Bell.*
LAUGHTER SPASMODIC– *Crocus Sat., Cupr Met., Ignat., Caust., Bell.*
WITH MENTAL ALIENATION–*Cupr Met., Stram., Bell., Croc Sat, Hyosyamus Nig.*

(c) PArts Particularly Affected

SPASMS OF THE HEAD, particularly–*Lycopodium, Caust., Cupr Met., Bell., Cicuta.*
SPASMS OF THE FACIAL MUSCLES–*Bell., Cham., Opium, Stram.*

SPASMODIC MOTION OF THE ARMS, particularly–
Cupr Met., Silicea, Stram.

SPASMODIC MOTION OF THE HANDS AND FINGERS, particularly–*Cupr Met., Ign.*

SPASMODIC MOTION OF THE LOWER LIMBS, particularly-*Cupr Met., Ign, Hyosyamus Nig.*

SPASMODIC MOTION OF THE FEET AND TOES–
Caust., Cupr Met., Lycopodium Clav., Silicea.

As suggested above it is best to commence the treatment with a dose of *Sulphur* 200, (single or divided), and then whether the disease originated in fright or not, a dose of *Ignatia 30* may be given. After this the particular medicines indicated by the symptoms most prominent at the commencement of, or during the attack, may be given in the *30th* potency at *weekly* intervals, and then in the *200th* potency at *fortnightly,* or longer intervals.

After the acute spasms are controlled in this way, the following medicines in the *200th* potency in the series :

Ignatia 200, Sulph. 200, Calcarea Carb. 200, Lycopodium Clav. 200, given at *monthly* intervals, help towards a cure of such cases.

If there are no special indications for any particular remedies, it is best to give the series of remedies in the following order–

Ignatia (or *Belladonna), Sulphur, Calcarea Carb., Lycopodium Clav.,* or *Sulphur, Causticum, Silicea* or *Cuprum Met.*

They may first be given in the *30th* potency at *weekly* intervals, and then followed in the *200th* potency at *fortnightly* or *longer* intervals.

This procedure helps to cure a large number of cases.

In cases of suppressed eruptions or ulcers, *Arsenicum Alb.*

and *Causticum,* and sometimes *Cuprum Met.* act to the best advantage.

Where paroxysms orginated in fright, *Ignatia, Hyoscyamus Nig.* and *Causticum* are particuarly called for.

5. CHOREA–ST. VITUS' DANCE

Definition

Chorea is essentially a disease of the nervous system, of a spasmodic nature. It is characterised by tremulous, irregular and in most cases, most ludicrous motions of all, or any of the voluntary muscles. These contractions are, to a certain extent, involuntary, they are more marked upon one side, usually the left, than on the other, they are without pain, and affect females more frequently than males, and occur chiefly with persons between six and fifteen years of age.

Causes

It is said to occur most frequently in children of a nervous, delicate and excitable temperament, some suppose it to be hereditary. No doubt, but that a disordered condition of the digestive system, as well as uterine diseases, predispose to the disease. Among the exciting causes may be mentioned, anything, which makes a forcible impression on the nervous system, strong mental emotions, such as fright is the most common, injuries to the nervous system, as fall upon the head and back, improper employment of lead, mercury etc., suppressed eruptions, discharges, particularly scold-head, itch, herpes, perspiration of the feet, etc. metastasis, or extension of rheumatism to the membranes of the spinal chord, second dentition, anxiety, concealed mental impressions and mental emotions, excited jealousy and envy, onanism, retained, or difficult, or suppressed menstruation.

DISEASES OF THE BRAIN AND NERVOUS SYSTEM

Symptoms

The attack is generally preceded by imperfect digestion, constipation, loss of appetite, and, in many cases, derangements of the menstrual function. These symptoms of disordered health are followed at first by slight irregular twitchings of the muscles of the face, or one of the extremities, and by degrees the spasmodic action more decided and general. Unlike other convulsive diseases, the patient does not loose consciousness, only, he is unable to do as he wishes, and has no control over his movements or actions. There is no pain and these violent and constant muscular contractions do not cause any fatigue. In choosing the appropriate remedies, the predisposing causes, such as, gastric derangements, uterine derangements, injuries to the nervous system etc., should be taken into account. The remedies are *Belladonna, Ignatia, Cocculus Ind., Colchicum, Hyoscyamus Nig., Pulsatilla, Nux Vomica,* and *Sulphur.*

In most acute cases, *Colchicum,* one dose every day for one week, followed by *Cocculus Ind.* in the same way for one week may prove useful. When the muscles of the face are principally affected give *Belladonna.*

Hyoscyamus Nig., when the convulsive movements are confined to the jaw or tongue, or when they affect single parts only, also when they interfere with the patient's swallowing, also when they are occcasioned by worms.

Nux Vom. or *Puls.,* especially, when the extremities are principally affected, and when the difficulty arises from the derangements of the stomach or womb.

Ignatia, when it is impossible to say what has occasioned the derngement, and when there are convulsive movements of the extremities and twitching of the corners of the mouth, also twitchings of single parts, or when there are occasional spasms of single muscles, here and there, in different parts of the system.

Sulphur, should the other remedies fail or afford partial relief.

***Administration of Remedies* :** Two globules of the selected remedy may be dissolved in one ounce of water and tea-spoon doses may be given three times a day. Doses may be repeated according to the susceptibility of the patient and the nature of the case.

CHAPTER-XXV

PARALYSIS

DEFINITION

It is an abolition of the faculty of exciting the normal function of the motor nervous apparatus and muscles. A mere diminution of voluntary motion, attended with a sense of fatigue, is termed *Paresis*. The latter may gradually pass into *Paralysis*.

CAUSES

Paralysis may arise:
- (*i*) From destruction of functional capacity of those parts of the cerebrum, or of the ganglia at the base of the brain, or of the cerebellum, in which volitional impulses are probably converted into motor excitations (*Central Paralysis*).
- (*ii*) From diminution, or abolition of the conductivity of the motor nerves, on any of their courses, from their origin in the brain and spine to their termination (*Paralysis of conduction*).
- (*iii*) From abolition of excitability and contractibility of the muscles (*Myopathic Paralysis*).

The causes are: *Wounds (Traumatic), diseases of parts* near the nerves, such as caries, enlarged glands, herniae, tumours, etc., *diseases of the nervous system,* such as neuritis myelitis, cerebral and spinal apoplexies, etc., *disturbances of the circulation,* such as thrombosis, venous stasis, etc., *poisoning of the blood by vegetable alkaloids,* such as ergot, nicotine, camphor, etc., and *metallic preparations,* such as ergot, nicotine, camphor, etc., and *metallic preparations,* such as, lead, etc., *chronic infectious diseases* and cachexia such syphillis, and scrofulosis, *acute diseases,* such as acute eruptions, erysipelas, typhoid fever, cholera, dysentery, etc., catching cold, *exhaustion of the nervous system* by forced marches, excessive venery, night watching, excessive mental exertions, etc., *reflex action* from some primary disease, injury or irritation of the nerves at periphery-reflex paralyses. Paralysis may *extend* over a single muscle, or a group of muscles, over one-half of the body (*hemiplegia*), usually caused by a lesion in the brain on the opposite side, though it may also, be of spinal origin, or over both halves of the body symmetrically, commencing usually in the lower extremities and spreading to trunk and upper extremities (*Paraplegia*).

Leading Indications

PARALYSIS OF THE EYELIDS–*Arnica Mont., Argencum Nit., Bell., Coccul Ind., Gelsemium, Plumb Met., Rhus Tox., Sepia, Spigelia, Zincum Met.*

PARALYSIS OF THE FACE–*Bell., Caust., Coccul Ind., Graph., Nux Vom., Opium.*

PARALYSIS OF THE TONGUE AND ORGANS OF SPEECH–*Aconitum Nap., Arnica Mont., Arsenicum Alb., Baryta Carb., Bell., Caust., Coccul Ind., Cuprum Met., Opium, Plumb.*

PARALYSIS OF THE ORGANS OF DEGLUTITION–*Bell., Caust., Coccul Ind., Cuprum Met., Gelsea, Silic.*

PARALYSIS OF THE BLADDER–*Arsenicum Alb., Bell., Gels, Natrium Mur., Opium.*

PARALYSIS OF THE RECTUM AND SPHINCTER ANI–*Caust., Opium, Phos., Sulph.*

PARALYSIS OF ALL THE LIMBS–*Arnica Mont., Arsenicum Alb., Gels, Mercurius Sol., Nux Vom., Rhus Tox.*

PARALYSIS OF THE UPPER EXTREMITIES–*Aconitum Nap., Arnica Mont., Bell., Calcarea Carb., Caust., Coccul Ind.,*

PARALYSIS

Lycopodium Clav., Mercurius Sol., Nux Vom., Rhus Tox., Sepia.

PARALYSIS OF THE RIGHT ARM AND LEFT LEG–*Terebinth.*

PARALYSIS OF THE HANDS–*Arsenicum Alb., Caust., Cupr Met., Natrium M, Rhus Tox., Ruta, Sil.*

PARALYSIS OF THE FINGERS–*Calarea Carb, Cupr Met., Natrium Mur., Secale Corn, Sil.*

PARALYSIS OF THE LOWER EXTREMITIES–*Alum, Arnica Mont., Bell., Bryonia, Coccul Ind., Kalium C., Mercurius Sol., Nux Vom., Phos., Plb Met., Rhus Tox., Secale Cor., Sulph.*

PARALYSIS OF THE FEET–*Arsenicum Alb., China off., Plumb Met.*

HEMIPLEGIA–*Alum, Anac, Argentum Nit, Arnica Mont., Bell., Caust., China off., Coccul Ind., Kalium Carb, Mercurius Sol., Phos. Ac., Plumb Met., Rhus Tox., Sepia, Stan.*

LEFT-SIDED HEMIPLEGIA–*Arnica Mont., Arsenicum Alb., Bell., Caust., Lach, Rhus Tox.*

RIGHT-SIDED HEMIPLEGIA–*Arnica Mont., Bell., Caust., Rhus Tox.*

PARALYSIS OF ONE AND SPASMS OF THE OTHER SIDE–*Bell., Lach, Stram.*

PARAPLEGIA–*Coccul Ind., Nux Vom., Secale Cor.*

PARALYIS IN CONSEQUENCE OF :

MENTAL EMOTIONS–*Arnica Mont., Ignatia, Natrium Mur., Stannum Met.*

BODILY EXERTIONS–*Arsenicum Alb., Arnica Mont., Rhus Tox.*

SPASMS–*Arsenicum Alb., Caust., Coccul Ind., Cupr Met., Hyosyamus Nig., Nux Vom., Plumb.*

APOPLEXY–*Arnica Mont., Anac, Baryta Carb., Caust., Cupr Met., Lach, Nux Vom., Plumb Met., Secale Corn, Stannum Met., Stram, Zinc Met.*

TAKING COLD–*Arnica Mont., Caust., Dulc., Colch, Mercurius Sol., Rhus Tox.*

GETTING WET–*Caust., Nux Vom., Rhus Tox.*

SUPPRESSION OF SWEAT–*Colch.*

ONANISM, SEXUAL EXCESS–*China off., Coccul Ind., Ferrum Met., Natrium Mur., Nux Vom., Sulph.*

RHEUMATISM–*Antimonium Tart, Arnica Mont., Baryta Carb., Bryonia Alb., Caust., China off., Coccul Ind., Gels, Lycopodium, Ruta, Sulph.*

INTERMITTENT FEVERS–*Arnica Mont., Arsenicum Alb., Natrium Mur., Nux Vom., Rhus Tox.*

TYPHUS FEVER– *Cupr Met., Nux Vom., Rhus Tox., Sulph.*

DIPHTHERIA–*Ars Alb., Gels, Lach, Natrium Mur.*

CHOLERA–*Cuprum Met., Secale Cor., Sulph, Verat Alb.*

SUPPRESSED ERUPTIONS–*Caust., Dulc., Hepar Sulp., Sulph.*

POISONING BY ARSENICUM–*China off., Ferrum Met., Graph, Hepar Sulp., Nux Vom.*

POISONING BY LEAD–*Cuprum Met., Opium, Platina.*

POISONING BY MERCURY–*Hep Sulp., Nitrium Ac., Staph, Stram, Sulph.*

Therapeutic Hints

Aconitum Nap., useful in every kind of paralysis. From congestion of spinal cord with numbness of the parts, facial paralysis accompanied with coldness from exposure to dry, cold winds,

PARALYSIS

especially in acute cases. Paraplegia with tingling.

Agaricus Mus., paralysis of lower limbs with slight spasms of arms, pain in lumbar region and sacrum, croswise affections.

Alum Met., paralysis from spinal diseases, loss of sensibility of the feet, inability to walk except with open eyes, and in the day time.

Anac., after apoplexy, loss of memory, imbecility of mind, loss of will.

Apis Mell., one side paralysed, the other twitching, cerebral origin.

Argentum Nit., parplegia from exhaustion.

Arnica Mont., in consequence of exudations within the brain or spine, in consequence of apoplexy, of concussions, of weakening diseases of protracted intermittent fevers and ischimas.

Arsenicum Alb., when associated with great prostration and neuralgic pains, also, in spinal affections with *gressus falinaceous*, and as an antidote to lead poisoning.

Baryta Carb., generl paralysis of old age, with loss of memory and trembling of limbs, also after apoplexy in old age, and especially in paralysis of the tongue. Facial paralysis of young people when the tongue is implicated.

Bell., apoplexy, congestion of the head, paralysis of the one, and the spasm of the other side of the body, paralysis of the face, locomotor ataxy.

Caulophyllum, paraplegia, in consequence of retroversion and congestion of the womb, after child-birth, with partial loss of sensation in the affected limbs, considerable emaciation, anemia and general debility.

Causticum, paralysis of face or tongue, or hemiplegia, with giddiness, weakness of sight, weeping mood, hopelessness, fear of death, drawing, lame feeling in the affected part, after exposure to severe cold winds, cararrhal and rheumatic conditions, suppressed eczema or other chronic eruption, apoplexy, the paralysis remaining after the patient has recovered, otherwise, *inability to select the proper word is an important indication.*

China off., after great loss of blood.

Coccul Ind., paralysis of the face, or tongue, or pharynx, paraplegia, rheumatic lameness, in weakened and nervous subjects, who are inclined to fainting fits and palpitation of the heart, also, when the paralytic affection originates in the small of the back, after taking cold, with cold feeling of the extremities and edema of the feet, likewise after apoplexy.

Colchic., after a sudden suppression of general perspiration, or of sweat of the feet by getting wet.

Conium Mac., paralysis of central origin, the sensation is little involved, and the tendency of the paralysis is to move from below upwards. Acute ascending paralysis. Paralysis of the aged.

Cuprum Met., after apoplexy, when there is congestion in the chest, strong palpitation of the heart, or slow, weak and small pulse, the eyelids keep closed and twitch; when opening the eyes, the eye balls move about, paralysis after cholera and typhus, paralysis commencing at the periphery, and progressing towards the centre.

Dulcamara, after taking cold (wet weather), and suppressed eruption, paralysis of the upper and lower extremities, and the tongue, the paralysed arm feels icy cold

Gel., loss of motion, but not sensation, paralysis of the organs of deglutition, and in loss of voice, following diphtheria, locomotor ataxia, paraplegia. *It is one of our best remedies in post-diphtheric and infantile paralysis.* Paralysis of the ocular muscles, drooping of the upper eyelids, the speech is thick, from paretic conditions of the tongue. Paralysis from emotions.

Graph., rheumatic, peripheric paralysis of the face.

Hepar Sulph., after mercurial poisoning.

PARALYSIS

Hyos Nig., after spasms.

Ignat., after great mental emotions and night-watching in the sick chamber, hysterical paraplegia.

Kalium Carb., trembling, paralytic weakness, with cramps in the fingers and hands, also, paralytic weakness in the hip joint.

Kalium Phos., after exhaustion of nerve power, after hysteria.

Lachesis, especially left side, awkward, stumbling gait, *gressus gallinaceus*, after apoplexy.

Mercurius Sol., rigidity and immobility of all the limbs, although they can be easily moved by others, indescribable malaise of body and soul, trembling of limbs and body, *paralysis agitans* (shaking palsy).

Natrium Mur., paralytic condition of the lower limbs, painful contraction of the ham-strings, after intermittent fevers, diphtheria, sexual excesses and violent fits of passion.

Nux Vom., incomplete paralysis of the face, arms, legs, with vertigo, weak memory, darkness before the eyes, ringing in the ears, loss of appetite, burning in the stomach, flatulence, vomiting after eating and drinking, consipation, especially in drunkards, after apoplexy, mental over-exertions. Paralysis of the lower extremities, contractive sensations and heaviness in the limbs. Paralysis of bladder, in old men.

Oleand., painless stiffness and paralysis of the limbs, insensibility of the whole body, or hyper-aesthesia, skin sore from the ordinary friction of the clothes, trembling of the knees when standing, and of the hands when writing, preceded by spells of vertigo a long time before paralysis develops itself.

Opium, paralysis and insensibility after apoplexy, in drunkards, in old people, retention of stool and urine.

Oxalic Ac., paralysis from inflammation of spinal cord, limbs stiff, paroxysms of dyspnea.

Phos., paralysis in consequence of spinal affections, after sexual excess, after confinement, tingling and tearing pain from the back, down into the limbs, *gressus vaccinus*.

Picric Ac., after tonic and clonic spasms, on standing, keeps legs wide apart, look steadily at objects, as if unable to make them out, limbs feel as if in an elastic bandage, particularly the legs, wasting palsy, progressive locomotor ataxia.

Plumbum Met., paralysis, with atrophy, is the watchword of *Plumb Met*. Wrist-drop, paralysis of the extensors. Paralysis due to sclerosis or fatty degenerations. Paralysis with contractions. Ptosis, heavy tongue, constipation, paralysis after apoplexy, with pale, dry, cold skin. Tremor followed by paralysis. Paralysis agitans (shaking palsy). *Plumb Met., Mercurius Sol., Zinc Met.* and *Hyoscyamus Nig.* are the principal remedies for paralysis agitans.

Psor., after debillitating acute diseases.

Rhus Tox., rheumatic, paralytic affections after getting sweat (*Dulc.*), and after great or unwonted muscular exertions, strainings etc., in consequence of typhoid processes, with painful stiffness, tearing, drawing and aching of the whole body; sometimes, with tingling and numbness of the parts, or continued cold feet for a long time, *worse* during rest, and when commencing to move, from washing in cold water, with every change of weather, *better* from dry heat near the stove, from continued gentle moving about, and flexion of the limbs.

Ruta, facial paralysis after catching cold.

Secale Corn., paralysis after spasms and apoplexy, with rapid emaciation of the affected parts, and involuntary discharges from bowels and bladder.

Silicea, paralysis of the left hand with atrophy and numbness in the fingers, paralysis of the legs, always worse in the morning, with heaviness of the head and ringing in the ears.

Stannum Met., hemiplegia, especially on the left side, with a feeling of heavy load of the affected arm, and corresponding side of the chest, and frequent night-sweats.

Stramonium, after convulsions, also paralysis of the one, and spasms of the other side of the body.

Sulphur, after typhus, exanthematic fevers, suppressed itch, or chronic eruptions and spasms, also when other remedies seem to fail.

Zincum Met., worse, after drinking wine, great restlessness of feet, after suppressed foot-sweat.

Terebinth., paralysis of right arm and left leg.

CHAPTER-XXVI

ANTERIOR POLIOMYELITIS

Definition

This affection has also been called 'Spinal Infantile Paralysis, Acute Spinal Paralysis of adults, Acute Atrophic Spinal Paralysis', and is marked by the following group of characterisitc symptoms–

It begins suddenly, usually with fever, with severe cerebral symptoms–deafness, coma, delirium, general convulsions, there is, very rapidly developed and complete paralysis, with entire relaxation of the muscles, this paralysis being of very variable distribution over the trunk of extremities, but generally in the form of paraplegia, there is an absence of any severe disturbances of sensation, no paralysis of the sphincters, nor bed-sores. There is malaise and general weakness, headache, drowsy, tongue furred, flushed face often, tender limbs, apprehensive, coryza often, nausea, vomiting and diarrhea often.

The disease may occur at all periods of life though it is by far the most frequent in children between the ages of one and four years.

If from the beginning of the initial fever, the indicated homeopathic remedy is given, the whole aspect of anterior poliomyelitis will can be very much modified, and the disease can be arrested before it develops into its full form. The treatment can be started at once, without waiting for a diagnosis of the name of the disease, which, in the case of this disease, can be done only when the paralysis actually manifests itself, and *the stage of prevention is already over.* Thus, homeopathy has a distinct advantage in the treatment of this much dreaded disease.

ANTERIOR POLIMOYELITIS

In the first stage, the remedies indicated are– *Aconite Nap., Apis Mell., Arsenicum Alb., Bell., Bryonica Alba, Caust., Cocculus Ind., Dulc., Gels, Lach, Lathyrus Sat, Mercurius Sol., Natrium Mur., Natrium Sulph, Nux Vom, Opium, Phos., Rhus Tox., Sulphur.*

Aconitum Nap., Bell. and Gels. are most likely to be indicated *for the first stage* in a large majority of cases.

If the sudden onset, rapid pulse, characteristic restlessness, anxiety and thirst are present, *Aconitum Nap.* will help to cut down the violence of the attack.

Belladonna, if the onset be rapid, with high fever, throbbing carotids, red face and eyes, with *dryness* of eyes, nose and throat (opp, of *Gels.),* severe throbbing headache, with aggravation of the patient's condition by touch, jar, motion and noise

Gelsemium, is the leading remedy for this disease, having a marked affinity for teh cells of the motor nerves, producing first congestion, and later destruction, causing paralysis. It covers very well the symptoms of flushed face, drowsiness, sneezing, irritation in nose and throat, and watery discharge from the nose, in addition to high fever. The onset is not as sudden as with *Aconitum Nap. and Belladonna.*

Rhus Tox., when getting wet or exposure to dampness is the exciting cause. It is considered very useful for paralysis of the lower extremities in acute as well as in chronic cases. Marked pain and restlessness are important indications. *Dulcamara,* is similar to *Rhus Tox.* in many respects, though not so suitable in chronic cases. *When the disease has passed the acute stage and ultimated in chronic Paralysis,* the following remedies are indicated :

Plumbum Met., has been much extolled for the later stages, the characteristic symptoms being a general paralytic state, preceded by sluggishness and paresis, the symptoms develop slowly and insidiously, progressive muscular atrophy, progressive paralysis, paralysed and painful parts wither. There is paralysis of both extensors and flexors, but it usually begins with the extensors, giving us the wrist drop. *Plumbum Met.* has a special affinity for the upper extremities, and has not been found useful for paralysis of the lower extremities. Paralysis may be preceded by tremor. Constipation, with hard, lumpy stools may be a high-ranking symptom. Retention or suppression of urine may be present.

Phosphorus, if and when the symptoms agree, should be considered, as it has an elective affinity for the brain and nerves and causes destruction (fatty degeneration) of these tissues.

Alumina, has paralysis of the lower extremities, especially of spinal origin, constipation requiring much straining to pass even a soft stool, formication of limbs, patient brushes his face, as if trying to remove a cobweb.

Lathyrus Sativus, presenting as it does a most striking picture of typical infantile paralysis, *"symptomatically, pathologically, and clinically",* should be considered to be a most effective *prophylactic* against the disease.

Dr. A. H. Grimmer of Chicago, Ice., claims that clinical application of this remedy as a prohylactic in many thousands of cases over a period of thirty years, in many epidemics, has registered *one hundred per cent. success.* For the purpose of immunizing, he suggests a dose of the remedy in the 30th or 200th potency, given about once every three weeks during an epidemic.

Curatively, its indications are– increases reflexes, tremulous, tottering gait, spastic paralysis, excessive rigidity of legs, cannot extend or cross legs when sitting, knees knock against each other when walking, toes do not leave the floor, heels do not touch floor, tips of fingers numb, urination frequent, involuntary, of he does not hurry up. Sir John Weir has cured cases with *Lathyrus Sativus, Curare and Physostigma* and has listed the following details which he has found useful in differentiating the remedies.

Lathyrus Sativus (Chick-pea). Affects the lateral and anterior column of the cord. Reflexes always increased. Paralytic affections of lower extremities. Spastic paralysis. Infantile Paralysis. Spastic gait. Cramp legs.

Curare (Arrow-poison), Muscular paralysis, without impairing sensation and consciousness. Paralysis of respiratory muscles. Arms weak and heavy, legs tremble. Reflexes are lessened or abolished, produces paralysis right deltoid.

Physostigma (Calabar bean). Spinal irritation, loss of motility, prostration, rigidity of muscles, pralysis. Depresses the motor and reflex activity of the cord, and causes loss of sensibility to pain, muscular weakness, followed by complete paralysis, although muscular weakness, followed by complete paralysis, although muscular contracility is not impaired. Poliomyelitis anterior. Crampy pains in limbs. Great prostration of muscular system.

CHAPTER-XXVII

NEURITIS

Neuritis is defined as inflammation of a nerve. Pathological symptoms include pain, tenderness, more or less impairment of function, sensory disturbances and in severe cases, of anaesthesia and even paralysis.

Neuralgia, on the other hand, simply means nerve pain. A typical neuralgic pain is defined as severe, darting or throbbing in character, intermittent, with sensitiveness of the skin. Generally there is relief from warmth and pressure.

Preceeding both neuritis and neuralgia, there is always some form of nerve irritation. Some cases are traumatic in origin, others toxic, still others are caused by nutritional deficiencies. Alcoholism and emotional stress are predisposing factors of considerable importance.

When the cause is traumatic, such local treatment must be instituted as the case may require. Fixation and rest of the affected part may be indicated. There is always more or less damage to nerve tissue in any injury, but the homeopathic remedy by matching the symptoms of motor and sensory disturbance will afford the maximum of relief, and restore function to the fullest extent possible.

Cases of nerve injury, associated with a bone or periosteal bruise, or where there are strained or over-stretched tendons, will respond to *Ruta*. Direct injury to nerves, in which the tactile sense is highly developed, will generally require *Hypericum*. This remedy is nearly always indicated following injury to the coccyx, also for bad effects following chilling of the buttocks and lower part of the back, as from sitting for a long time on a cold, damp bench or on the cold ground. This form of chilling in which there is damp, penetrating cold extending up the spine, is one of the important pre-disposing causes of poliomyelitis. Punctured wounds require

NEURITIS

Ledum Pal. and *Hypericum,* contusions and bruises require *Arnica Mont., Rhus Tox.* and *Calc Carb.* For injuries to the bloodvessels, for contusions to the eye, *Ledum Pal.,* for eye-strain. *Ruta, Apis Mell.,* for zig-zags in front of the eyes and aggravation from sunlight and other bright lights, *Natrium Mur.* (See Chapter XXVI for the leading indications).

Neuralgic pains in the stump of an amputated limb will generally be relieved by *Allium Cepa,* when the pains are fine, thread-like and shooting in character. *Ammonium Mur.* is often indicated after amputation of the foot, when there are tearing, stitching pains, worse in bed at night and better from massage. *Arnica Mont.* is the remedy following amputation through the fleshy parts of the arm or leg, when there is the sore, bruised feeling, and the history of considerable trauma to the muscular structure. *Hypericum* may be the remedy after amputation of the distal phalanx of any of the fingers following an accident, in which the tip of the finger has been chopped or cut off. Sharp, shooting pains will extend up the arm, the pain being almost intolerable and associated, perhaps, with a degree of shock, apparently out of proportion to the severity of the injury. *Phosphorus* is indicated after amputation in nervous, sensitive subjects, when there was excessive bleeding, during or following the operation, and a weak, all-gone feeling, with thirst for ice-cold drinks. *Staphysagira* has sometimes been used on a routine basis after amputation, but the indications are, what might be called, "clean-cut" cases with little or no contusion, and when the sensation, as of a knife cutting, persists long after the surgery.

A contusion causes local shock to the nerves in the involved area. A temporary paralysis results in an extravasation of blood from the capillaries into the surrounding tissues, then we have ecchymosis, bruise marks, or a black nail, if the injury is to the end of the finger. These effects can nearly always be prevented by giving immediate and adequate mechanical support to contused tissue, until the local efferent nerves recover from shcok, and at the same time suitable internal remedies as indicated above.

Neuritis involving the left shoulder and arm, after straining the heart from over-lifting or over-exertion, involvement of the Sciatic nerve, especially on the left side, aggravation in wet weather, from getting wet, and from dampness in general, require *Rhus Tox., Calcarea Carb.,* for the chronic effects in the traumatic field.

Bryonia Alba, following injury to the chest and ribs, with aggravation on the least motion, and relief from presssure, *worse* when taking a deep breath, raising arms or coughing. Suited to cases of both pleurisy and inter-costal neuralgia. Amelioration in either case by rightly strapping thej chest.

Carbo An., has the symptom, "easily sprained from lifting even small weights", also "great debility and easy spraining of the joints".Elderly people who are feeble, subject to colds, and when slight causes appear to produce unduly severe effects.

Dulcamara, sudden chilling when overheated, or sudden suppression of sweat from a cold wind, or in an air-conditioned room, when the outside temperature is in the nineties, will often cause neuralgia or even a neuritis, also, when there is a sudden, severe drop in temperature from hot and dry to cold and wet, in patients with a strong catarrhal disposition.

Causticum, following exposure to dry, cold winds, *Bell's* palsy, affecting especially the right side of the face, paralysis of single muscles, weakness of bladder, with inability to control the urine.

Psorinum, has an affinity for the nerve of supply to the deltoid muscle, and has cleared many cases in psoric constitutions, when the chronicity and recurrence are conspicuous features.

Silicea, following exposure to a draught, especially when perspiring, also for cases of neuritis following a suppressed foot-sweat.

Silicea, patients are better from warmth, and from wraping up the affected part.

NEURITIS

Arsenicum Alb., is a powerful remedy in neuritis, and more especially in the multiple neuritis of a severe type, with the characterisitic symptoms of burning, worse at night and relief by heat. It will suit especially the broken-down constitutions, anemic conditions and irritability, so often accompaniments of multiple neuritis.

Cimicifuga, indicated in alcoholic neuritis. *Ledum Pal.* and *Plumbum* are also recommended for the alcoholic variety, the latter being specially indicated in cases in which atrophy appears, no matter what the variety.

Phosphorus, also frequently indicated in the multiple variety.

Anemia predisposes to many cases of neuritis. Toxic causes include many of the acute affections, also malaria, gout, syphilis, lead poisoning and organic disease involving the cerebro-spinal axis. Dental caries and badly infected tonsils are responsible for some cases.

In treating neuritis, the root causes of the trouble should first be removed, before the indicated remedy is prescribed.

The general causes are:
- (*a*) Emotional stresses and conflicts.
- (*b*) Excesses and depletions.
- (*c*) Nutritional deficiencies.
- (*d*) Food toxemia.

The diet should first be corrected. In patients with gout, unless the diet is corrected in the first place, the trouble is bound to recur. Chronic lead-poisoning, or aluminium poisoning must be stopped. In a case of beri-beri, unless the nutritional deficiency is corrected, the indicated remedy will not act.

Tri-facial neuralgia (tic-dou loureux) will not respond to proper treatment, if there has been over-exposure to either the infra-red heat lamp or the ultra-violet, so called sun-lamp. Alcoholic injections and the X-ray have spoiled more cases than they have ever alleviated. Cases of excessive coffee drinking should also be treated first with *Nux Vom., Chamomilla,* and *Guarana* (a wonderful South American plant, recommended by Dr. Clarke), before the indicated remedies are given.

CHAPTER-XXVIII

DISEASES OF THE SKIN

1. ITCHING OF THE SKIN

If it is always commencing when underssing, *Nux vomica* or *Arsenicum Alb*.

If the itching always commences after the patient gets warm in bed, *Pulsatilla* or *Mercurius Sol*. if it continues the whole night, if this does not relieve, *Sulphur* may be given two days later, and continued daily till relief is obtained.

When the itching moves from one place to another on being scratched, *Ignatia*.

When the itching is accompanied by intense burning, *Rhus Tox.*, or *Apis Mell.*, or afterwards *Hepar Sulp*.

When the itching comes on in the day time, and arises from over-heating, *Lycopodium Clav*.

If any of the above remedies does not give relief in the first instance, one does of *Sulphur* taken morning and evening for a few days will give relief.

In addition to the use of the internal remedies, external application of coconut oil on the parts affected will be helpful.

2. ITCH, SCABIES

All eruptions, which appear on the outer surface of the body in the form of boils, itches, etc., are really the external manifestations of some deep internal constitutional troubles which nature, in her effort to clear the system of all poisons, throws them out on the surface of the skin, and helps us to rid ourselves of these poisons. In our attempt to get rid of these eruptions, we apply ointments or other external remedies, and in doing so, we may perhaps get temporary relief for the time being, but, on the other hand, we are really undoing the good work done by nature to help us to clear ourselves of these poisons, because these external applications have really the effect of throwing back these poisons inside the system and thus suppressing them. The consequence of this is, that as these poisons continue to remain in the system and affect the vital organs of the body, other diseases of various forms continue to appear from time to time and give trouble. The proper procedure will be, when these eruptions appear, to help nature and to take appropriate *internal* remedies, in order to clear the system of the remaining poisons and keep it free from disease-producing matter, and not apply and *external* remedies which have a contrary effect.

Among the many kinds of itch which trouble us, there is one caused by the presence of a very small mite or insect under the skin, where it makes its tracks and deposits its eggs, causing the eruption of little pustules. These tracks can be seen by careful observers, but not clearly visible to all. In the very beginning, it is possible to ged rid of the itch easily and without any danger, by outward applications. One simple method of external application which may be employed in our country is to make a decoction of margosa (neem) leaves and turmeric, and wash the itching parts with this decoction, or to apply margosa oil (neem oil) to those parts, or if the eruptions are extensive, *oil of lavender* may be got from a chemist, and may be applied *only over those parts which itch.*

In case these applications do not help because there are no mites present, it is advisable to take internal medicines.

Mercurius Sol., may be given for three days (one dose daily), with an interval of three days, and followed by *Sulphur* in the same way for three days, and then after an interval, *Mercurius* again for 2 or 3 days. If these don't help, and if the vesicles are small and dry, *Carbo Veg.* may be given on *alternate* days, if they contain pus, *Hepar Sulph,* morning and evening for a day, and then again waiting for a few days. it may be repeated again in the same way. If the pustules are large in size, *Mercurius Sol.,* for 3 or 3 days morning and evening, in watery solution, then *Sulphur* in the same way for 2 or 3 days, and then *Causticum* also in the same way.

If the eruptions don't develop after the external applicationof the lavender oil in the first place, then *Sulphur* may be given, and then *Calcarea Carb.* and *Sepia* at long intervals.

3. ECZEMA

It is an acute or chronic inflammatory, non-contagious disease of the skin, appearing in different forms and in different parts of the body. It is always of constitutional origin, and it is the action of the life force trying to drive the miasm from within the body, and throwing it out as an eczematous eruption upon the skin. As this is an attempt of nature to save the vital organs from the ravages of this destructive miasm, by throwing the disease to the surface, the proper method will be to give the anti-miasmatic internal remedies for the removal of the miasm which is the pre-disposing cause of the disease in the constitution and not to make use of any external ointments or medicaments which will produce the contrary effect of driving from back. The suitable remedy should be given, preferably in the higher potencies, and at long intervals, and the only external application permissible is the use of coconut oil which serves as a lubricant and keeps the skin smooth and free from irritation.

Irregularity of diet is also important and all those articles, which have a tendency to produce heat or cause irritation, should be avoided.

In selecting the appropriate remedy, the following should be borne in mind-
- (*a*)   The immediate or pre-disposing cause of the trouble.
- (*b*)   The constitution of the patient.
- (*c*)   The part of the body affected.
- (*d*)   The conditions or circumstances which increase the trouble or reduce it such as weather, locality, climate,etc.

Leading Indications

FOR THE RED ECZEMA AT THE ANUS, SCROTUM, PUDENDUM AND ON THE LIMBS, BACK OR NECK, WITH A LOT OF ITCHING AND BURNING–*Dulcamara, Rhus Tox., Mezereum, Graphites, Calcarea Carb., Sulphur.*

FOR ECZEMA ON THE HANDS AND FINGERS–*Mercurius Sol., Sepia and Sulphur.*

ECZEMA OF THE EAR–*Graphites, Mercurius Sol., Lachesis.*

ECZEMA OF THE NOSE–*Alumina, Graphites, Sepia.*

As most cases treated by alloathic doctors are given different preparations of sulphur, and external applications of sulphur or zinc ointments, it is always best to commence the treatment of such cases with doses of *Pulsatilla* 200 at weekly intervals so as to neutralise the effects of the sulphur preparations, till there is a change, and in several cases the trouble will be relieved, but in others even if there is no relief, the original trouble which was suppressed by allopathic medication will re-appear and give indication for the appropriate remedy. The indicated remedy may then be administered according to the symptoms.

Alumina, spare, dry, thin subjects, with mild, cheerful disposition, latent syphilitic patients who suffer with dry, scaly, itching *eruptions which are worse in winter,* itching *worse when warm in bed,* scratces until it bleeds, when it becomes painful, *craves*

DISEASES OF THE SKIN

starch, chalk, charcoal, indigestible things, habitual constipation.

Apis Mell., the erythematous eruption shows swelling and marked edema (complementary to *Natrium Mur.*), not to given after *Rhus Tox.*, eruptions worse on the face, lips, nose, ears throat, hands and feet, circumscribed spots that itch, burn and sting, skin often swollen, edematous, pale, waxy or dirty looking, deep red rash or dark red papules, *worse* in a *warm room* and *better by bathing* and *open air.*

Arsenicum Alb., deep chronic cases, skin like parchment, dry, rough, or dirty looking, child usually emaciated and suffering with some other deep chronic trouble. Thin, branlike vesicles *(Natrium Mur.)*, small, transparent, secreting a thin, watery exudation that excoriates the parts passed over, all eruptions itch intensely and pre accompanied with burning and smarting, discharge usually offensive, *better* by *warm applications* or *heat in general.*

It is one of our great eczema-asthma medicines, and like *Natrium Mur.* and *Sepia,* there is aggravation at the sea-side. An unquenchable thirst is another characteristic, urticaria with burning and restlessness. Poisoned wounds and ulcers, respond to *Arsenicum Alb.* when indicated. Sudden inflammations that rapidly take on a malignant look. Genital eruptions characterised by burning.

Agaricus Mus, eczema with burning, itching, pricking as from needles, electric-like stitches in the skin, small nodules deep in the skin, eczema *worse in the winter* and accompanied with chilblains, bright red erythema, with burning, biting, tingling, and intense itching.

Baryta Carb., tubercular diathesis, dwarfish children, who suffer with glandular enlargement, eczema of old people and drunkards. It is often followed well by *Tub., Psor., Syph.* Intolerable itching and tingling, *worse* by scratching and by thinking about it, parts red, excoriated, accompanied with much burning, erythematous eczema in the folds and flexures of the body.

Calcarea Carb., fair skinned, pale, weak, easily-tired women or children, chubby, fat babies who are deficient in bone, with an excess of flesh, large-headed children with pale skin, soft, flabby muscles and who are self-willed, cold, clammy hands and feet, eruptions, either dry or moist, yellowish thick crusts in seborrheic eczema of the scalp, latent syphilitic diathesis, discharges, light yellow, offensive, pus-like. Location, scalp, face, behind the ears, forearm.

Calcarea Phos., anaemic, dark complexioned people, dark hair and eyes, scrofulous children who are emaciated, weak and unable to stand alone, dry, crusty affections, tuberculous eczema, injured parts become the seat of eczematous eruptions. *Constitutional symptoms are the only safe guide in this remedy.*

Causticum, yellowish looking skin, eczema about the wings of the nose. Pustular eczema, with *burning* and *biting,* preventig sleep.

Dulcamara, phlegmatic, scrofulous constitutions. Vesicular eruptions on red, inflamed base, oozing a watery fluid. Impetiginous eczema of scrofulous children, who suffer with glandular enlargements, itching *worse* by *warmth,* from washing, *better* by *cold, worse* in the *winter* and in *cold and wet weather.*

Graphites, indicated in fair complexioned people inclined to *obesity* and *habitual constipation.*

The eczema is often accompanied with erysipelas, patients who never perspire, who normally have a thin, sensitive skin, who are always suffering from chapped hands, skin dry, greatly thickened, rough, horny, fissured, deep cracks that bleed easily, or *exude* a *watery, sticky fluid.* Eczema with *profuse, serous* exudation, *worse in wet or in snowy weather.* The favourite seats of the eruptions are on the hands, face, lips, behind the ears, joints and flexures of the body *(Tuberculinum, Petroleum, Psorinum, Hepar Sulp., Teucrium).*

DISEASES OF THE SKIN

Hepar Sulp., pustular and erythematous forms of eczema in torpid, lymphatic constitutions, persons with light hair and complexion, soft, flabby muscles, who are slow to act, who are *exteremely sensitive to cold,* croupous children, who perspire profusely, with unhealthy skin, slightest injury heals unkindly. Eczema often spreads by new papules appearing on the outer surface of the part affected. Eczema with profuse yellowish discharge and the parts very sensitive to touch, lesions red, raw, bleeding eaily, sensitive to cold and to touch, and bathed with a profuse yellowish purulent secretion, pustular or seborrheic eczema with soft, friable, yellow crusts, oozing a yellow pus, smelling like old cheese.

Lycopodium Clav., eruptions first vesicular then dry, humid, suppurating, full of deep rhagades, eczema of the face, genitals, any part of the body, covered with thick crusts, or bleeding easily, moist, scald head, or moisture behind the ears, eruptions have great tendency to ulcreate, itching worse at night while in bed, much belching with gastric distrurbaces.

Lachesis, eczema of the erythematous, pustular, vesicular and nodose forms. *Left-sided eczema, dark bluish erythema very sensitive to slightest touch,* dark bluish vesicular eruptions, burning itching with formication like ants, pruritis intense, almost driving the patient to distraction, *worse after sleep, parts very red and swollen and sensitive,* bluish coloured pustules with red streaks along the lymphatic vessels.

Mercurius Sol., eczema of the chest, forearms and legs, yellow cursts with inflamed areola, pustules exuding bloody, purulent secretion, skin dirty yellow, rough and dry, scaly, itching intolerable, *worse* at *night, by warmth of bed, better* in the *day-time and by cold,* eruption has *tendency to ulceration, to bleed* easily and is frequently *copper coloured.*

Mezereum, eczema rubrum in latent syphilitic patients, thick crusts oozing a bloody, purulent secretion, itching worse at night and by warmth, cold skin covered with white scabs, bleeds easily when touched.

Natrium Mur., find vesicular eruptions all over the body, with intense itching which is *worse by cold air* and *undressing,* vesicles dry up, leaving a thin crust, eczema raw, inflamed, discharging a corrosive fluid, *worse* in edges of hair, genitals, bends of the joints and flexure surfaces, low-spirited, despondent people with *tubercular taint* who crave *salt and sour things.*

Petroleum, eczema dry, scaly or moist, *disappearing in the summer* and *re-appearing in the winter or cold weather.* Like *Hepar Sulp.*, the slightest wound causes suppuration. Eczema fissure occuring on the hands, or behind the ears, a moist, purulent secretion, usually offensive, and bleeding easily, pustules burn and itch, eczema often accompanied with chilblains, *aggravation in the morning* and in open air, *itching* and *burning* often *accompanied with chilliness.*

Petroleum, is a deep acting drug, throwing the morbid matter to the surface, as anti-psoric drug working from within outward. Thus, deep-seated, long-standing, wasting diseases call for *Petroleum.*

Psorinum, eruption dry and scaly, moist or suppurating, low-spirited, despondent, unhopeful patients who dread the cold, skin dry, dirty looking, eczema of the scalp, bends and flexures of the body, behind the ears, in pale, peevish delicate children, discharges thin, fetid, excoriating, itching, *worse in the evening* and the *open air, better* by *warmth* and *by rest.*

Psorinum, is our most important skin remedy. It reaches down deeply into the life forces covering every organ, tissue, and mind. It is especially indicated in constitutions which are *'psoric',* that is, in those individuals who are subject to glandular and cutaneous affections and who fail to react to the apparently well-chosesn remedy.

DISEASES OF THE SKIN

Rhus Tox., dark erythematous eruption, more or less vesicular, thin, watery, dark colored and quite offensive secretion, hardness and thickening of the skin, dark, thin brown crusts, intense burning and itching, vesicles often contain a yellowish or straw coloured serum, location of eruption usually on the scalp, face, hands, lower extremities, genitals, *itching, worse by warmth, better by motion and rubbing.*

Sepia, dark complexioned, dark haired, delicate skinned women *eczema,* accompanied with pelvic or uterine disturbances, the lesions usually take on a brownish pigmentation or eruptions alternate with uterine affections, are worse during or after menstruation. Eruptions often assume a circular form or appear in rings, *better* by *warmth,* eruption worse in the flexures of the joints, dry, scaly, brownish patches.

Sepia, symptoms are definitely aggravated at the sea shore. The patient feels generally better from motion and exercise. There is a tendency to ptosis of the organs, with a "ball sensation" of the inner parts. Itching is marked on the hands and flexures, and all humid places. There is often herpes about the mouth and lips. Ringworm-like eruptions.

Sulphur, deeply psoric patients with dry, pimply skin, who never perspire, discharges usually scanty, frequently bloody, all eruptions accompanied with intense itching, which is worse at night and by warmth of bed, *scratching relieves the itching, but is followed by burning and smarting, scratches until* it bleeds, *stoop-shouldered patients who dread to stand or to take a bath,* who suffer from hot feet and from an empty gone feeling in the stomach between ten and eleven o'clock, relieved by eating, imperfectly developed or suppressed eruptions.

Sulphur, typifies inertia and relaxation of fiber, with feebleness of tone. His general appearance is slipshod and unkempt. He is often thin and stooped.

Syphillium, eczema following tertiary or latent syphilis, especially the pustular forms, pus yellowish-green, thick, ichorous, offensive, crusts dark green, even black, with oozing of ichorous, bloody pus, dry, scaly, brown or copper colored eruptions, brown, scaly patches in the bends of the elbows and flexures of the body, many cases cured, follows *Sepia* well, itching only slight, eruptions *worse* in *summer,* indicated in far, absent-minded people who have very little energy.

Thuja, sycotic patients, or after suppressed gonorrhea, *eczema following vaccination,* dirty brown skin, covered with itching vesicles, eruptions worse on covered parts, *moles and warty growths scattered over the body,* white, scabby, measly eruptions, biting, stinging after scartchinhg, follows *Medorrhinum* in suppressed gonorrhea.

Tuberculinum, adapted to light complexioned people, tall, slim, flat, narrow chested, with a family history of tubercular affections, melancholy, despondent, morose, takes cold easily, always chilly, symptoms ever changing, tubercular eruptions with greenish pus, oozing behind the ears, fiery red skin, with rawness and soreness in folds of the skin, eczema over the entire body, itching worse at night, intense when undressing *(Nat Mur., Arsenicum Alb., Hepar Sulp.).*

4. NETTLE-RASH–URTICARIA

Definition

Urticaria or Nettle-Rash, is a non-contagious eruptive disease, characterised by little, hard elevations, upon the skin, of uncertain size and shape, and generally of a red colour, with a whitish tinge, sometimes, however, there is little or no redness, and the elevated parts are even paler than the surface around them, more frequently, however, the elevated spots are partially red and partially white.

DISEASES OF THE SKIN

The eruption, on making its appearance, is attended with intense heat, tingling and itching in the spots.

Causes

Some persons have a constitutional pre-disposition to the disease, and the slightest error in diet, or the slightest derangement in the digestive function, is sufficient to bring on an attack. Children having a fine, delicate skin, are particularly pre-disposed to the attack, and in such cases slight gastric disturbance, a warm day, excessive clothing, dentition, or any slight disturbance is enough to bring on an attack.

Symptoms

The most frequent form of the disease in small children consists in large inflamed blothces of an irregular shape, being either round or oblong, appearing suddenly and preceded by very slight, if any, constitutional symptoms. In some cases, especially in older children, the eruption is preceded by headache, bitter taste in the mouth, coated tongue, nausea, vomiting and fever, particularly in cases in which it was induced by errors in diet and exposure to cold.

Another form of the disease which is preceded, for a few hours or a few days, by feverishness, headache, nausea, chilliness and languor, is where the blotches assume reddish and solid elevations, either round or oblong, often called wheals. This eruption, like the other forms, is attended with violent itching and burning. During this attack, the patient is usually more or less feverish, and suffers from headache, languor, loss of appetite, and other signs of gastric derangement.

Treatment

Aconitum Nap., if the eruption is preceded by much fever, with hot, dry skin, thirst, coated tongue, hard and quick pulse, restlessness and anxiety.

Pulsatilla, when the eruption has been produced by eating unwholesome food, and is attended by looseness of the bowels in the morning. This remedy is particularly suitable for females and persons of a mild temper.

Nux Vomica, when there is considerable gastric derangement with constipation, and when the eruption is excited by indulgenece in spirituous liquors.

Dulcamara, when excited by exposure to cold or damp, when occurring in wet weather, or when attended with some fever, bitter taste in the mouth, diarrhea at night, foul tongue, and violent litching and burning.

Rhus Tox., when arising from some peculiarity of constitution, in which the attacks are excited by some particular article of food.

Bryonia Alba, when the eruption has suddenly disappeared from the surface, and is followed by difficulty of breathing, pain in the breast, etc.

Belladonna, should be given when the eruption is attended by violent headache and red face, the children cry much, the patches are yellowish-red, and rubbing eases the itching.

Apis Mell., if the patches are bluish-red, or pale and transparent, *with much swelling, itching, stinging and burning,* rubbing cannot be borne at all, or if hard rubbing only gives relief, the children become angry easily.

Hepar Sulph, when attended by severe catarrhal symptoms, principally affecting the head and wrose on one side, if commencing on the arms and chest, *worse in the open air,* for persons of a violent, irritable temper.

Arsenicum Alb., if caused by eating unripe fruit, or in severe cases, worse at night, followed by a crup-like cough, also *after the disease has been suddenly suppressed.*

DISEASES OF THE SKIN

Calcarea Carb., when the eruption always appears *more after cold washing,* or *has been suddenly suppressed.*

Calcarea Carb., when the eruption always appears *more after cold washing,* or *has been suddenly repelled.*

Ledum Pal. will cure a majority of cases.

For chronic urticaria, give *Calcarea Carb.* and *Lycopodium Clav.*, in alternation every fourth day.

External applications of all kinds should be avoided in this as well as in other acute eruptive diseases, as their use is liable to cause a sudden disappearance of the eruption, which may have serious or fatal consequences.

5. ERYSIPELAS : ST. ANTHONY'S FIRE

Definition

Erysipelas, is a non-contagious disease, characterised by a deep-red rash, or superficial inflammation of the skin, which has the peculiarity of spreading from place to place, the part first attacked recovering while the neighbouring parts are becoming affected.

Aconitum Nap., is indicated in cases attended by much fever, hot, dry skin, thirst, etc.

Belladonna, is the principal remedy for this disease, when it is accompanied by acute shooting pains, heat and tingling, the redness commencing in a small spot and extending in rays, swelling. It is *particularly valuable in erysipelas of the face,* excessive swelling, so that the eyes are closed, and the features can scarcely be recognized, headache, thirst, hot, dry skin, restlessness and delirium.

Rhus Tox., if small or large blisters appear, or *Graphites.*

Graphites, eruptions oozing out a thick, honey-like fluid, erysipelas sometimes takes this form, and in such cases recurs again and again *(Sulph)*. erysipelatous, moist, scurtz sores ,or 'thin, sticky, glutinous, transparent fluid.'

Eradicates tendency to erysipelas andl so *Graphites 30*, may be given weekly as a prophylactic.

Bryonia Alba, when the disease attacks the joints, and the *pain is increased by the least movement. Sulphur* is sometimes requuired after *Bryonia Alba.*

Lachesis, if the blisters become *bluish.*

Apis Mell., if it *burns and stings,* and if the patients *do not like to be touched,* become ill-humoured, and *cannot bear the warm room.*

Pulsatilla, after *Rhus Tox.*, particularly in wandering erysipelas (when the redness disappears in one place to re-appear in another), and the skin is more of a *bluish-red,* also, in *erysipelas of the ear,* and likewise when the attacks follow some particular articles of food, *in persons pre-disposed to the complaint.*

Bryonia Alba and *Rhus Tox.* are also useful in cases of this kind.

Arsenicum Alb., when the erysipelas assumes a *blackish* hue, with a tendency to gangrene, accompanied by great prostration of strength.

Carbo Vegetablis, may follow *Arsenicum Alb.* in some cases.

Hepar Sulp., Mercurius Sol. and *Phosphorus* are important when the erysipelas ends in abscess.

Arsenicum Alb. and *Sulphur* in cases ending in ulceration.

To allay the itching and heat which is sometimes intolerable, cotton wool may be laid upon or wrapped around the affected part, or powdered starch may be dusted over the surface. *Wet or oily* applications *and washes of every kind should be avoided,* as they *always* aggravate the disease and may prove highly dangerous by suddenly repelling the eruption.

If erysipelas has been repelled, give *Cuprum Met.* It is also useful in cases where the erysipelas was at first slight, then disappeared and returned in a more violent form.

As a prophylactic, *Graphites 30,* weekly.

6. HERPES ZOSTER OR SHINGLES, HERPES CIRCINATUS OR RINGWORM

Definition

By the term 'Herpes' is meant, a peculiar, non-contagious, eruptive disease, characterised by an assemblage of numerous little vesicles or watery pimples, in clusters. These patches of vesicles are surrounded by more or less inflammation, or rather the vesicles are situated on an inflamed surface, and are separated from each other by portions of perfectly healthy skin. The fluid which fills the apex of each little vesicle is at first transparent and colorless, but soon becomes milky and opaque, and in the course of eight or ten becomes milky and opaque, and in the course of eight or ten days is entirely absorbed, or concretes into bran-like scales.

There are several varieties of herpes, those that are most common in children are *Zoster* or *Shingles,* and *Circinatus* or *Ringworm.*

Causes

The most common causes are digestive disturbaces, bilious disorders, of all kinds, sudden changes of temperature, suppressed perspiration, irregularity in diet, and local irritants.

The ringworm patches may appear in any part of the body, but most frequently upon the upper extremities and neck.

Shingles are generally preceded by constitutional symptoms, more or less severe, such as languor, loss of appetite, rigors, headaches, sickness and fever. The local symptoms are pungent and burning pain at the points, where the eruption makes its appearance.

Treatment

Ringworm yields easily under the action of *Sepia*.

One dose of *Sepia 200* may be given every night for three days in succession, and omitted for four days, and then repeated in the same manner.

If this proves insufficient, give *Rhus Tox.* once every third day, three doses, and follow with *Sulphur* in the same way. As soon as there is relief, further doses should be stopped.

Occasionally, it may be necessary to give the following remedies.

If there should be violent Itching–*Nitric Acid* or *Graphites*.

If the surface be scaly–*Sepia, Silicea* or *Sulphur.*

If it be moist or running–*Calcarea Carb., Graphites* or *Rhus Tox.*

For ringworm of the scalp, first give one dose of *Rhus Tox. 200,* every evening for three days, then omit for three days, and then repeat as before. If there is improvement, the doses may be taken at longer intervals until the cure is completed and then dropped. Should the eruption be moist and offensive, give *Staphysagria 200* in the same way as in the case of *Rhus Tox.,* and it may be followed after *Rhus Tox.* If these remedies don't give complete relief, one or two doses of *Arsenicum Alb.* will give better results.

If the eruption affects the scalp and face at the same time, give *Hepar Sulph* or *Calcarea Carb.*

When the glands of the neck become painful and swollen, give *Mercurius Sol.* or *Bryonia Alba.*

DISEASES OF THE SKIN

The only external application which will be useful is a solution of the same remedy which is taken internally. This may be prepared by dissolving eight or ten pills in a cupful of tepid water.

For *Zona or shingles, give Aconitum Nap.*, especially when, on the first breaking out of the eruption, there is languor, headache, pain in the chest, and fever, when these symptoms have subsided, *Rhus Tox.* will be the appropriate remedy and may be given in watery solution, every four hours.

If there should be nausea, and vomiting, give *Antimonium Tart.* every two hours till there is relief. When the fluid in the vesicles, becomes dark, give *Hepar Sulph., the same as Rhus Tox.* When there is great thirst, dry skin, with burning and uncomfortable restlessness, give *Arsenicum Alb.* Should the eruptive patches become ulcerated, give *Mercurius Sol., Lycopodium Clav., Sulphur* or *Sepia.*

If the above remedies don't give complete relief, a few doses of *Sulphur* will complete the cure.

7. WHITLOW–FELON

It is better to apply nothing but clothes, wet with cold or warm water, whichever agrees best, and *keep them wet day and night,* and take one of the following internal medicines.

Mercurius Sol., should be given in the commencement, and will often prevent the disease, from going on to suppuration.

Sulphur, taken after it, will in most cases complete the cure.

Hepar Sulp., is preferable when the pain becomes violent, throbbing, and the swelling increases. If this does not help at all, *Causticum* may be followed.

Silicea, if *Hepar Sulph.* helped somewhat, but when the pain in intense, and the swelling continues unabated.

Lachesis, in cases where the affected part is of a *deep red or bluish* colour.

Arsenicum Alb., if the sore becomes angry looking or *black, with burning pain.*

Sulphur and *Silicea,* administered alternately, at intervals of a week, will remove the tendency to a return of the disease.

8. PIMPLES ON THE FACE–ACNE

The remedies recommended for this disease are *Belladonna, Calcarea Carb., Carbo Veg., Sulphur, Nux Vom., Phosphoric Acid, Ledum Pal. and Sanguinaria.*

9. ABSCESSES

Definition

Abscess is a collection of pus or matter in any part of the body, resulting from inflammation, which may be either acute or chronic.

Causes

An abscess is not an original disease, but is always the result or termination of inflammatory action.

Some children have a hereditary dyscrasia, or constitutional taint-scrofula or some kindred disease-which dispose to the disorder.

Symtpoms

The *acute* form of abscess is preceded and accompanied by sensible and inflammatory action in the affected part, it is hot, throbbing and painful. At the commencement of the suppurative process that is, when the formation of matter takes place, there is a change in the character of the pain, as also in the appearance of

DISEASES OF THE SKIN

the skin. The pain which has previously been acute becomes dull and throbbing, and the skin changes from a red to a dull color. The tumour presents a somewhat conical shape, and the skin over its top becomes thin and of a dark color. At this point, if left alone, the abscess will burst, and allow its contents to escape.

In a *chronic* abscess, the inflammatory action is slow and almost imperceptible, and till the swelling reaches a big size, and becomes apparent, the presence of the abscess will not be known. an acute abscess readily heals as soon as the pus is freely discharged. Not so the chronic abscess, which takes a long time to discharge and so to heal.

Treatment

As abscesses do not always end in suppuration, but sometimes in resolution, that is, the inflammation and swelling subside, without the formation of pus, it is not always advisable to apply poultices, as this may cause it together, when it otherwise would not. Should a swelling appear anywhere upon the surface of the body, which we fear may terminate in an abscess, we should always try to bring about a resolution, that is, to cut short the inflammation before it reaches the point of suppuration. This can best be done by the internal administration of *Aconitum Nap.* and *Belladonna,* in alternation, and by the external application of cold water or cold mud poultice.

If this fails to arrest the disease, the next best thing is to hasten suppuration, and this may be done by the internal administration of *Hep Sulph. 6,* in watery solution, every four hours, and the external application of hot fomentations and poultices. This will help to open the abscess and discharge the pus. After the abscess has opened and matter has been freely discharged, the poultices should be discontinued and simple dressing applied. During this stage, the patient should take *Calcarea Carb. 30* or *Silicea 30.*

For hard and swelled glands on the neck, under the ears or chin, *Mercurius Sol.* and *Calcarea Carb.* are the principal remedies. The medicine should be given in watery solution every four hours.

10. BOILS

Definition

A boil consists of a round, or rather coneshaped, inflammatory, and very painful swelling, immediately under the skin. It varies in size from a pin's head to a lemon. It always has a central core, as it is called, and is common in strong and vigorous children. A boil always suppurates and sooner or later discharges its contents, the matter being at first mixed with blood, and afterwards composed of pus. A boil never discharges freely, and never heals until the core comes away.

Some persons have peculiar constitutional pre-disposition for boils, they also frequently follow after acute fevers, and other diseases.

Treatment

The treatment is about the same as that for abscesses. It is better to apply a poultice early and bring the tumour to a head as soon as possible, as the sooner the matter is discharged, the sooner the process of healing will begin.

Arnica Mont. 30 given internally lessens the pain and inflammation. It should be given in watery solution every four hours.

Should the boil be very red, hot and painful, give *Belladonna* once in three hours, either alone or in alternation with *Mercurius Sol.* When it is slow in coming to a head, give *Hepar Sulph 6.* After the tumour has broken, if the suppuration is excessive, give *Mercurius Sol.* and especially if there should be much swelling and hardness about the base of the tumour.

DISEASES OF THE SKIN

After the matter has been discharged, discontinue the poultice and apply simple dressing.

To eradicte the pre-disposition to boils, one dose of *Sulphur 200* may be taken weekly, for 2 weeks, and thereafter, two doses at fortnightly intervals will be enough.

11. CARBUNCLE

It is larger and harder than a boil, extends further, is of a livid hue and opens in several places, the patient suffers more, there is sleeplessness, prostration, want of appetite etc. After it is opened, there is no relief, and finally, portions of the skin and deeper parts slough.

It appears more frequently in old or debilitated persons, and generally appears on the back, near the spine or on the back of the neck.

Arnica Mont. 30 given from the beginning of the trouble may lessen the pain and prevent it altogether, if so, *Nux Vomica* will remove the remaining symptoms.

If, however, it develops, the best way to hasten the process of suppuration is to administer *Bryonia Alba 30* in watery solution in repeated doses, and in five or six days the tumour may begin to discharge. If action of this medicine appears to have ceased, then *Rhus Tox. 30* may be given in the same way and this will complete the cure in 8 to 10 days. If the malignant tumour, after previous allopathic treatment, secretes a badly coloured fluid, *Silicea 30* will give better results. If the tumour threatens to become gangrenous, and *Silicea* is not sufficient to prevent this, *Lachesis* and *Arsenicum Alb.* are the most effective medicines.

12. CHILBLAIN–FROSTBITE

For external application, plain white vaseline is the best but when this is not available, plain coconut oil may be used.

Pulsatilla, may be given when the skin assumes a deep red, bluish colour with pricking, burning pains, worse in the afternoon and evening, better by the cool air blowing on them Symptoms changeable, worse after menses and when getting warm.

Nux Vomica, when of a bright red colour.

Sulphur, when the above remedies are insufficient, also in deeply psoric patients with chronic dry skin.

Chamomilla, when, in addition to the itching and burning, there are acute pains in the affected part.

Arsenicum Alb., for acute, burning pains, also for the irritable, ill-conditioned ulcers which sometimes occur.

Belladonna, bright red, shining swelling of the part, very sensitive to touch, tingling and itching, *worse from touch.*

Agaricus Mus., acquired or *hereditary chilblains,* dark, purple or bright red blotches, *with a marked periodicity* of the appearance of the eruptions, electric-like shocks, pricking as of needles, redness of the part, with intense burning, biting, stinging and itching, indicated in light-haired people with lax muscle.

Petroleum, tubercular patients with moist chilblains, parts painfully swollen and red, pustules form, itch and burn like fire, chilly sensations throughout the body accompanying the itching. Chilblains of the hands, heels, toes, accompanied with moisture.

Rhus Tox., dark colored blothces with itching, burning, stinging, *worse* before storms or when getting wet. Chilblains with muscular pains throughout the body, the suffering is relieved by motion and gentle rubbing. Burning, stinging, smarting, itching, with fine vesicles appearing on a dark blue erythematous base.

Tuberculinum, in tall, slim, flat, narrow-chested people, who have a family history of tubercular affections, and whose symptoms are ever changing, who take cold easily, eruptions dry and scaly, itching intolerable, followed by long-lasting burning and smarting,

DISEASES OF THE SKIN

better by warm bathing. Obstinate chronic cases with tubercular history.

Psorinum, pale, emaciated, very psoric people, who worry and fret very much about their condition, who have unhealthy inactive skin, and who do not perspire, they are *extremely sensitive to cold,* dirty, tawny colored eruption, with fine scales over the surface, disappearing during the warm weather, but re-appearing during the cold, fingers and toes are so swollen that they can't flex them, with desquamation of fine scales. Suppressed cases are often reproduced by this remedy.

Local symptoms, intense itching, burning and biting, scratching until it bleeds.

13. CORNS

Corns are circumscribed hypertrophies of the epidermis, occurring more frequently about the small joints of the extremities.

They arise not only from tight boots and shoes, but also from a chronic disposition with some persons.

They may be reduced by the use of *Antimonium Crud., Arnica Mont., Bryonia Alba, Rhus Tox., Phosphorus, Lycopodium Clav., Phos. Acid.* and *Sulphur* according to temperament, constitution and other circumstances.

Relief may be got by bathing the feet in warm water and applying *Arnica Mont.* lotion.

If the corns pain much during change of weather, *Rhus Tox., Bryonia Alba* or *Calcarea Carb.* may be used according to the kind of weather.

14. WARTS

Warts are little papillomatous growth of sycotic origin, covered with hypertrophied layer of the epidermis.

There are several kinds of warts and the main point for consideration in giving the appropriate remedy is the *kind* of warts, viz., whether they are *fleshy, pedunculated* or *horny.*

FLESHY WARTS–*Caust., Rhus Tox.* or *Dulcamara.*

HORNY WARTS–*Calcarea Carb., Sepia, Antimonium. Crud, Thuja.*

PEDUNCULATED (FLAT-HARD AND BRITTLE) WARTS–*Caust., Lycopodium Clav.*

WARTS ON FACE–*Calcarea Carb., Caust.*

WARTS ON THE NOSE–*Caust., Thuja.*

WARTS NEAR THE NAILS, IF FLESHY–*Caust.*

WARTS OF THE HANDS AND FINHGERS–*Calcarea Carb., Sepia, Rhus Tox., Dulc., Thuja.*

WARTS ON THE BACK OF THE HANDS OR FINGERS–*Natrium Carb.,* and *Dulc.*

WARTS ON THE SIDES OF THE FINGERS–*Sep., Thuja, Calcarea Carb.*

FOR ISOLATED WARTS–*Caust., Natrium Carb., Calcarea Carb.*

FOR YOUNG GIRLS–*Sulphur, Sepia, Thuja.*

FOR SEVERAL KINDS GENERALLY–*Sulph, Dulc., Sepia, Thuja, Rhus Tox, Calcarea* and *Lycopopodium Clav.*

15. FALLING OUT OF THE HAIR

IF DUE TO THE USE OF MERCURIAL MEDICINES–*Aurum Met.,* followed by *Graphites* and *Hepar Sulph.*

SINGLE BALD SPOTS, ESPECIALLY BEHIND THE EARS–*Phosph.*

GREY HAIR IN YOUNG PEOPLE DUE TO GRIEF AND SORROW–*Phosph Acid.*

LOSS OF HAIR WITH MUCH ITCHING AND SCALES ON THE HEAD–*Lycopodium Clav., Bryonia Alba,* and *Calcarea Carb.*

IF THE HAIR WAS VERY DRY AND WILTED–*Kalium Carb.*

BALDNESS OF YOUNG PEOPLE–*Lycopodium Clav.,* also *Baryta Carb.*

FALLING OUT OF THE EYEBROWS–*Kalium Carb.* and *Graph.*

FALLING OUT OF THE WHISKERS–*Graph., Natrium M* and *Calcarea Carb.*

16. AFFECTIONS OF THE NAILS

Ingrowing Toe Nails, you may follow Hering's advice ('domestic Physician', pages 408 and 409) of scraping the nail in the middle with a sharp knife and afterwards not to trim them off on the side but in front, so that the depression is turned outwards. The soreness arising from the growing of the nails into the flesh may be healed, if sufficient lint soaked in a solution of *Tincture of Arnica Mont.* is introduced between the nail and the flesh and kept in place by a bandage, and the dressing renewed daily till the soreness is healed. If *Arnica Mont.* is not sufficient, and the ulceration had proceeded too far, *Sulphur 30* and then, the part is dressed with a lint dipped in the solution of two globules of the same medicine which is taken internally.

SOFT, PLIABLE NAILS–require *Graph.* and *Sulph.* Liability of the nails to *split–Silicea.*

BRITTLE NAILS–*Alumina, Silicea.*

THICKENING AND DISTORTION OF THE NAILS-
Graph., Silicea, Sulphur.

BADLY COLORED, YELLOW NAILS-*Sepia, Silicea, Sulphur, Graph., Nitricum Acid.*

HANGNAILS-continually forming, *Rhus Tox, Sulph., Calcarea Carb., Lycopodium Clav.*

17. BED SORES

These may frequently be *prevented* by placing an open vessel filled with water under the bed of the patient, renewing the water every day, or by bathing the red spots that threaten to become sore, with brandy. Wetting the sore places with *very cold* water, or applying wet cloths, accelerates the healing. If plain water alone does not suffice, a few drops of *Arnica tincture* may be dropped into the water and the same utilised as above.

If the parts become *gangrenous, China off.* 30 may be given internally, and the affected parts washed with a solution of the same medicine in a little water. When the wound is large, scraped sweet carrots may be applied to it.

18. LEUCODERMA

Definition

A disease characterized by the absence of the normal pigment matter of the skin. It may be congenital or acquired.

Symptoms

At first the patches are small, but they gradually increase in size. The disease spreads slowly, taking years to affect large surfaces. There is, as a rule, no impairment in the general health, except it be such mental conditions as would naturally develop from the disfigurement.

DISEASES OF THE SKIN

Treatment

Arsenicum Sulph flavum, has been found useful, and may be used in different potencies ranging from 30 to C.M. It has cured some cases of young persons and in recent cases, with the use of the higher potencies. In chronic cases of some years' standing, it has proved palliative, and arrested further development.

CHAPTER-XXIX

SOME GENERAL DISEASES

1. CHRONIC RHEUMATISM

Leading Indications

For pains excited or aggravated by the slightest chill– *Aconitum Nap., Bryonia Alba, Calcarea Carb., Dulcamara, Mercurius Sol.* or *Sulphur.*

When the attacks are excited by bad weather–
Calcarea Carb., Dulcamara, Rhus Tox., Lycopodium Clav. and *Hepar Sulph.*

When every change of weather causes a relapse–
Calcarea Carb., Silicea, Sulphur, Dulcamara, Rhus Tox. and *Lachesis.*

Rhus Tox. and *Bryonia Alba* are the two great remedies, the points of difference between the two are–

Rhus Tox.	Bryonia Alba
Restlessness and desire to move about continually, on account of the relief to the aches and pains.	Disposition to keep perfectly quiet, as moving causes an aggravation of all pains and yet sometimes pains force the patient to move.
Suitable especially for Rheumatism of *fibrous tissues, sheaths* of *muscles &c.*	Suitable for rheumatism of the *joints* and of *muscular tissue itself.*
Rheumtism from *exposure to wet* when over-heated and perspiring	Though a *Bryonia Alba* rheumatism may occur from these causes, this is not *specially* so, as in the case of *Rhus Tox.*

The great key notes of *Rhus* Tox are–
- (*a*) The pains are *worse* from sitting and from *rising from a sitting position,* or *on first commencing to move,* but continued motion, however relieves. The lumbago, however, is sometimes worse from motion.
- (*b*) The *stiffness* and soreness of the pains, also tearing pains, drawing paralyzed sensations, and even stitches.
- (*c*) The aggravation from damp weather are cold. Cold air is not tolerated, it seems to make the skin painful.
- (*d*) The relief of all the symptoms by warmth or warm applications.

Rhus Tox. has especial affinity for the *deep muscles of the back.* The sudden pain in the back known as 'Crick' is Met. well with this remedy. The *lower extremities* are also affected. It is also a remedy for the effects of over-exertion, such as sprains, wrenches etc., in the *fibrous tissues,* while *Arnica Mont.* affects the *softer structures.*

Bryonia Alba, the rheumatism of *Bryonia Alba* attacks the *joints* themselves, producing *articular* rheumatism, and also inflames the muscle tissue, causing *muscular* rheumatism. The muscles are sore, and swollen, and the joints are violently inflamed, red, swollen, shiny and very hot. The pains are *sharp, stitching* or *cutting* in character, and always *worse from the slightest motion.* Touch and pressure also aggravate.

Bryonia Alba, Ledum Pal, Nux Vom. and *Colchicum* are the four chief remedies having aggravation from motion.

Causticum resembles *Rhus Tox.* closely in many respects.

The points of difference are—

Causticum	Rhus Tox.
The restlessness of this remedy occurs only *at night*.	Restlessness all the time.
Rheumatism caused by *dry, cold, frosty air*.	Rheumatism from *damp, wet weather*.
Pains impel constant motion, which does not releive.	Motion relieves the patient temporarily.

The symptoms of *Causticum* are—

A *stiffness* of the joints, the tendons seem shortened and the limbs are drawn out of shape-it is a sort of *rheumatoid arthritis*. There is *relief from warmth*, as with *Rhus Tox.* There are drawing, musuclar pains and soreness of the parts on which the patient lies, much weakness and trembling, weakness of the ankle-joint, contracted tendons, and a sprained feeling in the hip joints.

Aconitum Nap., is often a useful remedy in the first stage of rheumatic fever, it is Homeopathic not only to the fever, but also to the local affections caused by the rheumatic poison.

Calcarea Carb., rheumatic affections caused by working in water. If *Rhus Tox.* fails, *Calcarea Carb.* will complete the cure. Gouty nodosities about the fingers are also present.

Dulcamara, a prominent remedy for rheumatism, made worse by sudden changes in the weather, especially when cold and damp. *Calcarea Phos.,* is also similar to this remedy, but *pains are especially in the back* and extending down the legs.

Arnica Mont. has rheumatism, resulting from exposure to *dampness, cold and excessive muscular strain combined.* The parts are sore and bruised. Rheumatic *stiffness* caused by *getting the head and neck wet is best* Met. with *Belladonna*.

SOME GENERAL DISEASES

Pulsatilla, has a tendency for the rheumatism to shift about, *wanering rheumatic pains being its main feature* (also *Kalmia, Bryonia Alba, Colchicum, Sulphur, Kalium Bichromicum* and *Kalium Sulph.),* *aggravtion* from *warmth, aggravation* in the *evening,* and *relief from cold.* The *knee, ankel* and *tarsal joints* are the seat of the trouble. There is restlessness the pains are so severe that the patient is compelled to move, and *slow, easy motion* relieves (also *Lycopodium Clav.* and *Ferrum Met.). Gonorrheal rheumatism (Thuja).* The joints are swollen and the pains are sharp and stinging, with a feeling of subcutaneous ulceration. *Kalium Bichromicum* is also a remedy for wandering rheumatism, but is *relieved* in a *warm room* (unlike *Pulsatilla).* Rheumatism dependent on *disturbance of the liver or stomach* finds its remedy in *Pulsatilla.*

Kalmia, another remedy for wandering rheumatic pains, is especially useful in rheumatism *affecting the chest,* or when *rheumatism or gout shifts from the joints to the heart, suppressed* in most cases by *external applications,* or allopathic remedies. It has also tearing pains in the legs, without swelling, without fever, but with great weakness, and in this symtpom of weakness, it resembles *Colchicum,* the pains about the chest in *Kalmia* cases shoot down into the stomach and abdomen. The muscles of the neck are sore and the back is lame, the rheumatic pains are mostly in the *upper parts of the arms* and *lower parts of the legs,* and are worse when going to sleep. *Inflammatory rheumatism, shifting from joint to joint, with tendency to attack the heart, high fever, excruciating pains, which are made worse by motion,* are the main features of *Kalmia.* In *valvular deposits, Kalima* and *Lithum Carb.,* are our foremost drugs.

Cimicifuga, its chief symptom is *great acting* in the *muscles,* right in the *fleshy part* (the belly of the muscles rather than the extremities), large muscles of the trunk rather than the small muscles of the extremities *(Nux Vomica).* Rheumatism *in the* muscles coming on suddenly and of great security, worse at night, and in wet and windy weather. There is great restlessness, but motion aggravates.

Colchicum, useful for *gout and rheumatism*. It has special affinity for fibrous tissues, tendons, ligaments and periosteum. It has also *shifting* rheumatism *(Pulsatilla, Kalima, etc.).* The pains are worse in the evening, the *slightest motion aggravates*, the patient is irritable, the pain seems unbearable. Sometimes useful when the rheumatism attacks the chest, with pains about the heart, and a sensation as if the heart were squeezed by a tight badage, there is great evening aggravation, the joints are swollen and dark red.

Colchicum, is specially useful for rheumatic affections in *debilitated persons*, those who are weak—*weakness being the characteristic*. It is also a remedy for the *smaller joints*.

Sanguinaria, inflames muscular tissue, giving a picutre of acute muscular rheumatism. The muscles are sore and stiff, with flying erratic pains in them or stitching. The *muscles of the back and neck are especially affected* by it. Its chief field is the *right deltoid muscle, described as a rheumatic pain in the right arm and shoulder*, worse at night or on turning in bed. It is so severe that the patient cannot raise the arm.

Phytolacca, useful in *syphilitc* cases. It is particularly useful in pains below the elbows and knees. There is stiffness and lameness of the muscles, the *pains* seem to *fly about*, are *worse at night* and are *especially aggravated by damp weather*. Rheumatic affections of the sheaths of the nerves, periosteal rheumatism or rheumatism ofj the fibrous tissues, rheumatism of the shoulders and arms, especially in syphilitic *cases*.

Silicea, is useful in treating *hereditary rheumatism*. the pains are worse at night, *worse* from *uncovering, better* from *warmth*.

SOME GENERAL DISEASES

Guaiacum, useful in the *chronic* forms of articular rheumatism where the joints are distorted with concretions or deposits. *One important symptom is the contraction of the tendons, which draw the limb out of shape,* worse on any motion, stiffness and soreness of the joints and soreness of the muscles also present. It follows *Causticum* very well.

Syphilitic or mercurial rheumatism, and gonorrheal rheumatism, where many joints are affected, they are rigid, hot swollen land painful, and the *contraction will be present,* the muscles seem too short.

2. LUMBAGO–PAIN IN THE LOINS AND BACK

Aconitum Nap., if accompanied by much fever.

Arnica Mont., if cuased by external injury, or by over-lifting, etc.

Bryonia Alba, when the pains in the back are very severe, compelling the patient to walk in a stooping posture, *aggravated* by the *least motion,* or *draught of air,* and attended with a general chilliness.

Nux Vomica, when the part affected feels as if bruised, or as after excessive fatigue, and when motion, and *particularly turning in bed aggravates the pain* (the patient has to sit up and then turn), also when accompanied by weakness, constipation and irritable temper.

Rhus Tox., when the pains are similar to those described under *Nux Vomica,* but are aggravated by rest.

Belladonna, may follow *Aconitum Nap.,* when the pains are *deep-seated,* and cause a heavinesss, gnawing, or stiffness.

Pulsatilla, when the pain resemble those mentioned under *Nux Vomica,* espcially in women or persons of a mild disposition.

Mercurius Sol., for pains described as above, but which are *much worse at night.*

3. SCIATICA

It is like lumbago, but the pain is more in the region of the hip-joint, shooting down the back of the thigh, and sometimes extending to the foot.

Aconitum Nap., when there is a numbness in the limbs or toes.

Colcocynth, is *particularly useful* in this affection, *especially* when seated in the *right hip*, or if excited by a fit of anger or indignation.

Rhus Tox., when the pains are *aggravated* by *rest*, and *better by motion*. It is the *best remedy for a combination of lumbago and sciatica*.

Nux vomica, when the pain is attended by a sensation of stiffness of contraction of the limb, also when *torpor with chilliness* is felt in the affected parts, constipation and sedentary habits.

Ignatia, for cutting pains, particularly on moving the limb.

Chamomilla, when the pains are worse at night, and attended with excessive sensitiveness.

Arsenicum Alb., in cases where the pains are acute and dragging, with a sensation of coldness in the part affected, also when the *pains* are *periodical*, it is also useful for weak or emaciated persons. It is *aggravated by cold*, but *relieved* momentarily by *warmth*.

Arnica Mont., due to over-exertion. The acute pains are followed by a sensation as if bruised.

Bryonia Alba has shooting pains, *worse from motion* and *relieved by hard pressure*. It is useful for sciatica of *rheumatic origin*.

Belladonna, with high inflammation, and the pains come on suddenly. There is neuritis, and the course of the nerve is sensitive, the pain is especially severe at night, the parts are sensitive to the

SOME GENERAL DISEASES

touch, the least concussion or a draft of air aggravates. Severe lancinating pains coming on in the afternoon or evening, has to change position often, worse from motion, noise, shock or contact, cannot bear the clothing to touch him. Relieved by letting the limb hang down, warmth and the erect posutre.

4. SLEEPLESSNESS

In most cases, when not the result of a disease, sleeplessness may be attributed to the manner of living. Some persons cannot eat anything in the evening, or but a little, without suffering from loss of sleep. Others cannot sleep soundly unless they have eaten something before going to bed. the most common causes of sleeplessness are the use of coffee and tea.

Exercise in the open air is one of the best preventives, but it must not be taken too late in the evening, or it will have a contrary effect. Drinking coffee and tea late in the evening by those who are not accustomed to it, and excessive use of these and at all tiems should also be avoided.

Belladonna, the sleepless conditions calling for *Belladonna* are due to *congestion,* sleep is extremely restless, as a rule it is interrupted by talking, startings, muscular jerkings and spasmodic motions, frightful images appear on closing the eyes and the patient, therefore dreads sleep. Children awake from sleep frightened. Often there is a violent throbbing in the brain which prevents sleep. The dreams found under *Belladonna* are frightful ones, and they constantly awaken the patient. It is probably our best remedy for insomnia due to cerebral hypremia, that is, it will be most often indicated *after the use of morphine* which produces cerebral hyperemia of a passive variety.

Belladonna, is most useful in restless sleep during dentition, child sleeps with eyes partially open, sudden starting, twitching, hot head and dilated pupils will indicate it.

Aconitum Nap., has intense anxiety and restlessness, fear of disaster of death.

Nux vomica, is especially the remedy for those who drink, too much, those who abuse coffee and tea, those who are subject to abdominal disorders and a sluggish portal circulation. Sleeplessness from mental overwork, from too close study, especially at night. The great characteristic of this remedy is that the patient is very sleepy in the evening, cannot keep awake, moreover the sleep is not sound or restful and the patient is awakened at night by anxiety and frightful dreams. He awakens at about three or four o'clock in the morning feeling somewhat refreshed, but soon sleeps again and awakens at the usual time feeling worse than ever. The morning sleep aggravates all the affections.

Pulsatilla, is sleepless in the evening, falling asleep very late, the sleep is restless, with frequent awakenings and troubled dreams. Sleeplessness after *quinine, iron, strychine, tea* or *chlorae.*

Sulphur, sleeplessness from nervous excitement, cutaneous irritations and external heat. The patient is drowsy all day and sleepless at night. Sleeps in "Cat Naps", wakes frequently. The slightest noise awakens, and it is difficult to get to sleep again.

Calcarea Carb., has long hours of wakefulness.

Hyoscyamus Nig., sleeplessness from nervous excitement, the brain is full of bewildering ideas and images. Sleeplessness from overworked minds and without apparent cause. After long illnessness and the brain cells are badly nourished, this remedy is very useful, specially useful for sleeplessness in children, who twitch, cry out frightened and tremble.

Hyoscyamus Nig., lacks the *anxiety* of *Aconitum Nap.,* the violence of *Belladonna,* the pessimism of *Nux Vomica,* and the stupidity of *Gelsemium.*

SOME GENERAL DISEASES

Gelsemium, for the insomnia of brain workers, for business men who pass restless nights, awaken early in the morning and worry over their business affairs. It is most useful also in a state of *alternate excitement and depression.*

It has also sleeplessness from emotional distrubances, and after evening company.

Bryonia Alba, is useful where the business cares of the day keep him awake.

Coffea, in cases where there is *exessive agitation of body and mind,* and where ideas force themselves on the mind. The patient is wide awake, without the slightest inclination to sleep, and all the senses are extremely acute, when excitement or good news, joys or night watching causes the insomnia.

It acts better in the 200*th* potency.

It is well suited to sleeplessness in children due to severe pain, and also for weak, nervous women. If the 30*th* potency does not act so well, the 200*th* will act better.

Opium, suits sleeplessness when the patient is *sleepy but cannot get to sleep,* is kept awake by hearing distinctly ordinary noises, such as the ticking of clocks and the crowing of cocks. *Great drowsiness* is characteristic of the remedy. The remedy also acts better in the 200*th* potency in older persons.

Arsenicum Alb., for the sleeplessness of *malnutrition,* where there is *general degeneration of the blood, and exhaustion of the nervous system.* Restlessness or anemic irritability.

China off., has sleeplessness from *exhausting diseases.* The mind is active and the patient indulges in castle building.

Phosphorus, sleeplessness following *intense mental overwork* and *anxiety,* coupled with *confusion, vertigo* and *pain in the head.*

Ignatia, has sleeplessness from *depressing news, recent grief,* causing a hyperemia.

5. SUNSTROKE

The following remedies are useful:

Glonoine (Nitro-glycerine), bad effects from being exposed inordinately to sun's rays. "For over-heating in the sun, or sun-stroke." Bursting headache, rising up from the neck. Great throbbing, sense of expansion as if head would burst. Cannot bear the least jar. Undulating sensation in head. Waves of heat, upwards, head feels larger. Congestions, blood tends upwards. Vessels (jugular, temporal) pulsate. Temporal arteries raised, felt like whipcord. Throbbing, constriction in neck, as if blood could not return from head. Sensation of strangulation in throat *(Lach.).* Whole head felt crowded with blood. All arteries in head felt as distinct as though they had been dissected out. Skull too small, brain attempting to burst it, even nausea, followed by unconsciousness. *Bell.* and *Glon,* both have the fullness, pain and throbbing, but that of *Glon* is more intense and sudden in onset, and subsides more rapidly when relieved. *Bell.* is better bending head back, *Glon.,* worse, *Glon.* has waves of pain, of blood, upwards. *Glon* has more disturbance of heart's action, *Bell.,* more intense burning of skin. Both have very red faces *(Mel.).*

Melilotus, fearful headaches, confusion of thought. Violent congestion to head. Violent, *throbbing* headache, relieved by nose-bleed. Most intense redness of face, with throbbing carotids.

Belladonna, also (with *Glon.)* sudden onset. Red flushed face, throbbing carotids, perhaps delirium, spasms, jerks and twitchings. Eyes staring, red, blood-shot : "when you put your hand on a *Bell.* subject, you want to suddenly withdraw it, the heat is so intense." Inflammation of the base of the brain and medulla from exposure to sun. *Bell.* covers all the symptoms to sun-stroke-

SOME GENERAL DISEASES

restlessness, vertigo, breathlessness nausea and vomiting, with frequent urination (even if only a few drops have accumulated), temperature high. Incontinence of urine and faeces. Stertor. Pulse rapid.

Acontum Nap., when there is much fear, restlessness, and anxiety. "Sun-stroke, especially from sleeping in the sun's rays." Head excessively hot *(Bell.),* with burning as though brain were moved by boiling water. Boiling and seething sensations. High fever, vertigo, face very red *(Bell., Stram., Melilot),* feels as if it has grown much larger *(Natrium Carb.), Tingling sensations exceedingly characteristic.* One of the remedies of apoplexy, of that apoplexy.

Gelsemium, from heat of sun in summer. Weakness and *trembling,* of any part, or the whole body. Headache begins in cervical spine, with bursting sensation in forehead and eyeballs, worse from heat of sun, sensation of a band around head, above eyes. Great heaviness of eyelids.

Lachesis, has also a reputation for sunstroke, or effects of sunstroke. "Paralysis depending on an apopletic condition of brain, after extremes of heat and cold." Face, dark red, *bluish,* bloated, as in apoplexy.

Great characteristic, worse from sleep. Sleeps into an aggravation. Dreads to go to sleep, because he wakes with such a headache. Rush of blood to head, weight and pressure on vertex. *Great sensitiveness to touch, especially throat and abdomen.*

Arnica Mont., apoplexy, loss of consciousness. Here the great characteristic in any sickness is *intense soreness and bruised feelings of the body. Everything on which he lies feels too hard.* Must move to get a new place, not yet sore. Heat of upper part of the body, coldness of lower face and head alone hot, body cool *(Camph.).*

Carbo Veg, ailments from getting overheated. Obtuseness, vertigo, heaviness of head, pale greenish face, cold, with cold sweat.

Vital force nearly exhausted. Complete collapse. Blood stagnates in capillaries, surface cold and blue. Air hunger.

Natrium Carb., chronic effects of sunstroke. Headache from slightest mental exertion, *from the sun,* even working under gets light. Inability to think. Feels stupid, comprehension slow, difficult. Head feels too large, as if it would burst *(Aconitum Nap.)*. Great debility from heat of summer. Aversion to and worse from milk.

Natrium Mur., sunstroke. Heat in head, with red face, nausea and vomiting. Rush of blood to head, headache, as if head burst *(Glon.)*. Heaviness occiput, draws eyes together. Blinding of eyes, *fiery zig-zag* charcteristic. Worse sun, worse seaside, worse summer.

Pulsatilla, ailments from heat of sun. Excessive vertigo. Headache with throbbing in brain. Even apoplexy, unconscious, face purplish, bloated, violent beating of heart. Pulse collapsed. *Puls.* is *worse,* sitting, lying, *better* walking in open air. *Puls.* is apt to be fearful.

In selecting the appropriate remedy for any case, it is not enough to take only the cause of the trouble and the ordinary symptoms, which follow, into account, but any prominent characteristic symptoms which may be present should also come into the picture for the purpose. To quote an example, Dr. Nash, when treating a mental case in a women of 30, who had been overheated in the sun, during an excursion, who feared she was lost and begged the doctor to pray with and for her, talked day and night about it, and would not sleep a wink, or let anybody else sleep, and said that her head was as big as a bushel, give *Glonoine, Lachesis, Natrium Carb.* etc., on the cause as the basis of the prescription, and all these proved useless. As *Stramonium* covered her prominent characteristic symptoms, viz., continuous talking on the same subject, it was given and she got normal in 24 hours and was saved the contingency of being sent to a Launatic asylum.

SOME GENERAL DISEASES

Note : A red or orange lining inside a hat, or along the spine in a coat, is said to protect from sunstroke.

A raw onion, kept inside a cap or turban, in touch with the top of the head, also affords protection.

6. CONVALESCENCE

Towards the end of acute diseases or prolonged illness, the recovery of the patient may be retarded for some reason or other, or after the recovery, there may still remain some symptoms which may prevent the early recuperation of the patient to normal health. It will be useful to indicate the remedies which will be necessary for the patient's early recovery and restoration to normal health.

Therapeutic Hints

Alstonia Sch. atonic dyspepsia and excessive prostration and debility following acute diseases. Characteristics are– empty gone sensation in stomach and sinking in abdomen, with debility. *A tonic after exhausting fevers.*

Anacardium, for neurasthenics who have a type of nervous dyspepsia, relieved by food, *impaired memory,* depression, and irritability, diminution of senses (smell, sight, hearing), aversion to work, lacks self confideence, irresistible desire to swear and curse. Empty feeling in stomach, *eating, temporarily relieves all discomfort.*

Arsenicum Alb., ravenous appetite, protacted case with mild delirium, anxiety and restlessness. *Great exhaustion after the slightest exertion.* Anemia and chlorosis. Degenerative changes.

Baptisia Tinct., lassitude and weakness of whole body, with indifference; disagreeable prostration, with soreness of muscles.

Calcarea Carb., easy relapses, interrupted convalescence. Great sensitiveness to cold, partial sweats. Desire for eggs.

Capsicum, persons of lax fiber, weak, diminished vital heat not much reactive force.

China off., marasmus, slow recovery, bilious vomiting and diarrhea.

Cocculus Ind., delayed convalescence, fever deeps up, faint feeling.

Cuprum Met., relapse from over-exertion of mind and body.

Fluoric Acid, unpleasant sensations running upward.

Guiacum, unpleasant sensations running downward.

Ignatia, hemi-crania, relapse from fright.

Kreosotum, obstinate vomiting.

Laurocerasus, lack of reaction in chest troubles.

Nux Vomica, relapse from anger, or from mental overexertion.

Psorinum 200, appetite does not return, or ravenous appetite, despair of recovery, prostration, sexual desire gone *(Phos.)*, weakening sweats, day and night. *Debility*, independent of any organic disease, especially the weakness remaining after acute disease.

Pulsatilla, cannot eat, everything tastes bitter, or ravenous appetite.

Rhus Tox., relapse from muscular over-exertion.

Selenium, chilliness, sensitiveness to least draught, lower limbs feel, as if paralysed, unpleasant sensation running upward.

Silicea, slow healing of bedsore due to cerebral lesions, of °inflammation of sacrum.

Sulphur, appetite does not return.

Valeriana, in nervous affectiosn remaining at a standstill *(Ambra Grisea)*.

7. EMERGENCIES–EUTHANASIA (Easy Death)

The question may be asked whether, in times of great suffering, Homeopathy can do anything to give immediate relief to the patient. While allopaths give morphine and other stupefying agents, which make the patients insensible to all sensations and give no real relief, Homeopaths prescribe suitable remedies which give ease and comfort to the patients, though a cure is not possible in desperate cases.

For consumptives in their last stage, when they have hectic fever, which so rapidly burns the patient up, the hot afternoon skin, the night sweat, the constant burning thirst, the red spot on the cheek, the diarrhea, the stool escapes when coughing, the intense fever in the afternoons, the constriction of the chest, suffocation, a dose of *Phosphorus* 1 M., but not repeated, will, after some initial aggravation, give him relief of the fever, and he will go on till death comfortably. If the patient has distressing suffocation, inward distress in the chest and stomach, streaming perspiration, great sinking, must have the clothing away from the neck, chest, abdomen, with ghastly countenance, a few doses of *Lachesis 200,* given, as often as may be required, will give prompt relief to the patient.

If he is covered with a cold sweat, and requires constant fanning, the abdomen is distended with flatus, and the breath is cold, he will require *Carbo Veg. 30,* in watery solution every hour. If this is given for 6 hours and then stopped he will pass away in peace.

If he gets severe pains in the abdomen in the last stage of mortification, he will require *Arsenicum Alb. 30* or *Secale Cor. 30* according to symptoms which will reduce the severity of the pains.

In the very last stage, when death is inevitable, *Tarentula Cub. 30* will ease his sufferings and take him to easy death.

8. COLLAPSE

The chief remedies in this condition are: *Carbo Veg., an almost "Corpse revivor".* Lack of reaction after some violent shock, some violent attack, some violent suffering. After surgical shock, collapse, and danger of dying of shock. Air-hunger, desire to be fanned, must have more air. Cold knees, breath cold, tongue cold, cold sweat, cold nose. Nose and face pinched, cadaveric, face very pale greysih yelow, greenish, corpse-like. May be distension of stomach and abdomen *(Colch.).*

Verat. Alb., wonderful coldness, coldness of discharges, coldness of body. *Profuse cold sweat, cold sweat on forehead. Fluids run out of body, produces watery discharges.* Lies in bed, relaxed and prostrated, cold to finger-tips, blue or purplish, lips cold and blue, face pinched and shrunken, sensation, as if the body were ice-water *(Arsenicum Alb.).* Head packed in ice, ice on vertex. *One of Hahnemann's great cholera medicines.*

Opium, from fright, shock from injury *(Arnica Mont.),* severe cases, rapid breathing, every breath a loud moan, face livid or pale, lips livid, cool, clammy skin, eyes fixed unequally, or, long slow expiration, cheeks blown out, or mouth wise open. Coldness extremities, or burning heat of perspiring body.

Characteristics, painlessness, inactivity and torpor. Increased excitability of voluntary muscles with decreased excitability of involuntary muscles.

Arnica Mont., from mechanical injuries *(Opium).* Concussion with unconsciousness, pallor, drowsiness. Cold surface, depressed vitality from shock. Stupor, with involuntary discharges.

Characteristic, while answering, falls into a deep stupor before finishing.

Camphor, coldness, blueness, *scanty sweat.* Scanty discharges (rev. of *Verat.).* "*Camph.* in heat, wants to be covered up, his coldness is relieved by cold, wants more cold. A troublesome patient to nurse, the more violent the suffering the sooner he is cold, and when cold, must uncover and be in a cold room, them a flash of heat and he wants covers on, wants hot bottles, and while this is being done, is cold again, and wants windows open, and everything cool. *Camphor* 6 or 30 will put him in a refreshed sleep.

Arsenicum Alb., the collapse of *Arsenicum Alb.* is marked by restlessness, and fear. *Prostration, with awful anxiety.* The prominent characteristics of *Arsenicum Alb.* are *anxiety, restlessness, prostration, burning* and *cadaveric odours.* "In bed first moves whole body, as prostration becomes marked, can only move limbs. At last so weak he lies quiet, like a corpse". Mouth black, parched and dry. Ceaseless thirst for small quantities often. "With his violent chills and rigors says, the blood flowing through his veins is like ice-water *(Verat Alb.),* then fever comes, and he feels that boiling water is going through his blood vessels."

Aconitum Nap., agonised tossing about. Excessively restless. Extreme anxiety *(Arsenicum Nap.).* Expression of fear and anxiety, especially *fear of death.* Condition *sudden* and *violent.* After exposure to cold, dry wind. Sits straight up and can hardly breathe, grasps throat, wants everything thrown off. Anguish with dyspnea as if boiling water poured into chest : warm blood rushing into the parts (comp. *Arsenicum Alb.). Arsenicum Alb.* comes far on in the condition, with *terrific exhaustion,* instead of *terrific violence.*

Antimonium Tart., asphyxia, from mechanical cases, as apparent death from drowning, from pneumonia, capillary bronchitis, etc., from accumulation of mucus, which cannot be expectorated. Impending paralysis of lungs. Drowsiness or coma, pale or dark-red face, blue lips, delirium, twitchings. Threat-like pulse.

Ammonium Carb., skin mottled, with great pallor. Face dusky, puffy. Lack of reaction, livid, weak and drowsy. Increasing shortness of breath, better cool air. Rattling in chest, but gets up little. Weak heart, causing stasis, dyspnea, etc., cold sweat, tendency to syncope. *"One of the best remedies in emphysema"*, edema of lungs, with somnolence from poison of blood with carbonic acid gas. Sputa thin, foamy, a dynamic state, with rattling of large bubbles in chest. Vehement palpitation with great pericardial distress, followed by syncope. Audible palpitation, great anxiety as if dying, cold sweat, involuntary flow of tears, loud, difficult breathing, with trembling hands. Angina Pectoris *(Latrodect mech)*. Exhaustion with defective reaction. Hysteria, symptoms simulate organic disease.

Carboneum Sulph., an important remedy for collapse. Frequent attacks of fainting, asphyxia. Violent headache till mind is affected. Sunken, staring eyes. Expression bewildered, as if demented. Pushed lower jaw forward, and gnashed with it against the upper, great thirst, great desire for beer. Colic about umbilicus, drawing navel in *(Plumbum Met.)*. Asphyxia from alcohol or coal gas. Feeling of heavy load hanging on back between scapulae. Sensation of vibration and trembling of whole body. Heard voices and believed he had committed a robbery. Sensation of a hole close by, into which he was in danger of falling.

Colchicum, sinking of strength as if life will flow out from motion or exertion. If he attempts to raise head, it falls back, mouth wide open. Tongue heavy, stiff (bluish, especially at base). Bruised, sore, sensitive, *nauseated by smell or thought of food.* Vomiting. Profuse diarrhea and passage of blood. Stools involuntary. Great distension of abdomen-tympanitis, restlessness, cramps in legs. Great prostration, skin cold, bedewed with sweat, cold sweat forehead *(Verat.)*. Respiration slow, but "without the fearfulness and dread of death of some remedies like *Aconitum Nap.*"

Crotalus Hor., rapidly becomes besotted, benumbed, putrid, semi-conscious. Prostration almost paralytic in character, skin yellow, pale, bloodless with blue spots. Rapid breaking down of blood vessels.

SOME GENERAL DISEASES

9. HOMEOPATHIC PROPHYLAXIS

Prevention is better than cure. So, if preventive medicines can give protection against epidemics, or any periodical visitations of diseases, they will certainly help people to ward off diseases when they do appear, and avoid sufferings which they entail. The effects of the allopathic vaccinations and serum injections and their after-effects have been dealt with in this chapter under para. 10. Homeopathy provides specific remedies for a number of diseases, which are easy to administer, effective in their action, and leave no after-effects.

Therapeutic Hints

AIR SICKNESS IN AVIATORS–*Bell.* 30

CAR SICKNESS OR SEA SICKNESS–*Nux Vom.* 30, *Petroleum* 30.

CHICKEN POX–*Puls.* 30.

CHOLERA–*Cuprum Met.* 30, *Veratrum Alb.* 30, *Sulphur* 30.

DIPHTHERIA–*Diphtherinum* 30.

ERYSIPELAS–*Graphite* 30.

HYDROPHOBIA–*Bell.* 30, *Cantharis* 30, *Stramonium* 30.

INTERMITTENT FEVER–*Arsenicum Alb.*, 30, *Chin Sulph* 30.

MEASLES–*Aconitum Nap.* 30, *Arsenicum Alb.* 30, *Puls.* 30, *Morbilinum* 30.

MUMPS–*Pilocarpine* 30.

THE PLAGUE–*Ignatia* 30.

POLIOMYELITIS–*Lathyrus sat.* 30 or 200.

PUS INFECTION–*Arnica Mont.* 30.

QUINSY–*Baryta Carb.* 30.

RAT OR CAT BITES AND BEE STINGS–*Ledum Pal. 30.*

SEPTIC CONDITIONS, VENOM INFECTION–*Arsenicum Alb. 30, Echinacea Tinct.*

SMALL POX–*Malandrinum 30, Variolinum 200.*

TETANUS–*Ledum Pal 30 or 200, Hypericum 30*

TYPHOID–*Baptisia 30.*

VACCINATION–*Thuja 30, Malandrinum 30.*

WHOOPING COUGH–*Drosera 30, Vaccin 30.*

10. VACCINATION

Vaccination, though it is commonly employed for the protection of children against small pox, has produced ill effects in a large number of cases. In babies and older children, the pustules began to increase in size, continued to emit serous matter, and increase the pain, and made the children very restless and uneasy, and did not heal for several months. In other cases, the children continued to have high fever, or diarrhea for a long time, while in others nervous affections, even convulsions, began to appear. In some cases, the after-effects continued for a long time, in the form of headache, asthma, epilepsy in later life, and all these were found to date from the original vaccination, and their subsequent repetition periodically as a matter of routine. Homeopathy has a number of remedies to replace Vaccination, and to afford sufficient protection against small pox, and thus avoid all the risks which vaccination engenders, and at the same time, to antidote vaccination and to remedy the after-effects of vaccination.

Therapeutic Hints

For the ill-effects, acute or chronic, on vaccination–*Apis Mell., Arsenicum Alb., Maland., Sil., Sulphur, Thuja.*

SOME GENERAL DISEASES

Thuja, a direct antidote to the vaccinal poison. In acute cases, wipes out the fever and eruption, and causes the pustules to disappear. In chronic cases, it acts like all chronic remedies, and is required to cure the many conditions of skin, nerve, etc., where the symptoms improve to a point, and then always recur, while the disease can be traced back to vaccination. *Thuja* will generally supply the deep stimulus that leads to a cure.

Malandrinum, nosode, prepared from 'grease' in horses. Very similar in symptoms and effects.

Silicea, the patient is feeble, lacks 'grit', shrinks from responsibility. Is chilly, sensitive to draughts, but enervated with very hot weather. Head sweats at night *(Calcarea Carb.),* sweaty, offenisve feet.

Sulphur, warm patient. Hungry for everything, for fats. Intolerant of clothing and weight of clothes. Kicks off bed clothes, puts feet out. Eruptions of every kind.

Arnica Mont., will also be necessary. Though it does not destroy the vaccination like *Thuja* and *Maland.* it has the amazing power of taking away pain, swelling and all inconveniences, while the process goes on to completion.

CHAPTER-XXX

EXTERNAL INJURIES, BURNS AND SCALDS

1. INJURIES

Arnica Mont., especially useful for injuries to soft parts, such as contusions, dislocations, bruises and sprains. It is also useful in injuries caused to any part of the body in accidents of any kind, such as concussion of the brain, spinal cord, fractures of limbs, crushing of fingers and the like. *Arnica,* is often indicated in stomach troubles following confusion to the abdomen. In these cases it is useful in the *30th* potency in the water solution for day or two. In injuries of long standing, it should be used in the *200th* potency, in single doses, at weekly or fortnightly intervals. *Arnica lotion* made by mixing a few drops of the tincture in a tumbler of water may be applied externally to the parts affected.

It may be followed by *Rhus Tox. 30* for the after-effects.

Rhus Tox., is the best remedy for sprains due to overlifting weights, stretching arms up high to reach things, several affections of the muscles of the back, and even the spinal membranes may be affected by sprains, or by exposure to cold or wet, by sleeping on damp ground, or in bed with damp sheets, and in all these cases *Rhus Tox. 30* will be useful. Even in injuries and strain of the voice in singers and speakers, it is useful.

Calcarea Carb., the chronic of *Rhus Tox.* in the traumatic field. Bad effects from over-exertion whether mental or physical. Strained and sprained feeling following hill or mountain climbing. Aggravation from ascending is characteristic. Worse from cold and dampness. Plethoric type with easy sweating tendency.

EXTERNAL INJURIES, BURNS AND SCALDS

Calendula 30, for deeper cuts or lacerated wounds, with soreness and pain, and also for wounds which have become suppurated. For best effect, it should be given internally and the lotion applied also externally.

Calendula lotion may be applied externally immediately after the cuts, till they are healed. The external solution should be diluted, one to four or six parts at least and used hot. Cold applications of whatever nature should never be applied to wounds.

Hypericum 30, for injuries to nerves and parts rich with nerves, such as the ends of the fingers and toes, the coccyx and spine or in open wounds that are exceedingly painful.

Bellis Perennnis, is especially suited to injuries to the blood vessels and following traumas to the coccyx, as in *Hypericum,* often called for in gastralgia from ice cold drinks taken when over treated, also for neuralgia after exposure to cold and wet when over-heated. As in *Arnica Mont.,* there is the sensation of bruised soreness. There is aggravation from cold and cold applications, and amelioration from continued motion as in *Rhus Tox.*

Ledum Pal. 30, for punctured wounds as from needles, nails or some sharp instruments, also useful for mosquito bites, bites of insects, astings and bites of rats or small animals, or for black and blue spots from blows or bruises. Punctured wounds of the extremities are best treated by cleansing the wound with *Calendula* solution and by giving internally *Ledum Pal. 30* or *200*. This is a more effective prophylaxis against prospective tetanus than the anti-toxin usually injected, and with no risk of unfavourable serum reaction. *Hypericum* may be required in extreme cases in which lymphangitis develops with red lines or streaks extending up the arm or leg.

Ruta 30, old sprains, bruises, pains in bones, joints and cartilages, such as sprains of the ankles and wrists. In strains of tendons, with weakness, loss of motion, and aggravation by change of weather and by damp weather, it is especially useful. It is also useful for eye-strains from close study, sewing etc., or from the abuse of spectacles, and may be used in the 200*th* potency fortnightly or at longer intervals.

Natrium Mur., when these are zig-zags in front of the eyes and marked aggravation from sun-light and other bright lights.

Apis Mell., for eye-strains when there is aggravation from heat and relief from cold.

Ammonium Mur., for the chronic effects of sprains, rightness if the tendons were too short, tense, sprained sensation in the groin with difficulty in walking erect, better in open air and from continued motion.

Symphytum, injuries to bone, such as bruises of bones or fractures, favours the formation of matter at the point of fracture to knit the bones and promote re-union, injuries of globe of the eye from blunt articles, if there is great pain in the eyeball itself. The remedy will act better in the *200th* potency.

Staphisagria 30, useful for clean cut wounds, and symptoms traceable to surgical operations, especially about the abdomen, when colic follows, wounds from glass, etc., where the pains are excruciating, rending and tearing, causing great agony.

Calcarea Phos., is an excellent remedy for promoting reunion of fractured bones, and is useful in repeated doses in the *6th* potency. It may be given twice a day for 3 days and repeated after an interval of 3 days.

For after-effects of surgical operations (see chapter XXVII- 'Neuritis').

2. BURNS AND SCALDS

In the case of burns, *Cantharis 30* may be given internally in watery solution, tea-spoon doses every two or three hours for 24 hours, and at the same time, apply externally *Cantharis tincture*

EXTERNAL INJURIES, BURNS AND SCALDS

to the parts affected. In cases of very old burns, *Causticum 30* should be given internally at *weekly* intervals.

3. EXTERNAL REMEDIES

CONCUSSIONS, BRUISES, DISLOCATIONS, FRACTURES, ETC.–*Arnica tincture.*

DEEP CUTS OR WOUNDS–*Calendula tincture* or *Hypericum tincture.*

BURNS AND SCALDS–*Cantharis tincture.*

A few drops of the tincture in the proportion of one to four or six may be mixed in a tumbler of water, and the solution applied externally. The solution should be applied hot in the case of deep cuts or wounds. Cold applications of whatever nature should never be applied to wounds.

4. STINGS

The stings of bees, wasps and scorpions may be treated be external application of *Apis Tincture* in watery solution, and internal administration of *Apis Mell. 30*.

5. FOREIGN SUBSTANCES IN THE EYE, EAR, NOSE AND THROAT

In the eye, no matter what has gotten into the eye, washing with cold water will always be beneficial.

Rubbing the eye only increases the irritation and therefore, should always be avoided. When lime, sand or ashes get into the eye, a little butter-milk is the best remedy. If a hard object or an insect has gotten into the eye, draw the eye-lids apart, and turn the upper one over the lower one a couple of times until it is felt that the substance is removed. If particles of iron have entered the eye and are fastened, bathe with *Arnica lotion*-ten drops in a tea drops in a tea-cupful of water, until you can have it extracted. Should there be much inflammation, take a few doses of *Aconitum Nap. 30.*

In the ear, insects sometimes find their way into children's ears, in such cases, lean the head to one side, and fill the ear, in which the insect is, with sweet oil. This will float it to the surface, when it can easily be removed.

If a bean or any other substance, which will swell by heat and moisture, gets into the ear, the best way to remove it is to make a hook by bending a hair-pin into the right shape. This should be cautiously introduced behind the substance, and an effort made gradually to remove it.

After the operation, wash the ear out with a lotion of *Arnica tincture* and give internally *Arnica Mont. 30* and *Pulsatilla 30.* Should there be fever and headache, give *Aconitum Nap. 30* or *Belladonna 30.*

In the Nose, foreign substances may be removed from the nose with a small pair of forecepts, or the same article recommended for the ear.

First, try to eject it by sneezing, which may be excited either with snuff, or by tickling the nose with a thread. Sometimes the obstruction may be pushed back so as to fall into the mouth. If these means fail, apply to a surgeon.

In the throat or windpipe, if a foreign substance lodges in the throat, first examine closely, and if within sight, endeavour to extract it with the fingers. If it is not visible, excite vomiting immediately by tickling the throat with the fingers, or by putting mustard powder far back upon the tongue.

Foreign substances have been removed from the windpipe by gently turning the patient upside down.

CHAPTER-XXXI

CONSEQUENCES OF SPIRITUOUS LIQUORS, COFFEE, TEA, TOBACCO, ACIDS, ETC

1. DRUNKENNESS

If a drunken man does not come to his senses, apply a cloth dipped into cold water, to the head, and give *Opium 30* in watery solution every fifteen minutes in teaspoon doses until the improves, if this fails, give *Aconitum Nap. 30* or *Belladonna 30*.

If children are made tipsy, or swallow brandy by accident, wash their head and abdomen with cold water, and give *Nux Vomica 30* in watery solution every fifteen minutes in tea-spoon doses. If they have fever, with restlessness, give *Aconitum Nap. 30*, and if not relieved, give *Belladonna 30*.

2. EFFECTS OF DRUNKENNESS

After drinking too much in the evening or night, if one feels unwell in the following morning, give *Nux Vomica*. For tedious headache, which has been caused, brought on after thinking or mental work, give *Calcarea Carb.*, if the patient is stout, or *Silicea* if he is thin. Do not repeat the dose until he is worse again, and if the repetition fails, give *Lachesis*.

For delirium in drunkards, in which one sees visions of animals or strange human faces, give *Opium 30* in repeated doses. If the face is flushed, the eyes are sensitive to light and there is throbbing in the neck, give *Belladonna 30*. For cold sweat on the face, *Veratrum Alb. 30*.

3. BAD EFFECTS OF COFFEE

For sleeplessness, headache, constipation and other troubles, *Nux Vom. 30*. If one wants to get over the coffee habit, *Nux Vom. 30* may be given in the evening for a few days, and repeated in the same way after an interval. For toothache following immediately upon drinking coffee, or in those accustomed to the use of cofee. *Chamomilla 30*.

4. BAD EFFECTS OF TEA

For indisposition from green tea, give *Coffea* or *Ignatia*, and if there is no relief in a few days, *China off*. For tedious complaints from the effects of tea, give *China off*.

5. TOBACCO

If persons unaccustomed to smoking have been made ill thereby, give *Pulsatilla 30*. If persons accustomed to smoking get sick in the stomach, give *Ignatia 30* or *Pulsatilla 30*. For bad effects of chewing tobacco, give *Pulsatilla 30, Nux Vomcia 30* or *Arsenicum Alb. 30*.

6. SPICES

For injurious effects caused by spices, such as pepper, ginger etc., give *Nux Vomica 30*.

7. SOUR THINGS

For bad effects, such as diarrhea, give *Nux Vomica 30*. For other troubles give *Arsenicum Alb. 30,* and for persons who have too much appetite and eat too much, give *Arsenicum Alb. 30,* and for those who have a craving for sweet things as a consequence,

Sulphur 30 may be used, for craving for acids or sour food, *Arsenicum Alb. 30,* if merely for sour drinks, *Bryonia Alba 30,* for disordered stomachs from acids, *Arsenicum Alb. 30* or *Lachesis 30,* for *diarrhea* from the use of acids and sour fruits, *Lachesis 30,* if from fruits merely, *China off. 30.*

CHAPTER-XXXII

EFFECTS OF INJURIOUS DRUGS IN GENERAL USE

1. OPIUM OR GANJA

For the immediate bad effects, give *Belladonna 30* in frequent doses in watery solution, tea-spoon doses every 2 or 3 hors. For chronic effects, give *Nux vomica 30,* followed by *Sulphur 30,* and then by *Plumbum Met. 200* or *Alumina 200.*

At some children who are brought up on small doses of these drugs become puny, sickly and often idiotic, *Plumbum Met. 200* or *Alumina 200* will be required to effect a change in them and cure them of these ill-effects.

2. HYDRATE OF CHLORAL

This preparation is employed by allopathic doctors generally to produce sleep in nervous patients, and in delirious cases. It is only a palliative and, if it is used for a long time, will produce serious bad effects. Large doses have produced death in a number of cases. For the immediate injurious effects, *Belladonna 30* should be given in repeated doses. For the chronic effects, such as increased wakefulness, shortness of breath, eruptions on the skin, give *Sulphur 200.*

3. QUININE

Quinine and its preparations are very largely employed by allopathic physicians for the treatment of fevers. Though they may give temporary relief, they have the effect of suppressing the fever and producing other serious results, which are difficult to expel from the constitution by any other means than the use of suitable Homeopathic remedies. The chief medicine, in most cases, is *Ipecacuanha*. Unless the effects of quinine which has been largely used in any case are removed, other troubles, which may have arisen in consequence, cannot be successfully treated. The other remedies, which will be necessary for the several troubles are :

For rheumatic pains, heaviness, prostration, soreness in all the limbs, drawing pain in the bones, great sensitiveness of every part of the body, when exercise, speaking, or blowing the nose, or loud sounds aggravate the pains, give *Arnica Mont*.

When there is constipation or diarrhea, and the body is cold with cold perspiration, *Veratrum Alb*. For jaundice, give *Mercurius Sol.,* and later, if required, *Belladonna*.

For heat in the face, determination of blood to the head, much pain in the head, face and teeth, *Belladonna*.

For ulcers of the legs, dropsy, short cough and shortness of breath, *Arsenicum Alb*.

For dropsy and other swellings, *Rhus Tox*.

For intermittent fevers–this has been dealt with under that head.

4. DIGITALIS

For the large use of *Digitalis,* even in small doses, for the treatment of heart complaints, and its dangerous consequences, give *Glonoine, Opium, Nux Vomica* or *Ignatia* according to symptoms. *Be careful not to give China off.*

5. MAGNESIA SALTS OR EPSOM SALTS

If the bowels do not move for twenty-four hours after their use, give *Nux Vomica*.

If the patient has violent pains, and particularly burning pains with fever, give *Arsenicum Alb.*

If there are sour smelling stools with colic, *Rheum,* and if this does not work, *Pulsatilla.*

6. CASTOR OIL

If the bowels do not move after the use of castor oil, give *Bryonia Alba.*

7. SULPHUR, IODINE AND IODIDE OF POTASSIUM

For the skin eruptions which appear after the use of sulphur spring-baths, or abuse of sulphur, give *Mercurious Sol.* or *Pulsatilla,* and later *Arsenicum Alb.* if they do not help.

For the bad effects of sulphurous vapors from the lighting of matchsticks, give *Pulsatilla.*

When patients suffer from the effects of Iodine, or have taken medicines containing Iodide of Potassium for coughs give *Hepar Sulph. 6.*

8. MERCURY

To counteract the effects of mercury in medicinal preparations containing this metal, such as calomel, Makharadwaj, yellow ointment for the eyes, etc., *Hepar Sulph.* 6 is useful, and may be given in a single dose or in 3 doses in watery solution, and after an interval of a week, it may repeated again in the same way. If no effect is produced, and if the improvement is slow, *Belladonna* may be given.

For complaints of the mouth and throat, for swelling of the tonsils and deafness, give *Hepar Sulp.* and later *Belladonna.*

For great sensitiveness to the weather, violent pains, particularly at night, worse when touched, great wekaness, when the patient has been much deibiltated by much purging and salivation, give *China off.*, and if this does not help, *Carbo Veg.*, particuarly if change of weather makes the patient worse.

If mercury had been taken for a long time, and the complaint is not completely removed, try *Sulphur.*

If a person has taken much mercury, and afterwards sulphur, or sulphur medicines, it will be well to give *Mercurius Sol.*, and then *Belladonna* or *Pulsatilla.*

When a person has taken much mercury, but no sulphur after it, and if *Hepar Sulp.* is not quite indicated, it is better to give *Sulphur.*

9. LEAD

Lead is often an ingredient in medicines such as white ointment, plasters, lotions, etc., which are used to dry up and cure eruptions, ulcers, bruises, burns and wounds. It is almost as poisonous, when applied externally, as if it were used internally, and produces constipation, colic, cough, and disease of the lungs. to remove these effects, give *Opium,* frequently repeated, or *Glonoine* followed by *Nux Vomica,* or *Belladonna,* and afterwards, if necessary, *Mercurius Sol.* or *Platina.*

10. ARSENIC

In medicines which contain *Arsenic Alb.*, such as Fowler's solution, which are mostly given in fever and ague, when the quinine will not cure, or for many skin diseases, or for cancers, applied both internally and externally, and aggravate the disease, give *Ipecac,* and if this does not effect some improvement, give *Hepar Sulp.*

11. IRON

Iron is frequently given in the form of steel drops, steel pills, bitter wine of iron etc., for intermittent fever, anemia, and complaitns of the lungs, but instead of curing these diseases it generally makes them much worse. Iron taken in large quantities, as a medicine, is as injurious as all the other metals, though it does not kill so rapidly. In case speedy relief is required, give *Pulsatilla* or *China off.*, and if they do not help, *Hepar Sulp.*, and after some time repeat the former medcines again.

CHAPTER–XXXIII

POISONING

The following tables give antidotes to the most powerful poisons-

1. POISONS

I. *Gases*

Poisons	Antidotes
Gas produced in places deprived of fresh air, such as privies, wells, etc.	Chloride of lime, vinegar or lemon juice.
Vapour of charcoal	Vinegar or lemon juice, and vapour of vinegar

II. *Acids*

Prussic Acid	Pouring of cold water to the spine and head, smelling salts.
Sulphuric, Muriatic, Phosphoric, Acetic acid and strong wine Vinegar	Tepid soap-studs, magnesia, chalk, powdered and mixed with water, wood ashes mixed with water, carbonate of potash of soda.
Nitric and Oxalic acids	Carbonates of Magnesia and lime.

III. Alkaline Poisons

Poisons	Antidotes
Pot and pearl ashes, Carbonate of Potash and Ammonia	Vinegar, lemon juice, and other vegetables acids, sour milk, olive or castor oil, mucilaginous drinks and injections.

IV. Metallic Substances

Arsenic	White of eggs with water, rust of iron, soapy fluid made with equal parts of lime water and coconut oil, sugar water, milk.
Corrosive sublimate, Copper.	White of eggs in water, sugar water, milk, starch from wheat flour.
Lead	Epsom salts, Glauber's salts.
Lunar Caustic	Common salt dissolved in water.
Tin	Sugar, white of eggs and milk.

V. Vegetable Poisons

Opium or Laudanum, Stramonium	Coffee, lemon juice or Vinegar.
Bitter almonds, peach kernels or peach leaves.	Smelling salts, coffee, cold applications.

2. POISONED WOUNDS

Sting and Bites of Animals

(*a*) STINGS OF BEES, ETC.–

In cases of great swelling, itching and great weakness, give *Apis Mell.*, sometimes when there is much pain, *Arnica Mont.* For the remaining symptoms, *Natrium Muriaticum.*

Mosquitoes may be drawn away by the smoke of brown sugar, strewn upon characola fire, after sometime, let the smoke pass out, and close the doors and windows. The bites of mosquitoes which pain severely are relieved by the application of lemon juice.

(*b*) BITES OF SNAKES–

The best plan is to apply heat *continuously* to the *part* bitten and around it, for three or four inches and not more, and smear oil around the wound, and when absorbed, renew it. Continue to apply heat until the patient begins to shudder and to stretch, if this should occur soon, continue the application for an hour if he can bear it, or until the symptoms of the poison give way. If these symptoms return, renew the application. After the wound has been thus treated rub into it *fine* salt and ashes. At the same time, the patient must be kept as quiet as possible.

Give inwardly, as soon as possible *salt water* or *garlic*. If bad symptoms appear, not withstanding, give wine or brandy, a few drops or half a tea-spoonful, every two or three minutes, until they disappear, but resume the treatment as soon as they reappear.

If the shooting pains grow worse, if they are in the direction of the heart, if the spot turns blue or spotted, or swells, if vomiting, giddiness or fainting follow, give *Arsenicum Alb.* in repeated doses, if there is improvement, stop further doses, and do not repeat until worse again. If several doses have produced no effect, give *Belladonna*. *Phosphoric acid* will sometimes remove the ramaining symptoms, and sometimes *Mercurius Sol.* or *Lachesis.*

(c) Bites of Mad Dogs—

The bite of a mad dog or of other rabid animals, should be treated in the beginning in the same way as snake bites. After the wound is treated as directed above., it should be allowed to heal quietly. Heat should be occasionally applied to the wound until the scar becomes of the natural color of the skin. It should be renewed whenever the wound appears hard, dark coloured, red or inflamed.

Vapour bath or hot steam bath is a very efficeint remedy.

To prevent convulsions, give *Hydrophobinum 30*, evening and morning *once a week*, until it produces fever, diarrhea etc. *Cantharis 3*, is also useful. If ulcers or eruptions should appear, no external application should be used, and they will disappear.

If the patient suffers already from hydrophobia, give *Belladonna* at every return of the convulsions. If, after sometime, the convulsions continue about the same way, give *Hyoscyamus Nig.*, if this fails, *Cantharis*.

When *putrid animal substances* have got into a wound, or pus-matter from ulcers of men or animals– give *Arsenicum Alb*.

If blood, pus or saliva of an animal affected with malignant splenic disease, glanders, etc., use *Arsenicum Alb*. and heat, as stated above.

For the bites of any angry animal, if pus or other diseased matter gets into a wound, it is best to expose your hands for five to ten minutes to as great a heat as you can bear, then wash them thoroughly in soap and warm water, and take *Arsenicum Alb*.

PART – III

PART – III

BIBLIOGRAPHY

Hahnemann	–	'Organon' (Fifth and Sixth Editions).
Do	–	'Chronic Diseases'.
Do	–	'Materia Medica Pura'.
William Boericke	–	Pocket Book of 'Materia Medica'.
Hering	–	'Condensed Materia Medica'.
Kent	–	'Materia Medica'.
Farrington	–	'Clinical Materia Medica'.
Kent	–	'Lectures on Homeopathic Philosophy'.
William Boericke	–	'A Compend of the Principles of Homeopathy'.
Garth Boericke	–	'Principles of Homeopathy'.
Allen	–	'Key Notes and Characteristics'.
Nash	–	'Leaders in Homeopathic Therapeutics'.
Do.	–	'Leaders in Respiratory Organs'.
Do.	–	'Typhoid Fever'.
Hering	–	'Domestic Physician'.
Jahr	–	'Forty Years' Practice'.
Do.	–	'Diseases of Females'.
Guernsey	–	'Obstetrics'.
Croserio	–	Do.
Minton	–	'Uterine Therapeutics'.

Do	–	'Diseases of Women and Children'.
Dewey	–	'Practical Homeopathic Therapeutics'.
Bell.	–	'Diarrhea'.
C. G. Raue	–	'Special Pathology and Therapeutics'.
Norton	–	'Ophthalmic Therapeutics'.
J. H. Allen	–	'Diseases of the Skin'.
H. C. Allen	–	'Therapeutics of Fevers'.
G. S. Raue	–	'Diseases of Children'.
H. C. Allen	–	'Materia Medica of the Nosodes'.
M.L. Tyler	–	'Pointers to common Remedies Nos. 1 to 8'.
Sir John Weir	–	'Samuel Hahnemann and his influence on Medical thought.'
A.H. Grimmer	–	'Homeopathic Treatment of Cancer' in the Journal of the American Institute of Homeopathy
W. H. Hay	–	'A New Era of Health'.
N. K. Banerjee and P.K. Banerjee	–	'Blood Pressure'.

APPENDIX-I

THERAPEUTIC INDEX

This index is only meant for quick use in urgent cases and is not, therefore, exhaustive. For full particulars, the chapters concerned should be consulted.

Where no specific potencies are mentioned, the medicines may be used in the 30*th* potency. The medicines should be administered in watery solution (two globules, No. 10 in one ounce of water) in tea-spoon doses and repeated at intervals, as advised according to the nature of the case. Where no intervals are mentioned the doses may be given twice a day (morning and evening). Single doses may be taken in globules dry on the tongue.

1. ABSCESS OR ATHERING—To reduce the pain and inflammation—*Arnica Mont.* 30, when there is throbbing pain and red swelling—*Belladonna* 30. When matter begins to form—*Hepar Sulph.* 6. When situated in the glands of the neck, or at roots of teeth—*Mercurius Sol.* 30. One dose every three hours. To remove a tendency to abscesses—*Sulphur* 30, on alternate days.

2. ACNE OR PIMPLES—Rough, dry, harsh skin, with 'black heads', *Sulphur* 30. In the young—*Carbo Veg.. 30.* Red pimples—*Ledum Pal.* 30. from sexual causes—*Phosphoric acid* 30. In women, with menstrual troubles—*Sanguinaria* 30.

3. APHATE, SORE MOUTH—When the disease first appears, especially if there is salivation and ulceration—*Mercurius Sol.* 30. If the swelling was due to the use of calomel or other mercurial preparations—*Carbo Veg.* 30, and then *Hepar Sulph.* 6, or *Nitricum Acid* 30. If not better, *Sulphur* 30.

4. APPENDICITIS—*Belladonna* 30 and *Mercurius Sol.* 30, in alternation, have proved useful in many cases, may be given every three hours.
5. APPETITE, LOSS OF—When caused by sedentary habits, late hours, over-indulgence in wine, or spirits—*Nux Vomica* 30. If from partaking of rich food, pastry, pork, etc. —*Pulsatilla* 30. After overloading the stomach—*Antimonium Crudum* 30. From illness, loss of fluids—*China off.* 30. Dose—Every three hours.
6. ASTHMA, for nocturnal paroxysms of suffocation, rattling, loose mucus, with mucus, and *breathing* out difficult, and with vomiting—*Ipecac.* 30. Must remain quiet—*Bryonia Alba.* 30. For suffocative wheezing, cold perspiration and small pulse—*Arsenicum Alb.* 30. Due to gastric disturbances—*Nux Vom.* 30. Worse in wet weather—*Natrium Sulph.* 30, *Dulcamara* 30. Sensation of dust in lungs—*Sulphur* 30.

   DIRECTIONS, give tea-spoon doses, every fifteen minutes to half an hour till there is relief, and then every two hours.
7. BACK-ACHE— catches on moving, better after some motion—*Rhus Tox.* 30. Associated with uterine trouble—*Sepia* 30. Violent and continuous—*Cimicifuga* 30. Dull and persistent—*Berberis Vul.* 30.
8. BARBER'S ITCH—Chief remedy—*Thuja* 30, also *tincture* may be applied externally.
9. BILIOUSNESS—Pain under right shoulder blade—*Chelidonium* 30. Yellow tongue, dirty complexion—*Mercurius Sol.* 30. Very irritable, liver region tender to touch—*Bryonia Alba.* 30. Caused by sedentary life, or too high living—*Nux Vom.* 30. Morning headache, white tongue, chalk-like stools—*Podophyllum* 30. Tea-spoon doses every hour till better.

THERAPEUTIC INDEX

10. BLADDER—Hot urine, painful, ill effects from retention—*Cantharis* 30. Frequent urging—*Apis Mell.* 30. Brick-dust sediment—*Lycopodium Clav.* 30. Bloody urine—*Terebinthina* 30. Urine passed involuntarily—*Causticum* 30. Dribbling, leaking—*Ferrum Phos.* 30.

11. BOILS—In repeated crops—*Arnica Mont.* 30. Swelling, with fiery-red inflammation and much throbbing pain—*Belladonna 30,* followed by *Mercurius Sol.* 30. After suppuration has commenced—*Hepar Sulph.* 6, which is also good to clear system, or tendency to the disease, and may be given in the 30*th* or 200*th* potency. A dose of the selected remedy every two hours.

12. BLOOD POISONING— From any cause—*Lachesis* 30. Teaspoon doses, every hour.

13. BONES— Caries—*Aurum Met.*30, Bone tumours—*Calcarea Flour* 30. Broken bones won't knit—*Symphytum* 30. Children's bones won't grow firm—*Calcarea Phos.* 6 and 30.

14. BRONCHITIS—at the onset—*Aconitum Nap.* 30 will generally check. Dry distressing cough, fever, *Belladonna* 30. Cough wich hurts head and whole body with painful respiration—*Bryonia Alba.* 30. Chest sore—*Mercurius Sol.* 30. Chronic cases—*Sulphur* 30, and later *Sulphur* 200 at long intervals.

15. BRUISES AND SPRAINS— *Arnica Mont.* 30 internally, and *Arnica lotion,* made with one part of the tincture to ten of cold water, applied externally to the part by means of cloth, when there is more of a sprain than bruise, *Rhus Tox* 30 internally, and *Hamamelis tincture* externally.

16. BUNIONS OR CHILBLAINS— Itching as from frosted feet—*Agaricus Muse.* 30. Caused by frosted feet—*Pulsatilla* 30. Externally—*Hamamelis* ointment, if suppurating or raw, *Calendula ointment.*

17. BURNS AND SCALDS, *Cantharis* 30 internally at first, and for after effects or later stages, *Causticum* 30 internally at first, and for after effects or later stages *Causticum* 30. *Cantharis tincture to be applied externally in solution.* If fever ensues—*Aconitum Nap.* 30, if suppuration takes place—*Hepar Sulph.* 6.

18. CATARRH—Coming on after exposure—*Aconitum Nap.* 30. With debility and then watery excoriating discharge—*Arsenicum Alb.* 30. Sneezing and running of clear water from nose—*Natrium Mur.* 30. Drooping of mucus back into throat—*Hydrastis* 30. Stringy mucus, ulceration—*Kali Bichromicum* 30. Dry catarrh—*Lycopodium Clav.* 30. Blowing out blood-streaked mucus—*Phosphorus* 30. Chronic cases, with thick yellow mucus—*Pulsatilla* 30, *Sulphur* 30.

    Doses.—Morning and evening till better.

19. CHILLS AND FEVERS— MALARIAL OR INTERMITTENT FEVER.

    MALARIAL FEVER. In beginning *China off.* 30 and *Ipecac.* 30 alternately every twelve hours, two doses of each.

    REGULAR ATTACKS :

    Back-aches, bone-pain, chill 7 to 9 a.m. thirst, but drinking causes nausea and vomiting bile—*Eupatorium Perf* 30. Fever long lasting, much sweat, nausea—*Ipecac.* 30. Chillness during heat, when uncovering—*Nux Vomica* 30. Chill, very long lasting, cold sweat, great exhaustion—*Veratrum Alb.* 30. Heat long lasting with great thirst, chill not clearly defined, comes on earlier each day (also dumb-ague)—*Arsenicum Alb.* 30. Chill always begins between shoulders—*Capsicum* 30. Chill, 10 to 11 a.m. bursting headache during heat—*Natrium Mur* 30. Red face during chill—*Gelsemium* 30. Pronounced ringing in the ears—*China off.* 30. In longstanding cases, where much quinine and other drugs have been taken—*Natrium Mur.* 30 and later *Natrium Mur.* 200.

Dose acts best if given after fever begins to subside.

20. CHOLERA, CHOLERA ASIATICA— for first symptoms of diarrhea during an epidemic, take *Sulphur* 30 in watery solution, tea-spoon doses, every fifteen minutes and this will generally check the disease. If however, rice-water discharges set in, then *Camphor tincture* or *Camphor* 6 may be taken. When cramps supervene, with cold extremities, *Veratrum* Alb. 30. If it fails, *Cuprum Met.* 30 follows next, especially indicated in cramps in calves of legs, for collapse, cols breath and ammost at points of death, *Carbo Veg.* 30 may still save the case. Should burning in stomach at any time be prominent, the case requires *Arsenicum Alb.* 30. Dose every fifteen minutes till the crisis pases. *Cuprum Met.* 30 may be taken as preventive.

21. COLDS— at the beginning of a cold, *Aconitum Nap.* 30 will, in most cases, be sufficient. For copious watery discharge from eyes and nose, excoritating the nostrils, with much burning, take *Arsenicum Alb.* 30. If not relieved soon, try *Mercurius Sol.* 30. If nose runs much during daytime, and is stopped at night, take *Nux Vom.* 30. One dose every two hours till better.

22. COLIC— for severe colic, causing the patient to double up and recurring at intervals, give *Colocynth* 30. For severe pains, better when being straight, but worse on bending double, give *Dioscorea* 30. For bilious colic, especially if brought on by violent anger, also for colic of children, give *Chamomilla* 30. This remedy may be followed after a few hours with *Nux Vom.* 30, or *Pulsatilla* 30. For abdominal neuralgia, *Belladonna* 30 will be found efficacious. Much accumulation of flatus as a constipated condition of the bowels. requires *Lyopodium Clav.* 30. If *Chamomilla*

should not help in bilious colic, give *Podophyllum*, which will also be of great value in painter's colic—One dose every hour till better.

23. CONSTIPATION—For persons of sedentary habits, afflicted with piles and headache, *Nux Vomica* 30, also if caused by coffee or dissipation. In habitual constipation, particularly if there is a tendency to hemorrhoids or uneasiness about the abdomen, give *Sulphur* 30. *Sulphur* 30 in the morning and *Nux Vom.* 30 in the evening, taken for some weeks, have cured several cases. If with metallic taste in the mouth, *Mercurius Sol.* 30, if with disordered stomach and headache, *Bryonia Alba.* 30, Hard black balls, no urging, *Plumbum Met.* 30. Of travellers, *Platina* 30. Frequent but ineffectual urging, *Causticum* 30. Great straining, *Sepia* 30. One dose three times a day.

24. CONVULSIONS— Face is blue, clenched hands, *Cuprum Met.* 30. Face flushed, *Belladonna* 30, face pale—*Zincum Met.* 30. When convulsions are frequent, *Cicuta Vir.* 30.

25. COUGHS— Barking, *Aconitum Nap.* 30, moist and loose, *Hepar Sulph.* 6, Hard, dry cough, *Belladonna* 30, worse at night, *Hyoscyamus Nig* 30, Hoarseness, raw feeling in the throat and pains in the chest, *Phosphorus* 30. For titilating, short dry cough, *Nux Vom.* 30. Obstinate cough, with copious expectoration, *Sulphur* 30. Dry, painful chest, *Bryonia Alba.* 30. Shaking cough, with sore throat and hoarseness, *Mercurius Sol.* 30. Cough worse on waking in the morning, with stringy mucus, *Kali Bich.* 30. Suffocating, spasmodic cough with rattling of much mucus in the chest, *Antimonium Tart.* 30. Cough with soreness in the chest and sweetish expectoration, *Stannum Met.* 30 with involuntary spurting of urine—*Causticum* 30. Nervous, more one coughs, more one has to, *Ignatia* 30.

DIRECTIONS.—One dose of the indicated remedy every three hours till better.

26. CROUP— Great thirst, hurried breathing, burning heat, dry cough—*Aconitum Nap.* 30. Much phlegm, rattling of much and loose cough—*Hepar Sulph.* 6. Loud, crowing cough, sawing respiration, accompanied with fits of choking, *Spongia. Aconitum Nap.* 30 may be given in watery solution every fifteen munutes, for a few doses, to be followed by *Hepar Sulph.* 6, every three hours, for a few doses, and then by *Spongia* 30 in the same way. Some physicians give these remedies every fifteen minutes in rotation till there is relief. The latter procedure may be followed in severe cases.

    If there is soreness in the chest, dry cough and headache, *Belladonna* 30. Dry croupy cough and true crop, especially in scrofulous children, *Iodum* 30.

27. CUT OR TORN WOUNDS— Bathe the part with a lotion made of *Calendula tincture,* twenty drops in a glass of water. Cuts, bring the edges of the wound together and secure them in place by strips of *Arnica Mont. plaster. Aconitum Nap.* 30 should be given internally if there be shock, or if fever comes on, and if much blood has been lost the resulting weakness will be greatly relieved by *China off.* 30. A dose of the selected remedy may be given every two hours.

28. DEBILITY— From illness, loss of fluids, or diarrhea—*China off.* 30. Nervous debility—*Phosphricum Acid* 30. Dose every four hours till better.

29. DEBILITY— Slow in teething, difficult—*Calcarea Phos.* 30. For pain and irritability of child in normal dentition—*Chamomilla* 30.

30. DIARRHEA— Painless, with weakness, undigested stool, *China off.* 30. Diarrhea of infants in summer, frothy,

yellowish—*Ipecac.* 30. Involuntary, *Aloe Soc* 30. Solid and fluid, *Antimonium Crud.* 30. Bilious diarrhea—Thirst, foul tongue, griping nausea, vomiting loss of appetite and irritaion, foul smelling—*Podophyllum* 30, follow if not better with *Mercurius Sol.* 30. From sudden change to chilly wet weather, *Dulcamara* 30, with gripings, *Chamomilla* 30. Severe with cramps and cold sweat, *Veratum Alb.* 30. Yellowish stools, coming out with a sudden gush, *Croton Tig.* 30. If the diarrhea is mostly in the morning, is of a chalky or yellowish appearance, occurring mostly in children, or if the appearance of stool changes almost with every evacuation—*Podophyllum* 30. Sour smelling stools of infants—*Rheum* 30.

DIRECTIONS—Give a dose (tea-spoon of a solution) of the indicated remedy with every evacuation, until relieved.

31. DIPHTHERIA—Throat intensely swollen, *Apis Mell.* 30. When nose bleed is prominent, *Crotalus Hor.* 30. Beginning in the left side. *Lachesis* 30, of right side—*Lycopodium Clav.* 30 Putrid Diphtheria—*Mercurius Cyanatus* 30.

32. DYSENTERY—If there is violent straining with bloody evacuations, mixed with mucus, clammy perspiration, shivering and the pain continuing even after stool, *Mercurius Sol.* 30. For similar symptoms, but wih griping colic, causing to bend double, *Colocynth* 30. For dysentery, with suppression of urine, give *Mercurius Sol.* 30. For small bloody stools, worse in the morning, with relief after stool—*Nux Vomica* 30. With burning thirst and prostration—*Arsenicum Alb.* 30.

DIRECTIONS—One dose of the indicated remedy in watery solution after every evacuation.

33. EAR-ACHE—In the majority of cases a few doses of *Pulsatilla* 30 will bring speedy relief. If relief is only partial, give *Mercurius Sol.* 30 after a few hours. If such attacks

are frequent and there is much discharge from the ear, give a few doses of *Sulphur* 30, night and morning, and continue the same medicines again. If these remedies fail, *Dulcamara or Rhus Tox.* may help.

34. ERYSIPELAS, (St. Anthony's Fire)—If there is burning heat swelling of the parts, redness, thirst, headache and restlessness, all more on the *right side, Belladonna* 30.

    If there are similar symptoms, but without thirst or redness, the so-called white erysipelas, give *Apis Mell.* 30. If the skin is covered with vesicles, with swelling, shining redness of the parts and restlessness—all more on the *left side* of the face, give *Rhus Tox. 30.*

    DIRECTIONS—Give one dose every two hours.

35. EYES—For simple inflammation, with much redness and fever, *Aconitum Nap.* 30. Grat sensitiveness to light, redness of the white of eye, dryness, pains around the eye and in the head. *Belladonna* 30. Severe aching pains in the balls, with but little apparent inflammation, great sensitiveness to light, profuse lachrymation and coryza, *Ignatia* 30. Granulated lids, *Graphites* 30. Eye lids agglutinated with profuse suppuration, *Mercurius Sol.* 30 and *Hep Sulph.* 6. Inflammation of the eyes with great swelling of the lids, *Apis Mell.* 30. Weakness of sight, also double vision, *Gelsemium* 30. Inflammation with profuse discharge, *Mercurius Sol.*30. Acrid tears, *Euphrasia off.* 30. Watery eyes, with agglutinated lids, yellowish pus, *Pulsatilla.* 30.

    DIRECTIONS—Give one dose every two hours.

36. FACE-ACHE OR NEURALGIA—If there is great in the face and redness, restlessness and irritation. *Aconitum Nap.* 30. Violent burning or tearing pain, worse at night, with great prostation. *Arsenicum Alb.* 30. For darting pains under the eye, running along the cheek-bone, aggravated by the

slightest movements, noise, warmth of bed, or a current of air, *Belladonna* 30. Insupportable pain and great excitability of the nervous system, *Coffea* 30. Violent rending and darting pains, Principally in the left side of the face, and extending to the ear, temples, nose and teeth, *Colocynth* 30. Pain "drawing", *Causticum* 30. *Spigelia* 30 has also cured many cases of intense neuralgic pains, when all else failed, especially where eyes are involved, or pains increase with day, and decline towards evening.

DIRECTIONS—Give a dose every half hour, until relieved.

37. FEET—Callosities—*Antimonium Crud.* 30. Offensive sweating. *Silicea* 30. Pain in heels, *Cyclamen* 30. soles burn, *Sulphur* 30. Cold and clammy, *Calcarea Carb.* 30. Chilblains. *Agaricus Mus.* 30. Cramps, *Cuprum Met.* 30. Fidgety feet, cannot keep them still, *Zincum Met.* 30. Weak ankles, give way at times, *Chamomilla* 30. Ankles swell, puffy, *Apis Mell.* 30.

38. FEVERS, simple or inflammatory— *Aconitum Nap.* 30, anguish with heat and shivering, *Arsenicum Alb.* 30, Scarlet, *Aconitum Nap.* 30 and *Belladonna* 30. Dull, stupid, apathetic, *Gelsemium* 30. High with throbbing and delirium, *Belladonna* 30. Skin dry, hot and burning without sweat, *Sulphur* 30.

DIRECTIONS—Give one dose every two hours.

39. FLATULENCE (WIND)— when arising from eating fatty or rich food, *Pulsatilla* 30. When there is distension and windy eructations, *Carbo Veg.* 30. Excessive accumulation of wind in the stomach which cannot be expelled either way, *Lycopodium Clav.* 30.

DIRECTIONS—Give one dose every two hours.

40. GRIPPE (INFLUENZA)— Loss of muscular power, shivering, feverish, dull, *Gelsemium* 30, pains of bone-breaking character, *Eupatorium Perf.* 30. Onset of disease

extremely sudden and malignant, epidemic grippe, extreme prostation, *Arsenicum Alb.* 30. Catarrhal symptoms prominent, nose swollen and much bad smelling perspiration, *Mercurius Sol.* 30. "Goose-Flesh" chills, creeping from feet up, or heat flushes upwards, muffled cough, *Sabadilla* 30. Limbs heavy, worse on motion, frontal headache, *Bryonia Alb. 30.* Premonitory chill, or fever, before disease is fully declared *Aconitum Nap.* 30, which may abort attack.

DIRECTIONS—A dose every half hour until better.

41. GUM-BOIL— for great heat, pain and swelling, *Aconitum Nap.* 30 followed by *Belladonna* 30. For considerable throbbing and pulsative pain, *Mercurius Sol.* 30. If suppurative stage supervenes, *Hepar Sul* 6, after the matter has matter has formed, give *Silicea* 30.

DIRECTIONS—Give one dose every two hours.

42. HEADACHE— throbbing, worse from light, noise or jar, *Belladonna* 30.

Awakes with headache, due to gastric troubles, alcoholic excesses or high living, *Nux Vomica* 30. Dull, heavy, listless, or going from nape of neck and settling over eyes—*Gelsemium* 30.

Splitting, frontal, every motion, even moving eyes causes pain, *Bryonia Alba.* 30. Daily headache. *China off.* 30.

Sick headache with blurred vision and sour and bitter vomit—*Iris Vers.* 30, with great nausea, *Ipecac.* 30, begins in morning, cannot tolerate light, or noise, *Sanguinaria* 30.

Nervous, neuralgic headache. If on left side, *Spigelia* 30, on the right side—*Silicea* 30, Head feels too large, *Argentum Nit.* 30, always better in open air—*Pulsatilla* 30.

DOSE—Every half hour till better.

HEADACHE, BILIOUS, commences with nausea, frequent vomiting of bile, bitter taste in throat, loss of appetite. headache, furred tongue, constipation—give three doses of *Mercurius Sol.* 30 two hours apart, if there is no relief, give three doses of *Nux Vomica* 30 at same interval.

If brought on by partaking of rich, fat food, give *Pulsatilla* 30 every two hours.

43. HEART-BURN—If occasioned by excesses in wine or spirituous liquors, *Nux Vomica* 30. Constant burning in throat with belching of wind, *Carbo Veg.* 30.

    Obstinate cases may be treated by *Calcarea Carb.* 30 and *Sulphur* 30.

    DOSE. Every hour till relieved.

44. HICCOUGH— the chief remedy is *Nux Vomica* 30. In obstinate cases try *Ginseng* 30.

45. HOARSENESS— from damp evening air, *Carbo Veg. 30.*

    Larynx rough and sore, *Phosphorus* 30. Complete loss of voice, *Causticum* 30. From over-straining the voice. *Arnica Mont.* 30.

    DOSE—Every four hours.

46. INDIGESTION OR DYSPEPSIA— *Nux Vomica* 30 and *Cocculus Ind.* 30 in alternation will relieve most temporary cases. Gas on stomach, flatulence and acidity, *Carbo Veg.* 30. Feeling of load on stomach, burning, bitter taste, water brash, *Bryonia Alba.* 30. Always better immediately after eating, *Anacardium* 30. Loss of taste, *Pulsatilla* 30.

    DOSE— at least half hour before each meal.

47. KIDNEY DISEASES— aching across loins, hot urine, *Cantharis* 30. Bloody urine, and painful pressure in kidneys, *Terebinthina* 30. Red sand in urine—*Lycopodium Clav.* 30.

    DOSE—Every half hour till better.

To prevent renal colic, give *China off.* 30 daily for three days, and, allowing three days' interval between each period, continue in the same way for one month. To allay pain of gall stones when passing, *Belladonna* 30 or *Calcarea Carb.* 30 every hour.

48. LIVER DISEASES— yellow tongue and skin, jaundice, liver sore to touch, *Mercurius Sol.* 30. Liver disorders from excesses of, or from taking too much allopathic or patent medicines, *Nux Vomica* 30. Torpid liver, *Podophyllum* 30. Pain under right shoulder blade, *Chelidonium* 30, liver spots, *Sepia* 30.

    DOSE—Every hour till better.

49. LUMBGO— sudden, knife-like pain, or soreness and stiffness, on attempting to rise from a seat, *Rhus Tox* 30.

    DOSE—Every half hour till better.

    In chronic cases, gives, give *Sulphur* 30 and then *Sulphur* 200 at longer intervals.

50. MEASLES— the disease comes on like a cold in the head. and after three or four days a small red eruption makes its appearance, first on the face, then on other parts of the body. If feverish symptoms are present, give *Aconitum Nap.* 30, every two hours, for a few doses, and then *Pulsatilla* 30, which is also a specific, every three hours. If any cough remains after these, *Sulphur* 30, once in two days in the mornings.

    A few doses of *Pulsatilla* 30 to those who are exposed, a dose daily will prevent the disease from spreading.

51. MIND— fear of any sort, anxiety, restlessness, *Aconitum Nap.* 30. For the 'blues', and complete mental break-down, *Kalium Phos.* 30. From grief, *Ignatia* 30. Suicidal inclination, black melancholy, *Aurum Met.* 30. May be given in the 200*th* potency after a few days, at intervals of a week to a fortnight.

52. MUMPS— consist of an inflammation of the large gland lying under and in front of the ears. It more frequently occurs in children and seldom attacks a person more than once, *Mercurius Sol.* 30 should be given first, and if much pain and redness supervenes, give *Belladonna* 30.

    The two remedies may be given in alternation every hour or two, according to the severity of the trouble, and the interval prolonged when better.

53. NERVOUSNESS— nervous debility, *Phosphoric Acid* 30. Dreads mental and physical exertion, *Silicea* 30. Brain fag, patient breaks down completely, men weep and give up, *Kalium Phos.* 30, nervous, cannot keep still, fidgety feet, *Zincum Met.* 30. Head weak, cannot think, backaches, imagines seeing faces in the dark, *Phosphorus* 30. Irritable, loses temper at slight things, everything goes wrong, insomnia, nightmares, angry at everything, *Nux Vomica* 30.

54. PILES— they are always constitutional, and generally accompanied by constipation. One dose of *Nux Vomica* 30 in the evening, followed by one dose of *Sulphur* 30 in the following morning, and continued for several weeks, will cure a large majority of cases. *Pulsatilla* 30 may be given, when much or mucus is discharged, with or without being mixed with blood. *Asculus Hip.* 3, for a sensation, as if a pricky lump were pressing upwards in the anus.

    Hamamelis 3 is the chief remedy for bleeding piles.

    DIRECTIONS—One dose, morning and evening.

55. RHEUMATISM— from exposure to dry cold—*Aconitum Nap.* 30. Bad cases marked by very tender, painful soles of feet, *Antimonium Crud.* 30. Where pain is almost unbearable, *Chamomilla* 30. In fleshy part of the muscles, *Cimicifuga* 30. Always worse from warmth, *Kalium Sulph.* 30,

Pulsatilla 30. Beginning in feet, *Ledum Pal.* 30. With creeping chilliness and much sweat, worse from warmth, *Mercurius Sol.* 30.

Stiff and sore, but better after motion, or pain drives one to motion, brought on by exposure, muscular rheumatism, *Rhus Tox. 30*, worse from motion, especially in the joints, *Bryonia Alba.* 30. In wrist, *Sabina* 30. In shoulders, *Ferrum Met.* 30.

DOSE—Every two hours till better. In all prolonged cases, a dose of *Sulphur* 30, once a week is good.

56. RINGWORM— a few doses a *Sulphur* 30, given morning and evening, may be sufficient. If after a week there is no improvement, give *Sepia* 30 in the same way, and then *Sepia* 200.

57. SCIATICA— in recent cases, *Colocynth* 30. Rheumatic sciatica, *Rhus Tox. 30*. If it gets worse at a given time every night, *Arsenicum Alb.* 30. Cases of long standing require *Sulphur* 30.

DOSE—Every hour.

58. SEA-SICKNESS— for a day or two before sailing, take *Nux Vomica* 30, a dose three times a day. After sailing, take it every fifteen minutes, if there is nausea or squeamishness. Where there is extreme nausea, the best remedy is *Tabacum* 30. For nausea, with inability to vomit, and vertigo, take *Cocculus Ind.* 30. For extreme weakness and prostration after an attack, take *Arsenicum Alb.* 30—a dose every two hours. *Petroleum* 30 is also recommended, particularly if there is much vomiting and constipation. *Glonoine* 30 *is the latest and one of the most successful remedies.*

59. SKIN DISEASES— harsh, dry, dirty skin, *Sulphur* 30, unhealthy, small hurts, suppurate and heal slowly, skin chaps easily,

Hepar Sulph. 6. Sticky scabby eruptions, coarse nails and inflamed old scars, *Graphites* 30. Turning brown or spotty, *Sepia* 30. Eruptions in hot weather *Sarsaparilla* 30. Cracked finger tips, *Petroleum* 30. Dry itching eruptions, *Staphysagria* 30. Red blotches that itch terribly, *Mezerium* 30. Greasy skin, *Natrium Mur.* 30.

60. SLEEPLESSNESS— sleepless restlessness of old age, *Aconitum Nap.* 30, chronic sleeplessness, *Opium* 30 *or* 200. Tired but cannot sleep, *Ambra Gris.* 30. With jerking, starting, unpleasant things appear, almost fears to go to sleep, *Belladonna* 30. In sickness, *Calcarea Carb.* 30. wakes early and cannot go to sleep again, *Sulphur* 30. In children *Chamomilla* 30.

61. SORE THROAT— inflammation with redness and dryness of the throat, much pain in swallowing, *Belladonna* 30. One dose every hour will generally suffice.

   When throat is raw, constant swallowing, glands swollen, breath offensive, *Mercurius Sol.* 30. For high fever, dry heat, great thirst and restlessness, difficulty in swallowing or speaking, burning or pricking sensation, *Aconitum Nap.* 30. Throat very dark red, *Phytolacca* 30. One dose every hour.

   Ulcerative sore throat with yellow patches, *Kalium Bichromicum* 30. Sore throat of smokers, *Capsicum* 30. See also 'Diphtheria'.

62. SPASMS OR CONVULSIONS OF CHILDREN— when excited by teething, give *Chamomilla* 30. When connected with disturbances of the brain and derangement of the nervous system, give *Belladonna* 30, every half hour, followed, if necessary after there hours, with *Ignatia* 30. As the spasm gets better, give medicine at longer intervals.

63. STOMACH DISORDERS— gastritis caused by cold drinks or getting chilled, *Aconitum Nap.* 30. Gastritis caused by ice-

cream, *Arsenicum Alb.* 30. Acidity of stomach, *Carbo Veg.* 30. Bitter stomach, water brash, *Bryonia Alba.* 30. Burning in stomach, *Arsenicum Alb.* 30. Disorders brought on by fat oily food, *Pulsatilla* 30. Wind on stomach, belching, *Lycopodium Clav.* 30. Cramps—*Cuprum Met.* 30. Gone feeling at pit of stomach —*Ignatia* 30. Vomiting of dark blood, *Hamamelis* 3 or *Ipecac.* 30. Disordered stomach showing white coating of tongue, *Antimonium Crud.* 30.

DOSE—Every hour.

64. TOOTHACHE— *Mercurius Sol.* 30 will give quick relief in majority of cases, especially in decayed teeth, if it falls, *Plantago* 30, is the next remedy. Toothache from anything warm taken into the mouth, *Chamomilla* 30. In teeth which have just been filled, *Arnica Mont.* 30. For abscess in teeth, *Silicea* 30.

65. VOMITING— if produced by eating over-rich food, *Pulsatilla* 30. If bilious or from weakness of the stomach, *Nux vomica* 30. Nausea and retching, sick at the stomach, *Ipecac.* 30. If it is accompanied by diarrhea and burning of the stomach, *Arsenicum Alb.* 30. Give a dose every two hours.

66. WARTS— fungus growths, pear shaped, and figwarts, *Thuja* 30, hands covered with warts, great crops of them, *Ferrum Picricum* 30.

DOSE—Once a day.

67. WATER-BRASH (acid rising)— If of an acid character and in cases of long standing, *Calcarea Carb.* 30—a dose morning and evening. If complicated with symptoms of dyspepsia or if brought on by excessive drinking, *Nux Vomica* 30. If from eating rich, fat food, *Pulsatilla* 30, *Carbo Veg.* 30 will also relieve a great many cases. *Arsenicum Alb.* 30 and *Phosphorus* 30 are also helpful. One dose every two hours until relieved.

68. WHOOPING COUGH— if child is full-blooded and of nervous temperament, flushed face, sudden violent whoop and no expectoration, give *Belladonna* 30, with much mucus on chest, *Antimonium Tart.* 30. Where coughing paroxysms go on almost to suffocation, and convulsion, *Cuprum Met.* 30. Disposition to retch and vomit, with nausea, *Ipecac.* 30. When case has run for some time, and is weakened, attack ends in retching and vomiting, *Drosera* 30. When exposed to disease, give *Pulsatilla* 30 as a preventive. Give a dose of the appropriate remedy after every fit of coughing. In chronic cases, *Corallium Rub.* 30 is useful.

69. WORMS— their presence is indicated by a pale face, picking of the nose, variable humour and appetite, grating of the teeth during sleep, hardness of the abdomen and constipation. *China off.* 200 is the main remedy in acute conditions. In chronic cases *Sulphur* 30 and *Calcarea Carb.* 30, weekly and then in the 200*th* potency, at fortnightly intervals.

DISEASES OF WOMEN

Menses, Retarded or Suppressed

Pulsatilla 30, in blondes, or where cause is from getting wet.

Belladonna 30, in the full blooded, suddenly suppressed, throbbing pains. *Sepia* 30 in brunettes, or dark complexioned persons, sick, headache, shivering, flushes of heat.

Caulophyllum 30, with menstrual colic.

Kalium Carb. 30, in young girls, scanty, acrid, pale, baggy under eyes.

Ferrum Met. 30, ashy greenish face.

Calcarea Carb. 30, fat and fair, sweat easily, subject to headache.

THERAPEUTIC INDEX

DOSE—Four times a day.

MENORRHAGIA—EXCESSIVE MENSTRUATION.

Belladonna 30, in the plethoric, hot discharge, pressing downward, bright red blood.

Platina 30, too early, dark blood those who mature too early, excitable sexually.

China off. 30, causing great weakness.

Ignatia 30, causing nausea.

Calcarea Carb. 30, takes cold easily, feet cold, clammy skin.

DOSE —Four times a day till better.

Dysmenorrhea—Painful Menstruation

Cimicifuga, especially in the rheumatic, ovaries and womb tender to the touch.

Belladonna 30, pressing, cutting, spasmodic pains, throbbing.

Sepia 30, Dragging down sensation, headache.

Pulsatilla 30, colic-like pains, vomiting.

Cocculus Ind. 30, sharp cutting pains in the abdomen, as from sharp stones. Increased by every movement, every breath, nausea unto fainting, discharge fitful, scanty and irregular, great vertigo.

Gelsemium 30, flushed face, congested eyes, very painful.

Calcarea Carb. 30, with nervous debility, pale face, clammy hands and feet.

Caulophyllum 30, cramp-like pains extending to bowels and rectum.

Collinsonia 30, when there is constipation and piles.

DOSE — Four times a day till better.

Sulphur 30, with any of the above remedies, where the case is more or less chronic.

Chlorosis—Green Sickness

Calcarea Carb. 30, with hectic fever and cough. *Ferrum Met.* 30 follows well after *Calcarea Carb.* 30, orin alternation with it.

Phosphorus 30, night sweats, diarrhea, form self-abuse.

Pulsatilla 30, mild, light-complexioned girls, shifting pains, always better in open air.

Natrium Mur. 30, where skin looks dirty, or greasy.

DOSE —Four times a day till better. Once or twice a week a dose of *Sulphur* 30, with selected remedy.

Leucorrhea, Whites

Pulsatilla 30, discharge thick and cream, sometimes burning. Alternate, *Calcarea Carb.* 30.

Sepia 30, discharge acrid, yellow, watery, with bearing down pains.

Mercurius Sol. 30, thick, greenish, and very corrosive, increased at night.

China off. 30, when very profuse and debilitating.

Kreosotum 30, smelling very offensive and causing itching and soreness.

DOSE —Four times a day till better.

An occasional dose of *Sulphur* 30 with the other remedies is beneficial.

Abortion or Miscarriage, Threatened Abortion

If there is a disposition to miscarriage, or if the patient had previously miscarried, as she approaches the period, she should lie on the bed, taking tea-spoon doses of *Sabina* 30, every fifteen, or twenty minutes in severe cases, every two hours in milder ones,

THERAPEUTIC INDEX

and when no danger is apprehended and in the early stages, every six or twelve hours, until the period is passed. If relief is not obtained in five or six hours, another remedy should be chosen. As preventive of this disorder, the principal remedies are *Sabina* 30, *Secale* Cor. 30, *Lycopodium Clav.* 30, *Calcarea Carb.* 30, *Sepia* 30.

APPENDIX–II

MATERIA MEDICA

(In Brief)

In order to help beginners to select the appropriate remedy, a brief 'MATERIA MEDICA' of the more important *Polychrest* remedies (medicines which are useful in may diseases) is appended, as in homeopathic practice, the name of the diseases is not the leading feature, but only its *general character and nature,* together with the *constitutional peculiarities* of the patient, only the *most important, and the general characteristics* of each remedy, are given along with their relationship with other allied remedies.

Aconitum Napellus

MONKSHOOD-PLANT—*Antipyretic and Anti-phlogistic.*

Fever, with hot dry skin, great thirst, anxiety or restlessness, all ailments brought on by exposure to *cold dry winds, or draughts. Fear is a very prominent symptom*—fear of a crowd, of going out, of anything. Restlessness, tossing about, anguish of mind and body, pain. Inflammation and congestion. Useful in all ailments that begin with a chill or shuddering, and fever. Dry cough. Worse, towards evening.

Its sphere is in the beginning of an acute disease and not to be continued after pathologic change comes, *Aconitum Nap.* should never be given simply to control the fever, not alternated with other drugs for that purpose. If it be a case requiring *Aconitum Nap.,* no other drug is needed, *Aconitum Nap.* will cure the case.

COMPLEMENTARY, to *Coffee,* in fever, sleeplessness, intolerance of pain, to *Arnica Mont.* in injuries, to *Sulphur* in all cases. *Sulphur* is *the chronic of Aconitum Nap.* and often completes a cure begun with *Aconitum Nap.*

ANTIDOTES, wine, vinegar, *Camphor, Nux Vomica.*

Alumina
Pure Clay—Mineral—Anti-Psoric.

Adapted to persons who suffer from chronic diseases, the *Aconitum Nap.* of chronic diseases. constitution deficient in animal heat *(Cal Carb.,Sil.).* Spare, dry, thin subjects, dark complexion, mild, cheerful disposition, hypochondriacs, dry, tettery, itching eruption, *worse* in winter *(Petr.),* intolerable itching of whole body when getting warm in bed *(Sulph.), scratches* until bleeds, then becomes painful. A very general condition is *dryness* of mucous membranes and skin, and tendency to paralytic muscular states. Old people, with lack of vital heat, or prematurely old, with debility. Sluggish functions, heaviness, numbness, and staggering, and the characteristic constipation, find an excellent remedy in *Alumina.* Dispositions to colds in the head, and eructations in spare, dry, thin subjects. Delicate children, products of artificial baby foods. abnormal craying for starch, chalk, charcoal, coffee or tea grounds, acids, indigestible things *(Psor). Potatoes disagree. Chronic eructations for years,* worse in evening. Constipation, no *desire for and no ability to pass stool, until there is a large accumulation (Melil.), great straining,* stool hard, knotty, covered with mucus, or soft, clayey, adhering to parts *(Plat.). Inactivity of rectum, even soft stool requires great straining (Anac., Plat., Ver Alb.).* Constipation, of nursing children, from artificial foods, of old people *(Lyc., Op.),* of pregnancy, from inactive rectum *(Sep.).* Has to strain at stool in order to *urinate.* Leucorrhea, *acrid and profuse, running down to the heels,* worse during the day time, better by cold bathing. After menses, *exhausted physically and mentally,* scarcely able to speak, *(Carb. an., Cocc Ind.).*

WORSE, in cold air, during winter, from eating potatoes, on alternate days, *at new and full moon.*

BETTER, in open air, from cold washing, damp weather.

RELATIONS, Complementary, *Bryonia Alba.*

Follows, *Bryonia Alba., Lach, Sulph. Alumina* is the chronic of *Bryonia Alba.*

SIMILAR TO, *Bar Carb., Con.,* in ailments of old people.

ANTIDOTES, *Ipecac., Cham, Bryonia Alba.*

Antimonium Crudum
*Black Sulphide of Antimony—Mineral—*Anti-Psoric.

The great characteristic of the remedy is a *white coated tongue, very white. Especially useful in disorders of the stomach from any cause, where the tongue is prominent.* Sore, cracked nostrils and corners in mouth, scurfy. Children *cannot bear to be touched, or even looked at, very fretful.* Nails split and are brittle, and soles of feet become very hard and sensitive for walking. Diarrhea and constipation alternate in old persons. Piles, with white of egg like exudation.

WORSE, after eating, cold bath, acids *after heat of sun of fire.*

SIMILAR TO, *Bryonia Alba., Ipecac., Lycopodium Clav., Puls.* in gastric complaints.

FOLLOWS WELL AFTER, *Puls., Mercurius Sol., Sulph.*

ANTIDOTIES, *Hepar Sulph.*

Antimonium Tartaricum
Tartar emetic (Metal).

Very useful for respiratory diseases, *rattling of mucus with little expectoration, has been a guiding symptom.* There is *much drowsiness, debility and sweat,* characteristic of the drug, which group should always be present, when the drug is prescribed. For diseases originating from exposure in damp basements and cellars. *Great sleepiness, or irresistible inclination to sleep, with nearly all complaints.* For bad effects of vaccination, when *Thuja* fails and *Silicea is not indicated.* In children's coughs, if *Antimonium Tart.* does not help, *Hepar Sulp.* acts better.

Worse, in damp, cold weather, lying down at night, warmth of room.

BETTER, cold open air, sitting upright, expectorating, lying on right side.

ANTIDOTES, *Puls., Sepia.*

Apis Mellifica

Poison of the Honey Bee

The striking key notes of this remedy are—burning, stinging pains and thirstlessness. Bulging out beneath the eyes. Extremely sensitive, when touched. Skin sometimes waxy-looking. drowsiness, intolerance of heat, better from cold water and open air. Has been successful, when the general characteristics are present, in hot, red swellings in any part of the body, ill effects of swallowing hot things, sore throat, nettle rash, dropsy, white swelling of knee, ophthalmia, erysipelas, and inflammation of kidneys. Affects right side—enlargement, or dropsy of right ovary, right testicle.

WORSE, after sleeping, closed or warm rooms, from getting wet, but better from washing the part in cold water.

BETTER, open air, cold water or cold bathing, when sitting erect.

COMPLEMENTARY, *Natrium Mur* disagrees, when used either before or after *Rhus Tox.*

Arsenicum Alb. and *Puls.*—follow *Apis Mell.* well.

ANTIDOTES, *Arsenicum Alb., Canth.*

Argentum Nitricum

Nitrate of Silver—Metal—Anti-sycotic.

Prematurely old children or adults, withered. Sight of high houses makes a patient dizzy, hurried feelings, very nervous. Headache, feeling as though the head expanded, which may also extend to body. Profuse purulent discharge from the eyes. Red tip of tongue with papillae, an indication in any disease. *Abnormal craving for sugar.* Catarrh of smokers. Inflammation of larynx in singers. *Belching accompanies most gastric ailments. Chilly, when uncovered, yet feels smothered, if wrapped up, craves fresh air.*

WORSE, cold food, cold air, eating sugar, ice-cream, *unusual mental exercise.*

BETTER, Open air, bathing with cold water.

For the effects of cauterizing with nitrate of silver, *Natrium Mur.*

ANTIDOTE, *Natrium Mur.*

The 200*th or 1000th potency in watery solution,* as a topical application in *Ophthalmia neonatorum,* has relived, when the crude silver nitrate failed.

It is useful for boy's complaints after using tobacco (*Arsenicum Alb., Ver Alb.*).

SIMILAR TO, *Natrium Mur., Nitricum Ac., Lachesis, Cuprum Met.*

Arnica Mont. Montana

Leopard's Bane (Plant).

This remedy, internally is prescribed for bad effects, either recent or remote, from all heavy blows, concussions, falls, and for the overstraining or overexertion of athletes, or labouring men.

Rheumatism following muscular strain. In diseases, the leading indications for this drug are sore, bruised and lame feeling, the bed seems to hard, foul eructations. Dyspeptic, cold face, body and feet cold. Sore throat from speaking, singing or shouting. Gout and rheumatism, *with great fear of being touched or struck by persons coming near him.*

Worse, least touch, motion, rest, wine, damp cold.

BETTER, *lying down, or with head low, motion (Rhus. Tox., Ruta).*

RELATIONSHIP, COMPLEMENTARY, *Aconitum Nap., Hyper., Rhus Tox., Ipecac.*

SIMILAR TO, *for soreness as if bruised, Bapt Tinct., China off., Phyt., Pyr., Rhus Tox., Ruta, Staph.*

Arnica Mont. follows well, after *Aconitum, Apis Mell., Ham., Ipec., Ver Alb.,* is followed well by *Sul Ac.*

In ailments from spirituous liquors or from charcoal vapours, *Arnica Mont.* is often indicated (*Am Carb., Bov.*).

In spinal concussion, compare *Hyper.*

ANTIDOTES, *Camph., Ign., Ipec.*

Arsenicum Album

White Oxide or Arsenic—Mineral—Anti-Psoric.

Among the leading general indications for this drug are prostration, restlessness, sudden sinking, extreme weakness, burning, great thirst, *worse* at rest and from cold.

A drug to be considered when attack of disease is *sudden and malignant.* Lips, mouth and throat dry, and stomach irritable. Breathing oppressed. Skin dry, scaly and burning. What *Aconitum Nap.* is to *simple fever, Arsenicum Alb.* is to *malignant.* Has been successfully prescribed in grippe, colds, excoriating the nose.

Thin watery, corrosive discharge, *ague, vomiting of drunkards, ophthalmia, burning eyes, asthma, neuralgia, inflammation of kidneys, diarrhea,* othorrhea, also stomach ills from green food, and skin diseases, in all these diseases where some of the leading indications are present, *especially, burning and thirst, Arsenicum Alb.* should be thought of in ailments from alcoholism, *ptomainc* poisoning, stings, wounds, chewing tobacco, ill effects from decayed food or animal matter, whether by inoculation, olfaction or ingestion, odour of discharges is *putrid,* in complaints that return annually (*Carbo Veg., Lach., Sulph., Thuja*). Anemia and chlorosis. Degenerative changes. Gradual loss of weight from impaired nutrition. Maintains the system under the stress of malignancy, regardless of location. Malarial cachexia. *Septic infections and low vitality.* Give quiet and ease to the last moments of life, when given in a high potency.

WORSE, after midnight (1 to 2 a.m. or p.m.), from *cold,* cold drinks or food, when lying on affected side or with head low.

BETTER, from heat in general (*reverse of Secale Corn.*) except headache, which is temporarily better by cold bathing (*Spig.*), burning pain better by heat, from warm drinks.

COMPLEMENTARY, *Rhus Tox., Carbo Veg. Phos., Thuja, Secale Cor.,* antidotal to lead poison.

ANTIDOTES, *Opium, Carbo Veg., China off., Hepar Sulp., Nux Vom., Ipec.*

Baptisia Tinctoria

Wild Indigo (Plant)

Chillness, with aching pains in head, back and limbs, weak, drowsy, confused, tongue brown, in fact, the beginning of typhoid, these are the leading characteristics of *Baptisia,* and taken in time this remedy will abort the disease. Foul diarrhea with no pain. Low forms of fever, with foul breath and conditions. Has also proved useful in chronic dyspepsia with above general characteristics. *Great muscular soreness and putrid phenomena always are present.*

(All the secretions are offensive—breath, stool. urine, sweat etc. In whatever position the patient lies, the parts rested upon feel *sore and bruised (Pyr. compare Arnica Mont.).*

WORSE, Humid, heat, fog, indoors.

SIMILAR TO, *Arnica Mont., Arsenicum Alb., Bryonia Alba., Gels.,* in the early stages of fever, with malaise, nervousness, flushed face, drowsiness and muscular soreness, when *Ars. Alb.* has been improperly given or too often repeated, in typhoid, *Baptisia* follows well. *Bryonia Alba.* and *Arsenicum Alb.* may be needed to complete the favourable reaction.

Baryta Carbonica

Barium Carbonate—Anti-Psoric.

This remedy is useful for children who are dwarfish, backward mentally and physically, do not grow and develop, with swollen abdomen, take cold easily and *always have swollen tonsils.* Children shy and averse to meeting strangers. Diseases of old men, when degenerative changes begin—Cardiac, vascular and cerebral,—who have hypertrophied prostate or indurated testes, very sensitive to cold, offensive foot-sweats, very weak and weary, must sit or lie down or lean on something. Often useful in the dyspepsias of the young who have masturbated and who suffer from seminal emissions, together with cardiac irritability and palpitation.

WORSE, while thinking of symptoms, from washing, lying on painful side.

FREQUENTLY USEFUL, before or after, *Psor., Sulph., and Tub.* After *Baryta Carb., Psor.,* will often eradicate the constitutional tendency to quinsy (inflammation of tonsils).

SIMILAR TO, *Alum, Calcarea Carb., Iod., Fluor Ac., Iod., Sil.*

INCOMPATIBLE, after *Calcarea Carb.*, in scrofulous affections.

Belladonna

Deadly *Nightshade* (Plant).

The general indications of *Belladonna* are very marked. Hot head, flushed face, bright with bloodshot eyes, and sometimes delirium, the pain accompanying inflammation in any part of the body is a *throbbing* one, whether of a boil or a headache. Throat sore, very red and dry. Worse from jarring, noise and light. A child well one moment, and down the next. Clinically useful in sore throat, scarlet fever, congestive headache, throbbing, blinding headache, congestion of brain, stiff neck, neuralgia, acute inflammation of the ears, erysipelas and sciatica. *Great children's* remedy (epileptic spasms followed by nausea and vomiting), corresponds to the symptoms of 'air-sickness' of aviators, and may be used as preventive. *Belladonna* stands for *violence* of attack and *suddenness* of onset.

No thirst, anxiety or fear with fever.

WORSE, from touch, motion, noise, draught of air, looking at bright shining objects (*Lys., Stram.*), after 3 p.m., night, after midnight, while drinking, uncovering the head, summer sun, lying down.

BETTER, rest, standing or sitting erect, warm room.

COMPLEMENTARY, *Calcarea Carb.*—*Belladonna* is the acute of *Calcarea Carb.* which is often required to complete a cure.

SIMILAR TO, *Aconitum Nap., Bryonia Alba., Cic, Gels., Glon., Hyosyamus Nig., Mel., Op., Stram.*

ANTIDOTES, *Camph., Coffee, Opium, Aconitum Nap., Hep Sulp., Puls.*

Bryonia Alba.

Wild Hops (Plant).

The key note to this remedy is *'worse from motion'*, where this is very marked, the remedy is plain in any disease. Another marked characteristic is *'better from pressure.'* Headache where one presses the head, cough when the head involuntarily is pressed on the chest, etc. Lips and mouth *parched with great thirst. Stitching pains in chest.* sensation of a stone in the stomach. Cough hurts head and chest. Constipation. *Bryonia Alba.* covers many every day ills. Clinically useful in frontal headache, water brash, bitter eructations, biliousness, pneumonia, pleurisy, acute rheumatism, joints hot and shiny, muscular rheumatism, pains in back, constipation, liver complaints, headache after every meal and hungry, yet no appetite.

Bryonia Alba. affects especially the constitution of a robust, firm fibre, and dark complexion with tendency to leanness and irritability. It prefers the right side, the evening, and open air, warm weather after cold days, to manifest its action most markedly.

Children dislike to be carried or raised. *Physical weakness, all pervading apathy. Complaints apt to develop slowly.*

WORSE, warmth, *any motion,* morning, warm food, hot weather, exertion, touch, cannot sit up, gets faint or sick or both, suppressed discharges of any kind.

BETTER, *lying on painful side, pressure, rest, cold things.*

COMPLEMENTARY, *Alumina, Rhus Tox.*

SIMILAR TO, *Bell., Hep Sulp.,* for hasty speech and hasty dinking.

AFTER BRYONIA ALBA., *Alum., Kalium Carb, Nux Vom., Phos., Rhus Tox., Sulph.*

ANTIDOTES, *Acontinum Nap., Cham, Nux Vom.*

Calcarea Carbonica

Carbonate of Lime—Anti-Psoric.

Especially indicated in rickety and scrofulous constitutions, inclined to obesity, sweaty head, cold damp feet, night sweats. Catches cold easily, acid stomach and diarrhea, always chilly, it may be indicated almost in any disease. Though incined to chilliness, the *Calcarea Carb.* Patient is prone to sweat of an unheathy nature in various parts, head, arm-pits, feet, etc. It also has a marked acid, or sour stomach. Clinically useful in scrofula, rachitis, goitre, headache with cold feet, eczema, hip disease, tumors, incipient consumption, dyspepsia, defective growth in children, maramus, soft bones and glandular affections. *A faded state, mental or physical, due to overwork, abscesses in deep muscles, polypi and exostoses.* Easy relapses, interrupted convalescence, persons of scrofulous type who take cold easily with increased mucous secretions, children who grow fat, are large-bellied, with large head, pale skin, chalky look, the so-called leuco-phlegmatic temperament, affection caused by working in water. Great sensitiveness to cold, partial sweats. Children crave eggs, and eat dirt and other indigestible things, are prone to diarrhea. *Calcarea Carb.* patient is fat, fair, flabby and perspiring and cold, damp and sour. This great Hahnemannian anti-psoric is a constitutional remedy *par excellence.*

WORSE, cold air, wet weather, cold water, from washing (*Antimonium Cr.*), morning, during full moon.

BETTER, dry weather, lying on painful side, (*Bryonia Alba., Puls.*).

RELATIONS, COMPLEMENTARY to *Belladonna which is the acute of Calcarea Carb.*

CALCAREA CARB. acts best, Before *Lycopodium, Nux Vom., Phos., Sil.* It follows, *Nit Ac., Puls., Sulph.* (especially if pupils are dilated), is followed by *Kali Bi.*, in nasal catarrh. According to Hahnemann, *Calcarea Carb. must not be used before Nit. Ac.* and *Sulph.*, may produce unnecessary complications. It is useful when *Pulsatilla* failed in school girls.

COMPLEMENTARY, *Bell., Rhus Tox., Lycopodium Clav., Sil.*

INCOMPATIBLE, *Bryonia Alba.*

In children it may be often repeated, but in aged people should not be repeated, especially if the first dose benefited. It will usually do harm.

ANTIDOTES, *Camph., Nit Ac., Sulphur, Nux Vom., Ipec.*

Calcarea Phosphorica

Phosphate of Lime.—Constitutional.

It is especially useful in tardy dentition, and troubles incidental to that period, bone disease, non-union of fractured bones and the anemias, after acute diseases and chronic wasting diseases. *Anemic children who are peevish, flabby, have cold extremities, and feeble digestion.* It has a special affinity where bones form sutures or symphyses, and all its symptoms are worse from any change of weather. *Numbness and crawling* are characteristic sensations, and tendency to perspiration and glandular enlargement are symptoms it shares with *Calcarea Carb.* Scofulosis, chlorosis and pthisis. Headache of school girls (*Natrium Mur. Psor.*).

WORSE, exposure to damp, cold, changeable weather, *melting snow,* mental exertion.

BETTER, in *summer, warm, dry atmosphere.*

RELATIONS, COMPLEMENTARY—*Ruta, Hepar Sulp.*

SIMILAR TO, *Carbo An., Calcarea flour., Calcarea Carb., Fluor Ac., Kalium Phos.,* to *Psor,* in debility remaining after acute diseases, to *Sil.,* but sweat of head is wanting.

ACTS BEST, *before Iod., Psor, Sulph.,* after *Arsenicum Alb., Iod., Tub.*

Cantharis

Spanish Fly (Animal).

Violent burning pains in bladder, and along urinary tract, with straining while urinating. Constant urging to urinate. Scalding urine. Urine passed in drops. Urine bloody. In gonorrhea, when there is intense sexual excitement with very painful erections. Chorde. sexual mania. Intense desire. Lumbago with kidney inflammation. The inflammations *Cantharis* produces (bladder, kindeys, ovaries, meninges, pleuritic and pericardial membranes) are usually associated with bladder irritation.

The *burning pain and intolerable urging to urinate* is the red strand of *Cantharis* in all inflammatory affections.

WORSE, from touch, or approach, urinating, drinking cold water or coffee.

BETTER, rubbing.

RELATIONSHIP—ANTIDOTES, *Aconitum Nap., Camph., Puls.*

SIMILAR TO, *Apis Mell., Arsenicum Alb., Merurius Cor.*

COMPLEMENTARY, *Camph.*

Carbo Vegetablis

Vegetable Charcoal—Anti-Psoric.

Sluggishness and stagnation of the blood, coldness of the body, bluish colour of flesh, slow digestion, veins livid, flatulence and offensive discharges—these are the broad lines of this remedy. Useful when illness dates from a particular event, "never well since".

A lowered vital power from loss of fluids, after drugging, after other diseases, in old people with venous congestions, states of collapse in cholera. Typhoid, these are some of the conditions offering special inducements to the action of *Carbo Veg*. The patient may be almost lifeless, but the head is hot, coldness, breath cool, pulse imperceptible, oppressed and quickened respiration and must have air, must be fanned hard, must have all the windows open. This is a typical state for *Carbo Veg*.

The patient faints easily, is worn out, and must have fresh air. Hemorrhage from any mucous surface. Very debilitated. Patient seems to be too weak to hold out.

Children fear ghosts at night. Nose-bleed, blood dark, patient cold, chronic hoarseness of bronchitis, asthma, old cases. Chronic dyspepsia, sour eructations, varicose veins tending to ulcers. hemorrhage from lungs, nose, bowels or bladder in the debilitated. *A good remedy to take occasionally, to preserve the general health.*

Worse, evening, night and open air, cold, from fat food, butter, coffee, milk, warm damp weather, *wine*.

BETTER, from eructation, from *fanning*, cold.

RELATIONS—COMPLEMENTARY, *Kalium Carb., Dros.*

Want of susceptibility to well-selected remedies (*Opium, Val.*).

COMPARE, *Opium*, with lack of reaction after well selected remedies fail to permanently improve (*Val.*)

Phos. in easily bleeding ulcers *Puls.*—bad effects from fat-foods.

China off., Plumb Met., in neglected pneumonia especially in 'old topers.'

Antimonium Tart., in threatened paralysis from inability to expectorate loosened mucus.

ANTIDOTES, *Camph., Arsenic Alb.*

Causticum

Hahnemann's Tinctura Acris Sine Kalium—Anti-Psoric.

Manifests its action mainly in chronic rheumatic, arthritic and paralytic affections, indicated by the tearing, drawing pains in the muscular and fibrous tissues, with deformities about the joints, progressive loss of muscular strength, tendinous contractures. Broken-down seniles. Restlessness at night, with tearing pains in joints and bones, and faint-like sinking of strength. This weakness progresses until we have gradually appearing paralysis. Local paralysis, vocal cords, muscles of deglutition, of tongue, eyelids, face, bladder and extremities. Coughing or sneezing accompanied by an involuntary spurt of urine, cough with inability to raise phlegm. All ills of bladder following too long a holding of the urine. Bed wetting of the young and old. General weakness of the bladder. Loss of voice. Drooping eyelids, or paralysis of same, feeling of sand in the eyes. Patient cannot pass stools while sitting, must stand. Neuralgia at every change of weather. Children are slow in learning to walk. Weak ankles. The skin of a *Causticum* patient is of a *dirty white sallow*, with warts, especially on the face. Emaciation due to diseases, worry etc. and of long standing.

Burning, rawness, and *soreness* are characteristic.

WORSE, dry cold winds, in *clear fine* weather, *cold air,* from motion of carriage, from getting wet or bathing.

BETTER, in *damp, wet weather, warmth.* Heat of bed.

RELATIONS—COMPLIMENTARY, *Carbo Veg., Petros.*

INCOMPATIBLE, must not be used before or after *Phos.,* always disagrees, *Coffea.*

COMPARE, *Arnica Mont.,* must swallow mucus, *Gels., Graph.,* in ptosis, hoarseness, *Rumex, Sulph.,* in chronic aphonia.

MATERIA MEDICA

Causticum antidotes paralysis from lead poisoning (bad effects of holding type in month by compositors), and abuse of *Mercurius Sol.,* or *Sulph.* in scabies.

It affects *the right side most prominently.*

ANTIDOTES, *Coffea, Nux Vom, Colo.*

Chamomilla

German Chamomille.

The chief guiding symptoms belong to the mental and emotion group, which lead to this remedy in many forms of disease. Especially of frequent use in diseases of children, where *peevishness, restlessness and colic* give the necessary indications. *Chamomilla* is *sensitive, irritable, thirsty, hot and numb.* Over sensitiveness from abuse of coffee and narcotics. *Pains unendurable,* associated with numbness. Night sweats. Child fretful, wants to be carried, wants things, and then does not want them, snappish. One cheek red and the other pale. Diarrhea and colic, green stools, like rotten eggs, during *period of dentition.* rheumatic pains that drive patient from bed, excessive restlessness and tossing, but no fear as under *Aconitum Nap.* Hot and thirsty. Wind colic Skin moist and hot. Sleeplessness of children.

WORSE, by heat, anger, evening, before midnight, open air, in the wind, eructations.

BETTER, from *being carried,* warm, wet weather.

RELATIONS—COMPLIMENTARY, follows *Belladonna* in diseases of children and useful in cases spoiled by the use of Opium or morphine in complaints of children, *Mag Carb.*

ANTIDOTES, *Camph., Puls., Nux Vom.*

COMPARE, *Bell., Bryonia Alba., Coff, Puls., Sulph.*

Chelidonium Majus

Celandine (Plant).

A prominent liver remedy, covering many of the direct reflex symptoms of diseased conditions of that organ. The jaundiced skin, and especially the *constant pain under inferior angle of right shoulder blade* (*Kalium Carb., Mercurius Sol.*—under the left, *Chenop., Sang.*), are certain indications, tongue yellow, bad taste in the mouth, jaundice, constipation, stools *hard, round balls like sheep's dung, especially* in enlargement of the liver. The great general lethargy and indisposition to make any effort is also marked. Gall-stones, with pain under the right shoulder blade. *Bilious complications during pregnancy.*

WORSE, right side, motion, touch, change of weather, very early in morning.

BETTER, after dinner, from pressure.

RELATIONS, *Chel.*, antidotes the abuse of *Bryonia Alba.*, especially in liver complaints.

Arsenicum Alb., Lycopodium Clav., Sulph., follow well, and will often be required to complete cure.

ANTIDOTE, *Cham.*

COMPARE, *Nux Vom., Sulph., Bryonia, Lycopodium Clav., Opium, Mercurius Sol.*

China off. (Cinchona)

Peruvian Bark (Vegetable).

Weakness and debility resulting from any drain on the system, *loss of blood or vital fluids,* nursing, diarrhea, etc. Pale face, sunken eyes with dark rings about them, sweats and headache. Hectic fever. Diarrhea from fruit, painless diarrhea. Affections that are worse every other day. *Chronic liver and spleen diseases.*

Dyspepsia with cold stomach. 'Bloodlessness'—Ringing in the ears. *Sensitive to touch, to pain, to drafts of air,* entire nervous system extremely sensitive.

WORSE, *Slightest touch, draught of air,* every other day, loss of vital fluids, at night, after eating, bending over.

BETTER, Bending double, hard pressure, open air, warmth.

RELATIONS—ANTIDOTES, *Arnica Mont., Arsenicum Alb., Nux Vom., Ipec.*

COMPLEMENTARY, *Ferrum Met.*

FOLLOWS WELL—*Calarea Phos.* in hydrocephaloid.

INCOMPATIBLE AFTER, *Dig, Sel.*

Is useful in bed effects from excessive tea drinking, when hemorrhage results.

Worm-seed (Vegetable).

The pre-eminent remedy for worms in children.

Child restless, jumps and jerks and cries in its sleep, is cross, does not want to be touched, face sometimes flushed and then pale, paleness about the mouth, bores its fingers into the nose or picks it, grinds its teeth, unnatural appetite. *Pain in shocks.* Skin sensitive to touch.

WORSE, Looking fixedly at an aboject from worms, at night, in sun, in summer.

RELATIONS, compare *Antimonium Crud., Antimonium Tart., Bryonia Alb., Cham., Sil., Staph.* in irritability of children. In whooping cough, after *Drosera* has relieved the severe symptoms. Has cured aphonia from exposure, when *Aconitum Nap., Phos., and Spong,* had failed.

Is frequently to be thought of, in children, as an epidemic remedy.

ANTIDOTES, *Camph.*

Cocculus

Indian Cockle (Vegetable).

For women and children with light hair and eyes, who suffer severely during menstruation and pregnancy, and for unmarried and childless women. The *Cocculus Ind.* condition is like the sickness that attacks some from riding in cars, or sea-sickness, consequently it is remedy for those conditions when they attack travellers, or for similar conditions when coming on without any apparent cause. Useful also, in headache in back part of head, vertigo, nausea, trembling of the hands, hands and feet frequently go to sleep. Affections caused by loss of sleep, night-watching, etc., and for *dysmenorrhea, difficult menstruation.* Great vertigo is nearly always present in *Cocculus Ind.* cases.

WORSE, eating, after loss of sleep of sleep, open air, smoking, riding, swimming, touch, noise, jar, afternoon, menstrual period. After emotional disturbances.

RELATIONS, compare, *Ign.* and *Nux Vom.* in chorea and paralytic symptoms, *Antimonium Tart* in sweat of affected parts. Has cured umbilical hernia with obstinate constipation, after *Nux Vom.* failed

ANIDOTES, *Coffea, Nux Vom.*

Coffea Cruda

Unroasted coffee (Vegetable).

Nervousness is the leading indication of this drug. It is to be considered in every case where the nervousness is not the result of coffee drinking. Great nervous agitation and restlessness. Extra sensitiveness characterises this remedy. Neuralgia in various parts, always with great nervous excitability and *intolerance of pain* driving to despair. *Unusual activity of* mind and body. Bad effects of sudden emotions, surprises, joy etc. Nervous palpitation. It will also relieve neuralgia following prolonged mental effort, and the peculiar toothache or toothache relieved by cold water. Headache, with excessive nervousness. Skin hypersensitive. *Coffee* is specially suited to tall, lean, stooping persons with dark complexions, temperament, choleric and sanuine.

WORSE, *excessive emotions* (joy), narcotics, strong odours, noise, open air, cold night.

BETTER, warmth, from laying down, holding ice in mouth.

RELATIONS, Complimentary, *Aconitum Nap.*

INCOMPATIBLE, *Canth. Caust., Cocc Ind., Ign.*

ANTIDOTES, *Aconitum Nap., Cham., Nux Vom.*

Colocynthis

Bitter Cucumber **(Vegetable)**—*Anti-Psoric.*

The keynote to '*Colocynths'* is— *Terrible cramps, or neuralgic colic, that causes the patient to bend double, or press the abdomen against something* in the endeavour to allay the extreme pain this colic may, or may not be attended with vomiting and diarrhea. It is also a remedy for crampy pains in the hip, and for facil and stomach neuralgia. It is especially suitable for irritable persons easily angered, and ill effects therefrom. Women with copious menstruation, and of sedentary habits. Persons with a tendency to corpulency. Sensations, cutting, twisting, grinding, contractions and bruised, *as if clamped with iron bands. Colocynth pains are always ameliorated by hard pressure on painful parts.*

WORSE, from anger and indignation.

BETTER, doubling up, hard pressure, warmth, lying with head bent forward.

ANTIDOTES, *Coffea, Staph., Cham.*

COLOCYNTH is the best antidote to lead poisoning.

COMPLEMENTARY, *Mercurius Sol.* in dysentery with great tenesmus.

COMPARE, *Dios., Cham., Cocc., Plumb Met., Magensia Phos.*

Cuprum Metallicum

Copper—Mineral—Anti-Psoric.

Spasmodic affections, cramps, convulsions, beginning in fingers and toes, violent, contractive and intermitting pain, are some of the more marked expressions of the action of *Cuprum Met.,* and its curative range, therefore, includes tonic and clonic spasms, convulsions and epileptic attacks. Chorea brought on by fright.

Nausea greater than in any other remedy. In Epilepsy, aura begins in knees, ascends to hypogastrium, then unconsciousness, foaming and falling. Symptoms disposed to appear periodically and in groups. Complaints begin on left side (*Lachesis*). Convulsions, blue face and clenched hands. Cramps in toes, fingers, calves, cramps of cholera. Wherever these conditions are present in whooping cough, cholera, diarrhea, chorea or any other diseases, *Cuprum Met.* is indicated. Intermittent fever with extreme coldness and cramps. Spasmodic asthma. *Bad effects of repercussed* eruptions (of non-developed, *Zinc.*) resulting in brain affections, spasms, convulsions, voiting, of suppressed footsweat (*Sil., Zinc Met.*), epilepsy, worse at night during sleep(*Bufo.*), about new-moon, at regular intervals (*menses*), from a fall, or blow upon the head, from getting wet.

WORSE, before menses, from voiting, contact, cold air, cold wind.

BETTER, during perspiration, drinking cold water.

RELATIONS—COMPLIMENTARY, *Calcarea Carb.*

ANTIDOTES, *Bell., Hepar Sulph., Camph.*

COMPARE, *Arsenicum Alb.* and *Ver Alb.* in cholera, *Ipecac.,* the vegetable analogue.

Ver. Alb. follows well in whooping cough and cholera.

Apis Mell. and *Zinc Met.* in convulsions from suppressed exanthems.

Drosera

Sun-dew **(Vegetable)—(*Constitutional*).**

Affects markedly the respiratory organs and was pointed out by Hahnemann as the principal remedy for whooping cough. *Drosera* can break down resistance to tubercle and should, therefore, be capable of raising it. Laryngeal phthisis is benefited by it. Phthisis pulmonum, vomiting of food from cough with gastric irritation and profuse expectoration. Pains about hip-joints. Tubercular glands. In whooping cough, the paroxysms follow each other so rapidly as to hardly give time for breath. Tickling cough, beginning as soon as one lies down. Sensation of feather in larynx. Chronic coughs.

WORSE, after midnight, lying down, on getting warm in bed, drinking singing, laughing.

RELATIONS—COMPLIMENTARY, to *Nux Vom.*

FOLLOWS WELL, after *Samb., Sulph., Ver Alb.*

IS FOLLOWED BY, *Calcarea Carb., Puls., Sulph.*

COMPARE, *China off., Coral., Cup Met., Ipec., Samb.* in spasmodic coughs, often relives the constant, distressing night-cough in tuberculosis.

ANTIDOTES, *Camph.*

Dulcamara

Bitter-Sweet—Anti-Psoric.

The leading indication for this remedy is the modality—*All complaints worse from, or caused by, a change from warm to cold, wet weather, or especially aggravated by cold, wet weather*, on this it can be prescribed with considerable assurance of good results, thus making it cover quite a large number of diseases, such as colds, aching limbs, rheumatism, coughs, catarrh, diarrhea, back-ache, stiff neck, urticaria etc. It is to the *wet, cold*, what *Aconitum Nap.* is to *dry, cold*. It has a specific relation also to the skin, glands and digestive organs, *mucous membranes*, secreting more profusely while the skin is inactive. The *rheumatic troubles* induced by *damp cold* are aggravated by every cold change, and somewhat relieved by moving about. Results from sitting on cold, damp ground. Icy coldness. One-sided spasms with speechlessness. Paralysis of single parts. Congestive headache, with neuralgia and dry nose. Patients living or working in damp, cold basements (*Natrium Sulph.*). Eruptions on hands arms or face around the *menstrual period*.

WORSE, at night, from *cold* in general, *damp, rainy weather*, suppressed menstruation, eruptions, sweat.

BETTER, from moving about (*Fer Met., Rhus Tox.*), external warmth.

RELATIONS—COMPLIMENTARY TO, *Baryta Carb., Kalium Sulph.*

INCOMPATIBLE WITH (should not be used before or after) *Belladonna, Lachesus.*

FOLLOWS WELL, after *Calcarea Carb., Lycopodium Clav., Rhus Tox, Sep.*

SIMILAR TO, *Mercurius Sol.*, in ptyalism, glandular swellings, bronchitis, diarrhea, susceptibility to weather changes, night pains, *Kalium Sulp.*, the chemical analogue.

USEFUL for the bad effects or abuse of *Mercurius Sol.*

ANTIDOTES, *Camph., Cupr Met.*

Eupatorium Perfoliatum

Boneset (Plant).

Known as 'Bone-set' from the prompt manner in which it relieves pains in limbs and muscles that accompany some forms of febrile disease, like malaria and influenza. *Breakbone fever, Grippe. Chills and fever, chill from 7 to 9 a.m.,thirst before and during chill and during fever* when the *characteristic bone symptoms* are present. *Eupatorium Perf.* acts principally on the gastro-hepatic organs and bronchial mucous embrane. Cachexia from old chronic, bilious intermittents. Worn-out constitutions. Sluggishness of all organs and functions. *Bone pains,* affecting back, head, chest, limbs, especially the wrists, as if dislocated. *Bruised feeling, as if broken, all over the body (Arnica Mont., Bellis Per., Pyr.).*

Painful soreness of eye-balls, coryza, aching in every bone, great prostration in epidemic influenza (*Lac. Can.*).

WORSE, Periodically.

BETTER, by conversation, by getting on hands and knees.

RELATIONS, is followed well, *by Natrium M.* and *Sepia.*

COMPARE, *Chel., Pod., Lycopodium Clav.,* in jaundiced conditions. *Bryonia Alba.* is the nearest analogue, having free sweat, but pains keep the patient quiet, while *Eup Perf* has scanty sweat and pains make patient restless.

Euphrasia

Eyebright (Plant).

Manifests itself in inflaming the conjunctival membrane especially, producing profuse lachrymation. Patient is better especially, producing profuse lachrymation. Patient is better in open air. Catarrhal affections of mucous membranes, especially of eyes and nose, profuse *acrid lachrymation,* with profuse *bland coryza* (reverse of *All.C.*). Worse, evening, hawking up of offensive mucus. *Menses,* painful, regular, *flow lasting only one hour,* or late, scanty, short, lasting only one day (*Bar. C.*).

Amenorrhea, with catarrhal symptoms of eyes and nose, profuse acrid lachrymation.

WORSE, in evening, indoors, warmth, from light.

BETTER, in dark.

RELATIONS, similar to, *Puls.* in affections of the eyes, reverse of *All C,* in lachrymation and coryza.

ANTIDOTE, *Puls.*

Ferrum Metallicim

Iron—Metal—(Constitutional).

Best adapted to young, weakly persons, anemic and chlorotic, when the face is habitually, or greenish pale, yet who flush easily to a fiery red from emotions or exertion, cold extremities, *oversensitiveness,* worse after any active effort, weakness from mere speaking or walking, though *looking* strong. *Pallor* of skin, mucous membranes, face, alternating with flushes. The *rushes of blood to the head in these weak ones is its key note.* There may also be hemorrhages of blood from various parts of the body. Blood watery. Chill, with red face and cold feet. Diarrhea, undigested stools, painless and sometimes involuntary, and sometimes while urinating. Cough only in daytime, (*Euphr Off.*), relieved by lying down, better by eating. Menses pale and watery. Oppression in the chest.

WORSE, at night, rest, especially while sitting still, after cold washing and over-heating.

BETTER, *walking slowly about, in summer.*

RELATIONS—ANTIDOTES, *Arsenicum Alb., Hep Sulp.*

MATERIA MEDICA

Complimentary, to *Alum., China off.*

China, the vegetable analogue, follows well in nearly all cases, acute or chronic. Should never be given in syphilis, always aggravates the condition.

Ferrum Phosphoricum

Phosphate of Iron (*Metal*)

In the early stages of febrile conditions, it stands midway between sthenic activity of *Aconitum Nap. and Bell.*, and the asthenic sluggishness and torpidity of *Gels.* The typical *Ferrum Phos.* subject is not full blooded and robust, but nervous, sensitive, anemic, with the false plethora and easy flushing of *Ferrum Met.* Prostration marked. and face more active than *Gels.* Pulse soft and flowing, no anxious restlessness of *Acononitum Nap.* Susceptible to chest troubles. Bronchitis of young children. In acute exacerbation of tuberculosis a fine paliative of wonderful power.

The remedy for first stage of all febrile disturbances and inflammations before exudation sets in, especially for catarrhal affections of the respiratory tract.

Ferrum Phos. 3, increases hemoglobin. In pale, anemic subjects, with violent local congestions, hemorrhages, bright from any orifice.

Worse, at night and 4 to 6 a.m., touch, jar, motion, right side.

Better, cold applications.

Relations, *Aconitum Nap., Gels., China off.*

Gelsemium

Yellow jasmine (Plant).

The guides to this valuable remedy are, *low forms of prostration, weakness, torpor, drowsiness, with trembling of* hands and body, muscles almost refuse to do their duty, so weak and stupid is the patient. The trembling is not that of a chill, but of *weak muscular power.* Headache, dull and tired heavy eyelids. Fever, but never pronounced, little thirst, where there is a *chill,* there is shaking but little coldness. Slow pulse, tired feeling, mental apathy. Paralysis of various groups of muscles about the eyes. Throat, chest, larynx, sphincter, extremities, etc. Post diphtheritic paralysis. *Muscular weakness.* Complete relaxation and prostration. Lack of muscular co-ordination. General depression from heat of sun. Sensitive to a falling barometer, cold and dampness bring on many complaints. Clinically useful in grippe, where chills run up the back, aching all over, desire to hug the fire, sneezing, etc. Useful in colds contracted in hot weather. Writer's or piano player's cramp. Paralysis of single parts. Nervous affections of cigar makers. Intermittents, and states of low vitality. Cerebro spinal meningitis. slow pulse of old age.

WORSE, damp weather, fog before a thunderstorm, emotion or excitement, *bad news, tobacco smoking, when thinking of his ailments,* at 10 a.m.

BETTER, bending forward, by profuse urination, open air, continued motion, stimulants.

RELATIONS—compare, *Baptisia Tinct* in threatening typhoid fever, *Ipecac.* in dumb ague, after suppression of quinine.

ANTIDOTES, *China off., Coffea.*

Glonoine

Nitro-Glycerine (Chemical).

Great remedy for sunstroke and its after effects, congestive headaches, hyperemia of the brain from excess of heat or cold, inter-cranial, climacteric disturbances, or due to menstrual suppression. *Surging of blood to head and heart.* In menstrual suppression. In headache characterised by a furious throbbing. The throbbing seems to involve the neck and body. *Sensation of pulsation throughout the body. Pulsating pains.* Epilepsy, rush of blood to head. Threatened apoplexy. *Pulsating neuralgia. A peculiar mental symptom* is that well-known places seem strange, or patient forgets where he lives.

WORSE, *in sun,* exposure to sun's rays, gas, open fire, jar, stooping, having hair cut, stimulants, lying down, from 6 a.m. to noon, left side.

RELATIONS—ANTIDOTES, *Aconitum Nap.*

COMPARE, *Amyl Nit., Bell., Opium, Stram.*

Black Lead—Powerful Anti-Psoric.

The guides to this remedy are chiefly oozing, moist, *sticky* and scabby eruptions, ugly inflamed scars, that will not heal, old oozing sores and thick ugly or brittle nails. Moist eruptions on eyelids. Cracks and fissures on hands. Constipation with large stools, or brown foul diarrhea. Sticky eruption around anus. This is *especially useful in patients who are rather stout, of fair complexion with tendency to skin affections and constipation, fat, chilly and costive, with delayed menstrual history, take cold easily.* It will clear up many ills when the above conditions are more or less present, such as eczema, nasal catarrh, erysipelas, chronic sore throat, gastralgia, seminal weakness etc.

WORSE, warmth, at night, during and after menstruation.

BETTER, in the dark, from wrapping up.

RELATIONS—ANTIDOTES, *Nux Vom., Aconitum Nap., Arsenicum Alb.*

COMPLEMENTARY, *Caust., Hep Sulp., Lycopodium Clav.*

Grahpites follows well, after *Lycopodium Clav., Puls.,* after *Calc.,* in obesity of young women with large amount of unhealthy adipose tissue, follows *Sulph.* well in skin affections, after *Sepia* in *gushing* leucorrhea.

SIMILAR TO, *Lycopodium Clav., Puls. in menstrual troubles.*

Hamamelis Virginica

Witch Hazel (Plant).

It is adapted to venous hemorrhage from every orifice of the body—nose, lungs, bowels, uterus, bladder. Venous congestion, passive, of skin and mucous membranes, phlebitis, varicose veins, ulcers, varicose with stinging pricking pain, hemorrhoids. "Its the *Aconite* of the venous capillary system". Great value in open painful wounds, with weakness from loss of blood. *After operations, supersedes the use of morphine.* Chronic effects of mechanical injuries.

WORSE, warm, moist air.

RELATIONS—COMPLEMENTARY, *Ferrum Met.* in hemorrhage and the hemorrhagic diathesis.

ANTIDOTES, *Arnica Mont.*

COMPARE, *Arnica Mont., Calen.,* for traumatic, and to hasten absorption of intraocular hemorrhage.

Hepar Sulphuris Calcarea

Hahnemann's Cacium Sulphide—Constitutional.

Especially suitable for scrofulous and lymphatic constitutions, who are inclined to have eruptions and glandular swellings. The *Hepar Sulp.* patient is extremely sensitive to cold air, must be wrapped up, takes cold easily, very sensitive to touch and to all impressions, and has an unhealthy skin, *very prone to suppuration from the slightest scratch.* Useful in chronic catarrh when nose stops up every time patient goes out. In coughs, loose and rattling, though little mucus comes up, croupy, difficult breathing. Asthma that is better in damp weather. Sensation of splinter in throat.

Dyspepsia with craving for sour things. Inability to entirely empty bladder, urine difficult of expulsion. In quinsy, when suppuration is threatening. Boils, abscesses, run-rounds, felons. *Chilliness, hypersensitiveness, splinter-like pains, craving for sour and strong things are very characteristic. Feeling as if wind were blowing on some part.* After abuse of mercury.

WORSE, from cold air, uncovering, eating or drinking cold things, lying on painful side (*Kalium Carb., Iod.*), touching affected parts, abuse of mercury.

BETTER, warmth in general (*Arsenicum Alb.*), wrapping up warmly, especially the head (*Psor., Sil.*), *in damp wet weather (Caust., Nux Vom.—reverse of Natrium Sulph.).*

RELATIONS—COMPLEMENTARY, to *Calendula* in injuries of soft parts. *Hepar Sulp.* antidotes, bad effects of *Mercury* and other metals, Iodine, Iodide of potash, cod-liver oil, renders patient less susceptible to atmospheric changes and cold air.

COMPARE, the psoric skin affections of *Sulphur* are dry, itching, better by scratching, and not sensitive to touch, while in *Hepar Sulp.* the skin is unhealthy, suppurating, moist, and extremely sensitive to touch.

ANTIDOTES, *Bell., Cham., Sil.*

Hyoscyamus Niger

Henbane (Plant).

It causes a perfect picture of *mania of a quarrelsome and obscure character.* Convulsions, spasms, all the muscles twich or jerk. *Suspicion is a marked mental symptom.* Sleep unrefreshing from crowded dreams, things running through the mind. Its symptoms also point to weakness and *nervous agitation,* as in typhoid and other infections, with *coma vigil. Tremulous weakness and twitching of tendons.* Diseases with increased cerebral activity but *non-inflammatory in type*—hysteria or delirium tremens, in delirium. *Hyoscyamus Nig.* occupies a place midway between *Belladonna* and *Stramonium,* lacking the constant cerebral congestion of the former and the fierce rage and maniacal delirium of the latter. Spasms, without consciousness, very restless, *every muscle in the body twitches, from the eyes to the toes* (with consciousness, *Nux Vom.*), dry *spasmodic* night coughs, *worse when lying down, relieved by sitting up* (*Drosera*).

WORSE, at night, during menses, mental affections, after eating, when lying down.

BETTER, stooping.

RELATIONS—COMPARE, *Bell., Stram.* and *Verat Alb., Phos.,* often cures lasciviousness, when *Hyos Nig.* fails.

Follows, *Bell.,* in deafness after apoplexy.

Antidotes, *Bell., Camph., China off.*

Ignatia Amara

St. Ignatius Bean (Plant).

Produces a marked hyperesthesia of all the senses, and a tendency to clonic spasms. Mentally, the *emotional element is uppermost, and co-ordination of function is interfered with.* Hence, one of the chief remedies for hysteria. It is especially adapted to the nervous temperament—women of sensitive, easily excited nature, dark, mild disposition, quick to perceive, rapid in execution. Rapid change of mental and physical condition, opposite to each other. Great contradistinctions. *The superficial and erratic character of the symptoms is most characteristic. Effects of grief and worry. Cannot bear tobacco.* Pain in small, circumscribed spots. *The Plague.*

Fever, with no thirst, intermittent chill, relieved by external heat. During fever, patient wants to be covered.

Sore throat, relieved by swallowing. Feeling as of a lump in throat, abnormal brooding sorrow, and grief, weak feeling at pit of stomach, melancholia, hysteria, merriment followed by tears. twitching. Headache as of a nail driven in through the side. Prolapsus of the rectum, afraid to strain at stool. Sciatica recurring in cold weather. *Ignatia* bears the same relation to the diseases of women, that *Nux Vom.* does to sanguine bilious men.

WORSE, from *tobacco, coffee,* brandy, contact, motion, strong odours, mental emotions, grief, in the morning, open air, after meals.

BETTER, warmth, hard pressure (*China off.*), change of position or walking, when eating.

RELATIONS— INCOMPATIBLE, *Coff., Nux Vom., Tab.* The bad effects of *Ignatia* are antidoted by *Puls., Cham., Cocc Ind.*

COMPLEMENTARY, *Natrium Mur.*

ANTIDOTES, *Puls., Cham., Cocc Ind.*

Ipecacuanha

Ipecac.-root (Vegetable).

The principal feature of this remedy is its *persistent nausea and vomiting,* which form the chief guiding symptoms, tongue apt to be clean, *stomach seems to be relaxed and hangs down,* sick headache, pain over one eye, dry spasmodic cough and wheezing breath. Clinically useful in vomiting, sick stomach, diarrhea, cough with gagging and retching, spasmodic asthma, whooping cough, hemorrhages of bright red blood, and intermittent fever. Especially indicated in fat children and adults, who are feeble and catch cold in relaxing atmosphere, warm, moist weather. Spasmodic affections.

WORSE, winter and dry weather, warm, moist, south winds, (*Euph.*), slightest motion.

RELATIONS—COMPLEMENTARY, *Cuprum Met., Arnica Mont.* Is followed well—by *Arsenicum Alb.,* in influenza, chills croup, debility, cholera infantum, by *Antimonium Tart.*, in foreign bodies in larynx.

SIMILAR TO, *Puls., Antomonium Carb.* in gastric troubles.

ANTIDOTES, *Arsenic Alb., China off., Arnica Mont.*

Kali Bichromicum

Potassium Bichromate—Mineral—*Anti-Syphilitic.*

The special affinities of this drug are the mucous membrane of stomach, bowels and air passages, bones and fibrous tissues, characterized by *tough, stringy or ropy,* mucus, or discharge from any part, ulceration in nose with plugs of mucus that form as fast as removed, ulceration in mouth, skin and eyes yellow, tongue yellow, kidneys, heart and liver are also affected. Useful in chronic rheumatism of the cold variety, or in fat persons, dyspepsia of beer drinkers, the ills of excessive fat, bronchitis, asthma, yellow mucus in eyes, catarrh, croup, etc, *for pain in small spots in various parts of the body.* Blotched face, diphtheria, ulcerated sore throat. Symptoms are worse in the morning, *pains migrate quickly,* rheumatic and gastric symptoms alternate. *Perforation of the septum.* Chronic atonic catarrh. Polypus. Dilatation of stomach and heart.

WORSE, heat of summer, hot weather.

BETTER, from heat, skin symptoms are better in cold weather (reverse of, *Alum.,* and *Pet.*).

RELATIONS, COMPARE, *Brom., Iod., in croupy* affections.

AFTER, *Canth.,* or *Carb. Ac., has* removed the scrapings in dysentery, *Iod.,* in croup, when hoarse cough, with tough membrane, general weakness and coldness are present, *Calarea Carb.,* in acute or chronic nasal Catarrh.

Antimonium Tart. follows well in catarrhal affections and skin diseases.

ANTIDOTES, *Arsenicum Alb., Lach.*

Kalium Carbonicum

Potassium Carbonate—Mineral—*Anti-Psoric and Antisyscotic.*

The weakness characteristic of all potassium salts is seen specially in this, with soft pulse, coldness, general depression and *very characteristic stitches,* which may be felt in any part of the body, or in connection with any affection.

All Kali pains are sharp and *cutting,* nearly all are better by motion. *Never use any salts of Potash where there is fever.* Sensitive to every atmospheric change, and *intolerance of cold weather.* One of the best remedies following labour, for consequent debilitated states. *Early morning aggravation is very characteristic.* Fleshy, aged people with dropsical and paretic tendencies. *Sweat, back-ache and weakness.* Throbbing pains. Tendency to dropsy. Tubercular diathesis. Pains from within out, and of stinging character. "Giving out" sensation. Fatty degeneration. Stinging pains in muscles and internal parts. Pain in small spots on left side. *Cannot bear to be touched.* Starts when touched ever so lightly, especially on the feet. Great aversion to being aone (*Arsenicum Alb., Lycopodium Clav., desire to be alone—Ign., Nux Vom.).* Bag-like swellings between the upper eyelids and eyebrows. *Feels badly, a week before incnstruation, back-ache, before and during menses.*

WORSE, in cold weather, in morning about three o'clock, lying on left and painful side.

BETTER, in warm weather, though moist, during day, while moving about.

RELATIONS—COMPLEMENTARY, *Carbo Veg.* (lowness of vitality may suggest a preliminary course of *Carbo Veg.* to nurse up recuperation to the point that *Kalium Carb.* Would come in helpfully). Follows *Nux Vom.* often in stomach and bladder troubles.

COMPARE, *Bryonia Alba.*, *Lycopodium Clav.*, *Natrium M.*, *Nitricum Ac.*, *Stan.*

FOLLOWS WELL, after, *Kalium Sulp.*, *Phos.*, *Stan Met.* (in loose rattling cough). Will bring on the menses, when *Natrium Mur.*, though apparently indicated, fails—Hahnemann.

ANTIDOTES, *Camph.*, *C off,*.

Lachesis

Surukuku Snake Poison* (Animal)—*Constitutional.

Like all snake poisons, *Lachesis* decomposes the blood, rendering it more fluid, hence a hemorrhagic tendency is marked. Purpura, septic states, diphtheria and other low forms of disease, when the system is thoroughly poisoned and the prostration is profound. *The modalities are most important in guiding to the remedy.* Ills beginning on left side, as of throat, patient cannot bear anything close around the throat or waist, always awakens from sleep worse. Clinically useful, in diphtheria, headaches' that always come on from exposure to the sun, ears full of pasty wax, horribly offensive diarrhea, hemorrhages of dark blood, blood poisoning, gangrene, depraved boils, and ulcers, bad blood. Also useful in suffering at climacteric (change of life). Trembling of drunkards. Fistula of anus. All symptoms, especially the mental, *worse after sleep, or the aggravation wakes him from sleep,* sleeps into the aggravation, unhappy, distressed, anxious, sad, worse in morning on awaking. Epilepsy, comes on during sleep (*Bufo.*), from loss of vital fluids, onanism, jealousy.

WORSE, *after sleep,* (*Kalium Bich.*). *Lachesis* sleeps *into* aggravation, ailments that come on during sleep (*Calcarea Carb.*), left side, in the spring, warm bath, pressure or constriction, hot drinks, closing eyes.

BETTER, appearance of discharges, warm applications.

MATERIA MEDICA 579

RELATIONS—COMPLEMENTARY, *Hep Sulp., Lycopodium Clav., Nitricum Ac.*

INCOMPATIBLE, *Acet Ac., Carb. Ac.*

Antidotes, *Arsenicum Alb., Mercurius Sol.*, heat, alcohol, salt.

In intermittent fever, *Natrium Mur.*. follows *Lach.* well when type changes.

Lycopodium Clavatum

Club Moss (Vegetable)—*Anti-Psoric, Anti-Syphilitic and Anti-Sycotic.*

In nearly all cases where *Lycopodium Clav.* is the remedy, some evidence of urinary or digestive disturbance will be found. *Lycopodium Clav.* is adapted more especially to ailments gradually developing, functional power weakening, with failures of the digestive powers, where the function of the liver is seriously disturbed. *Atony, malnutrition, deep-seated, progressive, chronic, diseases. Emaciation, presenility.* Ascites, in liver disease.

The general characteristics of this remedy are as follows:—

Grumbling fermentation in abdomen with much flatulence, though very hungry, a few mouthfuls of food produce a feeling of satiety, bloated, constipation with painful urging, *complaints go from right to left, worse from 4 to 8 p.m.*, red-sediment in urine, sleeps after eating and awakes worse, *mental torpor.* It is one of the deep acting chronic disease remedies and, if the above generals correspond, may be useful in dyspepsia, water brash, constipation, liver and urinary troubles, stomach diseases, heart-burn, eczema, chronic lung troubles, diphtheria, bone-pains, piles, puny children, old men's troubles, diphtheria, bone-pains, piles, puny children, old men's troubles, impotence, etc.

WORSE, right side, from right to left, from above downward, 4 to 8 p.m. (*Hell Nig.* from 4 to 9 p.m., *Col., Magnesium Phos.*), from heat or warm room, hot air, bed.

Warm applications, except throat and stomach which are better from warm drinks.

BETTER, by *motion* after midnight, from warm food and drink, on getting cold, from being uncovered.

RELATIONS—COMPLEMENTARY, *Lycop.* acts with special benefit after *Calcarea Carb. and Sulph. Iod., Graphites, Lach., Chelid.*

BAD EFFECTS, of onions, bread, wine, spirituous liquors, tobacco smoking and chewing (*Arsenicum Alb.*).

It is rarely advisable to begin the treatment of a chronic disease with *Lycopodium Clav.* unless clearly indicated, it is better to give first another antipsoric.

Lycopodium Clav., is a deep-seated and long acting remedy and should rarely be repeated after improvement begins.

ANTIDOTES, *Camph., Puls., Caust.*

Mercurius Solublis

Hahnemann's Soluble Mercury (Mineral)—Anti-syphilitic and Anti-Sycotic.

Every organ and tissue of the body is more or less affected by this powerful drug, it transform healthy cells into decrepid, inflamed and necrotic wrecks, decomposes the blood, producing a profound anemia. This malignant medical force is converted into useful life-saving and life-preserving service, if employed Homeopathically, guided by its clear cut symptoms. The lymphatic system is especially affected with all the membranes and *glands,* and internal organs, bones. etc. When you find spongy, bleeding gums, flabby, moist unhealthy mouth and tongue, offensive breath, tonsils more or less swollen, chilliness towards evening, much oily sweat. Which does not relieve, slimy cough, unhealthy moist skin, nose red, swollen and sore, hoarseness, *Mercurius Sol.* is the remedy. Clinically useful in jaundice, torpid liver, rheumatism, mumps, quinsy, sore throat, diarrhea, dysentery (stool, slimy, bloody, with colic and fainting) colds, coughs, night sweats, diseased eyelids, leucorrhea, stiff neck, raw throat, when generals as above, are more or less in evidence. The chief remedy for *toothache from decayed teeth, and for loose teeth from diseased gums.* Also the chief remedy for syphilis, if recent.

WORSE, at night, wet, damp weather (*Rhus Tox.*), lying on right side, perspiring, warm room and warm bed. *Mercurius Sol.* is *worse* by heat of, but *better* by rest in bed.

RELATIONS, follows well, after *Bell., Hep Sulp., Lach., Sulph.,* but should not be given after *Silicea.*

If given in low potencies hastens. rather than aborts suppuration.

The bad effects of *Mercurius Sol.* are antidoted by *Aurum Met., Hep Sulp., Lach., Mezer, Nit Ac., Sulph.,* and by a high potency of *Mercurius Sol.,* when the symptoms correspond.

COMPARE, *Mezereum,* its vegetable analogue, for bad effects of large doses, or of too frequent repetition. Ailments from sugar, insect stings, vapours of arsenic or copper. Diseases occurring in winter.

Mercurius Corrosivus

Corrosive Sublimate—Mineral—*Anti-syphilitic and Anti Sycotic.*

This salt leads all other remedies in tenesmus of the recessant, and is not relieved by the stool. The tenesmus often involves the bladder as well. The keynote to the remedy in bowels and bladder is, *Tenesmus, i.e., a painful straining in the effort to evacuate them.* The stools are scanty, bloody and painful, with burning in anus and bladder, dysentery, bloody flux. A remedy also for syphilitic affections of skin and bones. Dyspepsia, with aversion to warm food. Nightly bone-pains. Albuminuria in early pregnancy (*Phos.,* later and at full term).

WORSE, evening, night, acids.

BETTER, while at rest.

Natrium Muriaticum

Common salt—Mineral—*Anti-Psoric.*

A great remedy for certain forms of intermittent fever, anemia, chlorosis, many disturbances of the alimentary tract and skin, paleness and emaciation. Heart fluttering. Headache, throbbing, of a chronic nature, especially associated with constipation. Headache of school girls from sunrise to sunset. *Colds with much sneezing,* and clear, watery secretions. Cold sores or fever blisters. Tongue *mapped, with red insular patches, chills* and fever, followed by intense headache. Skin dry and harsh, or else greasy. Morbid coldness. Backache. Chronic cracking sounds in the ears when moving jaws. Hang nails. Ophthalmia, with profuse discharge. Nightly bone pains. excessively sore, red eyelids. Heart-burn always after eating. *Great emaciation, losing flesh, while living well,* emaciation, most notable in neck. Great liability to take cold. *Dry mucous membranes.* Constrictive sensation throughout the body. *Great weakness and weariness.* Oversensitive to all sorts of influences. Abnormal craving for salt. Urticaria, acute or chronic, over whole body, especially after violent exercise (*Apis Mell., Calcarea Carb., Hep Sulp.*), heavy, difficult speech, *children slow in learning to talk and walk.* Intermittents, *Paroxysms at* 10 *or* 11 *a.m., old chronic, badly treated cases especially after suppression by quinine,* headache, with unconsciousness during chill and heat, sweat relieves pains.

WORSE, at 10 or 11 a.m., at the seashore, or from sea air, heat of sun or stove, mental exertion, talking, writing, reading, lying down.

BETTER, in the open air (*Apis Mell., Puls.*), cold bathing, *going without regular meals,* lying on right side (on painful side, *Bryonia Alba., Ign., Puls.*).

RELATIONS—COMPLEMENTARY, to *Apis Mell.*, acts well before and after it. *Natrium Mur* is followed by *Sepia* and *Thuja.* Cannot often be repeated in chronic cases without an intercurrent, called for by symptoms. *Should never be given during fever paroxysms, but only when they begin to subside.* If vertigo and headache be very persistent, or prostration be prolonged after *Natrium Mur., Nux Vom.* will relieve.

ANTIDOTES, *Arsenicum Alb., Phos.*

Natrium Sulphuricum

SODIUM SULPHATE—MINERAL—*ANTI-SYCOTIC* (*CONSTITUTIONAL*).

A liver remedy, especially indicated for the so-called hydrogenoid constitution, where the complaints are such as are due to living in damp houses, basement, cellars, *are worse, in rainy weather,* water in any form, *feels every change from dry to wet,* cannot even eat vegetables or fruits growing near water, nor fish. Always feels *better in warm, dry air.* Clinically, it has been found a valuable remedy for *spinal meningitis,* head symptoms *from injuries to head,* and mental troubles there from. Every spring, return of skin affections. Tendency to warts. Fingers and toes affected. Chronic gout (*Lycopodium Clav.*). Liver sore. Expectoration and exudation yellowish or greenish-yellow. Bilious. Stomach sore. *Chronic asthma, worse in wet weather, or hereditary asthma in children* (constitutional remedy).

WORSE, damp basement or dwellings, damp weather (*Dul.*), rest, lying down.

BETTER, dry weather, pressure, sitting up (cough), changing position (but better in wet weather, *Caust.*), open air. Must change position frequently but it is painful, and given no relief (*Caust.*).

RELATIONS, *Natrium Mur.* and *Sulphur* which are very similar, *Thuja* and *Mercurius Sol.* in syphilis and sycosis occurring in hydrogenoid constitutions.

COMPLEMENTARY, *Arsenicum Alb., Thuja.*

Nux Vomica
Poison-nut (Vegetable).

It is the *greatest of polychrests,* because the bulk of its symptoms correspond, in similarity, with those of the commonest and most frequent of diseases. It is frequently the first remedy, indicated after much dosing, establishing a sort of equilibrium of forces and counteracting chronic effects.

Nux Vom. is pre-eminently the remedy for many of the conditions incident to modern life. The typical *Nux Vom.* patient is rather thin, spare, quick, active, nervous and irritable. He does a good deal of mental work, has mental strains and leads a sedentary life, found in prolonged office-work, overstudy, and close application to business with its cares and anxieties. All these things involve the use of a great deal of allopathic or proprietary medicines, abuse of tea or coffee, or alcoholic liquors, indulgence in rich and stimulating fods, and *Nux Vom.* is their remedy to start with in every case. Headache of high livers, and from alcoholic drinks, from sprees. Impaired appetite, dyspepsia, bilious, liver out of order, in constipation, frequent but ineffiectual desire to pass stool, *"never-get done"* feeling. Cold in the head, stopped up in warm room, better out of doors. Piles. Back-ache. Wakes up with headache. Neuralgia recurring in the morning. OVERSENSITIVE *to external impressions, to noise, odours, light or music, trifling ailments are unbearable* (*Cham.*), every harmless word offends (*Ign.*). Alternate constipation and diarrhea (*Sulph.*), (*Ver Alb.*), in persons who have taken purgatives all their lives. Repugnance to cod or to cold air, chilly, on least movement, from being uncovered, *must be covered in every stage* of fever—chill, heat or sweat. Menses, too early, profuse, lasts too long, or keeping on several days longer, with complaints at onset and remaining after, every two weeks, irregular, never at right time, stopping and starting again (*Sulph.*), during and after, *worse* of old symptoms.

WORSE, *morning, waking at 4 a.m., mental exertion,* after eating or over-eating, touch, noise, anger, spices, narcotics, dry weather, in cold air.

BETTER, in evening, while at rest, lying down and in damp wet weather (*Caust.*).

RELATIONS—COMPLEMENTARY, *Sulphur* in nearly all diseases, *Sepia.*

INIMICAL, *Zinc Met.,* must not be used before or after.

FOLLOWS WELL, after *Arsenicum Alb., Ipec., Phos., Sep., Sulph.*

IS FOLLOWED WELL, by *Bryonia Alba., Puls., Sulph., Nux Vom.* should be given on retiring, or better, several hours before going to bed, it acts best during repose of mind and body.

ANTIDOTES, *Coff. Ign., Cocc Ind., Puls.*

POPPY (Vegetable).

Especially adapted to children and old people, diseases of first and second childhood (*Baryta Carb.*), person with light hair *lax* muscles, and *want of bodily irritability, Want of susceptibility to remedies, lack of vital reaction, the well chosen remedy makes no impression* (*Carbo Veg, Laur, Val.*). *All complaints, with great sopor, painless, complains of nothing, wants nothing, and are accompanied by heavy, stupid sleep, stertorous breathing. Sweaty skin.* Opium lessens voluntary movements, contracts pupils, depresses higher intellectual powers, lessens self-control and power of concentration, judgment, stimulates the imagination, checks all secretions, except that of the skin. Diseases that originate from fright. Constipation, of chidren, of corpulent, goodnatured women (*Graph.*) from inaction or paresis, no desire, from lead-poisoning, stools hard, round black balls (*Chel., Plumb., Thuja*), faeces protrude and recede (*Sil., Thuja*). *Opium* renders the intestines so sluggish that the most active purgatives lose their power (Hering). Persistent diarrhea in those treated with large doses of the drug. (Lippe.)

WORSE, during and after sleep (*Apis Mell., Lach.*), while perspiring, from warmth, stimulants.

BETTER, from cold, constant walking.

RELATIONS—ANTIDOTES, for *poisonous doses, strong black coffee, Nux Vom., Kalium permangenicum 2x dilution,* for potencies, *Camphor, Coffee, Calcarea Carb., Hepar Sulp, Sulph.*

When symptoms correspond, the potencies may antidote bad effects of opium drugging.

Chronic opium poisoning, *Ipec., Nux Vom.*

Berberis is useful to counteract opium habit.

Petroleum

Crude Rock-oil—Mineral oil—*Anti-Psoric.*

Adapted to scrofulous diathesis, irritable, quarrelsome persons (*Nux Vom.*), who suffer from catarrhal conditions of the mucous membranes, gastric acidity and skin eruptions. Very marked skin symptoms, acting on sweat and oil glands. Ailments are worse during the winter season. Ailments from riding in cars, carriages or ships. Lingering gastric and lung troubles. Chronic diarrhea. *Long-lasting complaints* follow mental states—fright, vexation, etc. Cracked hands and fingers, full of bloody chaps, finger-tips fissured, gouty, stiff finger joints, herpes in knees, cold feet tender, cracking joints. *Winter eczema,* i.e., always worse then. Headache every morning. Seeming gauze before eyes. Raw and red behind ears. Itching, moist scrotum. *Burning corns, bunions and chilblains.*

WORSE, carriage riding (*Cocc Ind.*), during a thunderstorm, in winter (*Alum.*).

BETTER, warm air, dry weather, lying with head high.

RELATION, one of our best antidotes for lead poisoning. The skin symptoms are worse in winter, better in summer (*Alum.*), if suppressed, causes diarrhea.

ANTIDOTES, *Nux Vom., Coccul Ind., Aconitum Nap.*

COMPLEMENTARY, *Sepia.*

Phosphorus

Phosphorus—Mineral—*Anti-Psoric.*

Tall, slender persons, narrow chested, with thin, transparent skin, weakened by loos of animal fluids, with great nervous debility, emaciation, amative tendencies, seem to be under the special influence of *Phosphorus.* Great susceptibility to external impressions, to light, sound, odours, touch, electrical changes, thunder-storms. *Suddenness* of symptoms. sudden prostration, faints, sweats, shooting pains, etc. Blood broken down, watery—every small wound, or ulcer, bleeds freely, fatty degeneration with anemic condition, softening or atrophy of brain and spinal chord, burning heat. Restlessness, especially about twilight, does not want to be alone. Catarrh, in which mucus with blood is blown from nose. Face pale, bloated, waxy colour. *Must eat often—Wants cold things. Anus seems to be wide open and stools ooze forth.*

Oppression on chest, hoarseness, sputa yellow, blood streaked or rust coloured.

Clinically, useful where above generals are in evidence, in caries of bones, liver diseases, atrophy of nerves, ulcerations, catarrh, polypi, kidney diseases, chronic diarrhea, constipation, sexual organs, diseases of the chest, fevers and hemorrhages.

Worse, touch, physical or mental exertion, twilight, warm food or drink, change of weather, from getting wet in hot weather, evening, *lying on left or painful side, during a thunder-storm, ascending stairs.*

Better, in the dark, lying on right side, from being rubbed or mesmerized, from cold food, cold water, until it gets warm, cold, open air, washing with cold water, sleep.

Relationship— Complementary, *Arsenicum Alb., Lycopodium Clav., Silicea.*

Incompatible with *Caust.*, must not be used before or after.

Phos. removes the bad effects of Iodine and *excessive use of table salt,* antidotes the nausea and vomiting of chorform and ether.

Follows well, after *Calcarea Carb.* or *China off.*

Antidotes, *Nux Vom., Camph, Coffea.*

Hahnemann says, "Acts most beneficial when patient suffers from chronic loose stool or diarrhea.

Phosphoric Acid

Phosphoric Acid—Mineral—*Anti-Psoric.*

Best suited to persons of originally strong constitutions, who have become debilitated *by loos of vital fluids,* sexual excesses (*China off.*), violent acute diseases, chagrin or a long succession of moral emotions, as grief, care, disappointed affections. Ailments, from care, grief, sorrow, home-sickness (*Ign.*), sleeply, disposed to weep, night-sweat towards morning. Nervous debility, with mental depression, gloom and hopelessness, nervous debility, from excessive sexual indulgence, self-abuse or loss of vital fluids, cold, clammy skin, pimples on face, frequent desire to urinate. Watery painless diarrhea, diabetes, phosphates in urine, emaciation, weakness, pain in back, cough, weakness in chest, acid dyspepsia. Cerebral typhoid, *complete apathy and stupor,* intestinal hemorrhage, blood dark.

WORSE, exertion from being talked to (*Stann Met.*), loss of vital fluids, sexual excesses.

BETTER, from keeping warm.

RELATIONS, compare, *Phos., Puls., Sil., Mur. Ac.,* (in typhoid).

Phos. Ac. acts well before or after *China off.* in profuse sweats, diarrhea, debility, after *Nux Vom.* in fainting after a meal.

ANTIDOTE, *Coffea.*

Psorinum

A product of Psora—Nosode-Anti-Psoric.

Especially adapted to the psoric constitution. In chronic cases, when well selected remedies fail to relieve or permanently improve, (in acute diseases, *Sulphur*) when *Sulphur* seems indicated but fails to act. *Psorinum* is a cold medicine, wants the head kept warm, *wants warm clothing,* even in summer *extreme sensitiveness to cold.* Debility, independent of any organic disease, especially the weakness remaining after acute disease. *Lack of reaction,* when well chosen remedies fail to act. Scrofulous patients. *Secretions have a filthy smell.* Profuse sweating. Cardiac weakness. Skin symptoms very prominent. Often gives immunity from cold-catching. Easy perspiration when walking. Syphilis, inherited and tertiary. Offensive discharges.

Hungry in the middle of the might, must have something to eat (*Cina., Sulph.*). Quinsy, tonsils greatly swollen, not only relieves acute attack, but *eradicates the tendency.*

Profuse perspiration after acute diseases, *with relief of all suffering* (*Natrium Mur.*). Asthma, dyspnea, *worse,* in open air, sitting up, better, *lying down and keeping arms stretched jar apart* (Rev. *of, Arsenicum Alb.*) despondent, thinks he will die. *Hay Fever,* appearing regularly every year the same day of the month, with an asthmatic, psoric or eczematous history. (Patient should be treated the previous winter to eradicate the diathesis and prevent summer attack). Skin, abnormal tendency to receive skin diseases (*Sulph.*). Eruptions *easily suppurate* (*Hep Sulp.*), *dry, inactive, rarely sweats, dirty look* as if never washed, coarse, greasy, as if bathed in oil, bad effects from suppression by sulphur and zinc ointments.

WORSE, coffee, *Psorinum* patient does not improve while taking coffee, changes of weather, in hot sunshine, from cold, *Dread of cold.*

BETTER, heat, warm clothing, even in summer.

RELATIONS—COMPLEMENTARY, *Sulphur* and *Tuberculinum.*

Is followed well by, *Alum., Hep Sulp., Sulph., Tuber.*

After—*Lactic Ac.,* in vomiting of pregnancy.

After, *Arnica Mont.* in traumatic affections of ovaries.

Sulphur follows *Psorinum* well, in mammary cancer.

Pulsatilla

Wind flower—Plant—(*Anti-sycotic*)—*Constitutional.*

The disposition and mental state are the chief guiding symptoms to the selection of *Pulsatilla.* It is pre-eminently a female remedy, especially for mild, gentle, yielding disposition, sad, crying readily, weeps when talking, *changeable,* contradictory. The patient seeks the open air, always feels better there, even though he is chilly. Mucous membranes are all affected. *Discharges thick,* bland, and *yellowish green.* Often indicated after abuse of Iron tonics, and after badly managed measles. Symptoms ever changing. Thirstless, peevish and chilly. When first serious impairment of health is referred to age of puberty. Great sensitiveness. Menstrual difficulties in women, irregular menses, uterine spasms, ills brought on by wet feet. Warm room, and bed clothes, oppress. Chronic affections following measles clinically useful in very many diseases, mostly adapted to lymphatic temperaments and light-haired persons, dyspepsia, water brash. Catarrh, loose coughs, passive diarrhea, gouty, shifting pains, rheumatism in joints, styes, gummed eyes, earache, catarrhal deafness, inflammation of testicles, hydrocele, varicose veins, irritation of prostate, chilblains, neuralgia, worse from warmth, dysmenorrhea. Ills of pregnancy generally. Antidote to too much iron and quinine. Lies with hands above head.

WORSE, *in a warm, close room, evening, at twilight,* on beginning to move, lying on the left, *or on the painless side,* very rich, fat, indigestible food, pressure on the well side, if it be made towards the diseased side, warm applications. *Heat (Kalium Sulp.).*

BETTER, *in the open air,* lying on painful side (*Bryonia Alba.*), cold air cool room, eating or drinking cold things, cold applications (*Kalium S*).

RELATIONS—COMPLEMENTARY, *Kalium Sulp.* (its chemical analogue), *Lycopodium Clav., Sil., Sul Ac.*

Silicea is the chronic of *Pulsatilla,* in nearly all complaints, follows, and is followed by *Kalium Sulp.*

One of the best remedies with which to begin the treatment of a chronic case (*Calcarea Sulph.*). Patients, anemic or chlorotic, who have taken much iron, quinine, tonics, even years before, ailments from abuse of chamomile, quinine, mercury, tea-drinking, sulphur.

FOLLOWS WELL, after *Kalium Bi., Lycopodium Clav., Sep, Sil., Sulph.*

ANTIDOTES, *cham., Coff., Ignatia, Nux Vom.*

Rhus Toxicodendron

Poison Oak—Vegetable—*Contitutional.*

Adapted to persons of a rheumatic diathesis, bad effects of getting wet, especially after being over-heated, ailments from spraining or straining a *single part,* muscle, or tendon *(Calcarea Carb., Nux Vom.),* over-lifting, particularly by stretching high up to reach things, lying on damp ground, too much summer bathing in river or tank, affects the fibrous tissue, especially *(Rhod.—Serous, Bryonia Alba.)* the right side more than the left. Cannot lie still, pain or uneasiness, makes patient move, turn or toss, pains worse from cold. Rheumatism, especially from getting wet. Lumbago, the chief remedy. Pains brought on by sprains. Muscles, sore and stiff. Rheumatic pains in back and shoulders. Vesicular eruptions, burning, itching, and tingling, erysipelas, eczema. Influenza, with aching bones and restlessness. Jaws painful, and crack when chewing. A remedy for ills following cold, wet weather. Heart troubles of athletes. Headache in wet weather. *Septicemia.* Tongue, *triangular red tip.* Diarrhea, *with beginning typhoid,* involuntary, with *great exhaustion,* tearing pain down the posterior part of limbs during stool.

WORSE, during sleep, cold wet rainy weather, at night, especially after midnight, from getting wet while perspiring, *during rest.*

BETTER, warm, dry weather, wrapping up, warm or hot things, *motion, change of position, moving affected parts.* The great characteristic of *Rhus Tox.* is that, with few exceptions, the pains occur and are *worse during repose and are better by motion. Sepia,* often quickly relieves itching and burning of *Rhus Tox.,* the vesicles up in a few days.

Rhus Tox., poisoning is antidoted by the *similimum,* the potentized remedy given internally, also *Bell., Bryonia Alba., Coffea, Sulphur.*

RELATIONS—COMPLEMENTARY, *Brynoia Alba., Calcarea Carb., Fluor Acid., Phytol.* (Rheumatism).

INIMICAL, *Apis Mell.*, must not be used before or after.

COMPARE, *Arnica Mont., Bryonia Alba., Rhod., Natrium Sulp., Sulph.*

Sabina

Savine (Plant).

Chronic ailments of women, arthritic pains, tendency to miscarriages, especially at third month. *Music is intolerable, produces nervousness, goes through bone and marrow (causes weeping—Thuja).*

Drawing pains in small of back—from sacrum to pubes, in nearly all diseases. Ailments, following abortion or premature labour, *hemorrhage from the uterus, flow partly pale red, partly clotted, worse from least motion (Sec Corn.),* often relieved by walking, *pain extending from sacrum to pubes.* For profuse flow from female genital organs, as in hemorrhage, after labour, etc. for threatened abortion. Swelling of wrist and toe joints. Gouty women. *Violent pulsations.* Wants windows open. Discharge of blood between periods, with sexual excitement. Retained placenta from atony of uterus, intense after-pains (*Caul., Sec Corn.*).

WORSE, from least motion, heat, warm air.

BETTER, in cool, fresh air.

RELATIONS—COMPLEMENTARY, to *Thuja.*

FOLLOWS, *Thuja* in condyloma and sycotic affections.

COMPARE, *Calcarea Carb., Croc Sat., Mill., Sec Corn., Trill.*

ANTIDOTES, *Puls., Camph.*

Sanguinaria

Bloodroot (Vegetable).

It is a right-sided remedy pre-eminently, and affects chiefly the mucous membranes, especially of the respiratory tract. Habitual sick headache, american sick headache, nausea and vomiting of bitter stuff, pains apt to rise with the sun and decline with it, and to begin in back of head and spread forward. Headaches *return at the climacteric,* every seventh day (*Sabad., Sil., Sulphur*). *Climacteric ailments,* flushes of heat, and leucorrhea, burning of palms and soles, compelled to throw off bed clothes, painful enlargement of breasts, *when Lachesis and Sulphur fail to relieve.* Also *loose cough with especially bad smelling sputa and breath, circumscribed red cheeks. Phthisis. Sudden stopping of catarrh of respiratory tract, followed by diarrhea. Rheumatic pain in the right arm and shoulder (left. Fer Met.),* cannot raise the arm, worse at night.

WORSE, sweets, right side, motion, touch.

BETTER, acids, sleep, darkness.

RELATIONS—Complementary, *Antimonium Tart.*

COMPARE, *Bell., Iris., Mell.,* in sick headache, *Lach., Sulph.,* in climacteric affections, *Chel., Phos., Sulph.,* in chronic bronchitis or latent pneumonia. As a dynamic remedy for the anaesthesia of opium.

Secale Cornutum

Ergot (Vegetable).

Adapted to women of thin, scrawny, feeble, cachectic appearance, irritable, nervous temperament, pale, sunken countenance. Very old, decrepit, feeble persons. Hemorrhage, continued oozing, thin fetid, watery black blood, the slightest wound causes bleeding for weeks (*Lach., Phos.*). *Debility, anxiety, emaciation, though appetite and thirst may be excessive. Cold surface of the body, yet patient does not want to be covered.* Cramps, numbness and crawling. Blue rings about the eyes. Cholera infantum, baby looks shrivelled as an old person. Dry and senile gangrene. Threatened abortion, especially at third month (*Sab.*), prolonged bearing down, forcing pains. *During labour, pains irregular, too weak, feeble or ceasing, everything seems loose and open but no expulsive action, fainting.*

After-pains, too long, too painful, hour-glass contraction.

Pulse-small, Rapid, contracted and often intermittent.

WORSE, heat, warm covering.

BETTER, cold, uncovering, rubbing, stretching out limbs.

RELATIONS—COMPARE, cinnamon in post-partum hemorrhage, it increases labour pains. controls profuse or dangerous flooding, always safe, while ergot is always dangerous.

SIMILAR, to *Arsenicum Alb.* but cold and heat are opposite.

RESEMBLES, *Colchicum* in cholera morbus.

ANTIDOTES, *Camph., Opium.*

Sepia

Cuttle-fish—Animal—*Anti-Psoric* (Constitutional).

Diseases of women, especially those occurring during pregnancy, child-bed and lactation, or diseases attended with sudden prostration and sinking faintness, yellow complexion, bearing down sensation, dragging pains, labour like pains, as though something would come out, prolapsus. "Ball" sensation in inner parts. Pains extend down to back, chills easily. Tendency to abortion. Hot flushes at menopause, with weakness and perspiration. Upward tendency of its symptoms—all pains are from below up. Acrid leucorrhea.

All pains better from warmth. Irregular menses. Child wets the bed in first sleep. Chronic gleet. Yellow bridge across the nose. Liver spots. Chronic nasal catarrh. Goneness and faintness in stomach. Sensation of weight to rectum, oozing moisture. Humid spots at bend of knees. Tettery eruptions. Ringworm. Scaly eruptions on legs. Skin itches in spots. Headaches, with perspiration of feet and at arm-pits.

Dyspepsia with craving for sour things. Yellow colour about the mouth. Toothache in pregnant women. Caries of the bones. Tubercular patients with chronic hepatic troubles and uterine reflexes.

WORSE, in afternoon or evening, washing, laundry work, dampness, left side, after sweat, cold air, before a thunder-storm, (*Psor.*).

BETTER, by *violent exercise,* pressure, warmth of bed, hot applications. Many symptoms, especially those of head, heart and pelvis, are both worse and better by rest and exercise. It antidotes mental effects of over-use of tobacco, in patients of sedentary habits who suffer from over-mental exertion.

RELATIONS—COMPLEMENTARY, *Natrium Mur.*

INIMICAL TO, *Lach.,* should not be used or after, to *Puls.,* with it should never be alternated.

SIMILAR TO, *Lach., Sang.,* in climacteric irregularities of the circulation.

FREQUENTLY indicated after, *Sil., Sulph.*

ANTIDOTES, *Aconitum Nap.,* vinegar.

A single dose often acts curatively for many weeks.

Silicea

Pure Silica—Mineral—*Anti-Psoric.* (*Constitutional*).

Adapted to the nervous, irritable, sanguine temperament,

persons of pale face, weakly with lax muscles, constitutions which suffer from deficient nutrition, not because food is lacking in quality or quantity, but from imperfect assimilation, (*Bar. Carb., Calcarea Carb.*), over-sensitive, physically and mentally. In cases of suppuration, after active discharge has ceased. Patient very weak, lack of nerve power, lack of vital heat. Takes cold easily, wants head wrapped up. Foot-sweat with very offensive odour. Ills following external suppression of foot-sweats. Scrofulous diathesis. external suppression of foot-sweats. Scrofulous diathesis. Chronic headache.

Abscesses, especially in teeth, fistula. Hip-joint disease.

Abscess of lungs. Head-sweats. Vaccination sores.

Chronic inflammation of the ears. Spinal irritation. Caries of the bones. *Ill effects of vaccination, suppurative processes. Intolerance of alcoholic stimulants. Ailments attended* with pus formation. Epilepsy. *Want of grit, moral or physical.* Promotes expulsion of foreign bodies from the tissues,—needles, bone splinters, etc.

WORSE, *during new moon,* cold, during menses, uncovering, especially the head, *lying down.*

BETTER, warmth, especially from wrapping the head, all the symptoms, except gastric, which are better by cold food (*Lycopodium Clav.*). *Silicea* is the chronic of *Pulsatilla.*

RELATIONS—COMPLEMENTARY, *Thuja, Puls., Fluor Ac., Mercurius Sol.* and *Silica* do not follow each other well.

COMPARE, *Hep Sulp., Kalium P., Pic Ac., Calcarea Carb., Phos.*

FOLLOWS WELL, by *Hep Sulp., Fluor Ac., Lycopodium Clav., Sep.*

ANTIDOTES, *Camph., Hep Sulp.*

Spgelia

Pinkroot (Vegetable).

It is an important remedy in pericarditis (inflammation of the membranous sac around the heart), and other diseases of the heart, with violent palpitation and great pain. It is adapted to anemic, debilitated subjects of rheumatic diathesis, and to scrofulous children with worm troubles. Has marked elective affinity for the eye, heart and nervous system. Neuralgia in the eyes, cannot move them on account of violent pressive pain. Sharp pain back of eye-balls. Neuralgia of the face very severe, parts swell. Parts feel chilly. *Very sensitive to touch.* A touch sends shudder through the entire frame. Worse, during the rainy weather. Neuralgic headaches, feeling as though head were opening. *Neuralgia of bowels. A great remedy for neuralgia in any parts.*

WORSE, from touch, motion, noise, turning the eyes, *from every shaking, motion or concussion.*

BETTER, lying on the right side with head high (*Arsenicum Alb., Spong.*).

RELATIONS, compare, *Aconitum Nap., Arsenicum Alb., Cact., Dig., Kalium Carb., Spong., in heart affections.*

ANTIDOTES, *Puls., Camph.*

Spongia Tosta

Roasted sponge.

A remedy especially useful in the symptoms of the respiratory organs, cough, croup etc., heart affections, and often indicated for the tubercular diathesis, especially adapted to diseases of children and women, with light hair, lax fibre, fair complexion, swelling and induration of glands, *Goitre. Exhaustion and heaviness of the body, after slight exertion, with rush of blood to chest, face. Anxiety and difficult breathing. Croup (with Aconitum Nap.),* cough dry, and breathing sounds as if a saw were being driven through a board, sometimes near suffocation. In cases where patient awakes with sense of suffocation, cough, and anxiety, cannot lie on back without smothering sensation. Chronic hoarseness.

WORSE, ascending, wind, before midnight.

BETTER, descending, lying with head low.

RELATIONS, *Spongia follows well, after Aconitum Nap., Hep Sulp.,* in cough and croup, when dryness prevails, after *Spong., Hep Sulp.,* when mucus commences to rattle.

COMPARE, *Arnica Mont., Caust., Iod., Lach.*

ANTIDOTE, *Camph.*

Staphsagria

Stavesacre (Vegetable).

Nervous affections, with marked irritability, diseases of the genito-urinary tract and skin, most frequently give symptoms calling for this drug, for the mental effects of onanism and sexual excesses, very sensitive to slightest mental impressions. Ill effects of anger and insults. *Sexual sins and excesses. Very sensitive.* Mechanical injuries from sharp cutting instruments, *post surgical operations. Craving for tobacco.* Teeth turn black and *decay on edges* (at the roots, *Mez., Thuja*), cannot be kept clean, toothache, painful to touch of food, or drink, but not from biting or chewing. *Styes on eyelids, leaving hard nodosities.* Extreme hunger even when stomach is full of food. pain in the back, spermatorrhea with sunken features, guilty, abashed look, weak, relaxed, nervous weakness. Eczema, yellow crust with acrid moisture, figwarts. Mind dwells unhealthily on things sexual, memory weak, moody, shuns the opposite sex. "*Lunacy of masturbation*" nightmare. Lice seem to get on children in spite of cleanliness. *All ills which can be traced to masturbation.*

WORSE, mental affection, from anger, indignation, grief, mortification, loss of fluids, tobacco, onanism, sexual excesses, from the least touch on affected parts.

BETTER, after breakfast, warmth, rest at night.

RELATIONS, compare, *Caust., Col, Ign., Lycopodium Clav., Puls.* and *Staph.* act well after each other.

Caust., Col, Staph. follow well in the order named.

ANTIDOTE, *Camph.*

INIMICAL, *Ranun, Bulb* either before or after.

Stramonium

Thorn-apple (Vegetable).

The entire force of this drug seems to be expended on the brain, though the skin and throat show disturbance. Adapted to ailments of young plethoric persons (*Aconitum Nap., Bell.*), especially children in chorea, mania and fever delirium. Delirium, loquacious, talks all the time, sings, raves, delirium is more furious, the mania is more acute. *Desires light and company, worse in the dark and solitude,* afraid in the dark, hallucinations, sees animals and all sorts of things, chorea, muscles of the face are *distorted. Eyes wide open, prominent, brilliant, pupils widely dilated, insensible. Stammering.* Nervous asthma, fears almost to draw breath. *Painlessness characteristic with most complaints.*

WORSE, *in dark room, when alone,* looking at bright or shining objects, after sleep (*Apis Mell., Lach., Op., Spong.*), when trying to swallow.

BETTER, *from bright light,* from company, warmth.

RELATIONS, *Stramonium often follows, Bell., Cup., Hyos., Lycopodium Clav.*

In metrorrhagia from retained placenta, with characteristic delirium, *Secale Corn.* often acts promptly, when *Stram.* has failed (with fever and septic tendency, *Pyr.*). After overaction, from repeated doses of *Bell.* in whooping cough.

ANTIDOTES, *Bell., Tabac., Nux Vom.*

Sulphur

Sublimated Sulphur—*Anti-Psoric.*

This is *the great Hahnemannian anti-Psoric.*

Its action is centrifugal—from within outward—having an elective affinity for the skin, where it produces heat and burning, with itching, made worse by the heat of the bed. Inertia and relaxation of fibre, hence feebleness of tone characterizes its symptoms. *Ebullitions of heat, dislike of water, dry and hard hair and skin, red orifices, sinking feeling of stomach, about 11 a.m., and cat-Nap. sleep, alwats indicate Sulphur* Homeopathically.

Characteristics are—dirty habits, hates to wash, heat on top of head, flushes of heat, burning palms and soles, orifices of body red, dry dirty, itches and burns, eyes burn—in fact, *itching and burning may be anywhere, with attendant scratching which makes the place burn the more. A great remedy where skin diseases have been 'cured'* (and in fact really suppressed) *by external means,* and ill-health follows bringing back the eruptions and betters the health. Discharges, from all outlets, burning, offensive smell of body. Clinically an aid in a vast number of diseases, scrofula, skin diseases, rheumatism, ophthalmia, piles, constipation, diarrhea, fevers, dyspepsia, wherever the general characteristics given above are present. A few doses of the remedy in the spring tends to keep the health good.

When carefully selected remedies fail to act, especially in acute diseases, it frequently arouses the reactionary powers of the organism and brings about a cure. In chronic cases, in beginning the treatment, a few doses of a high potency are necessary to neutralise the effects of previous medications, and to prepare the ground for the cure of the trouble, if it is the real remedy, or for the indication of the appropriate remedy which will be necessary for a cure.

WORSE, at rest, *when standing, warmth in bed,* washing, bathing, in morning, at 11 a.m., night, from alcoholic stimulants, periodically.

BETTER, *dry, warm weather,* lying on right side (rev. of *Stann.*), from drawing up affected limbs.

RELATIONS—COMPLEMENTARY, *Aloe Soc., Psor.*

Ailments from the abuse of metals generally.

COMPATIBLE, *Calcarea Carb., Lycopodium Clav., Puls., Sars, Sep.*

Sulph., Calcarea Carb., Lycopodium Clav., or Sulph., Sars., Sep. frequently follow in given order.

Sulphur is the chronic of *Aconite,* and follows it well in pneumonia and other acute diseases.

Mercurius Sol. and Calcarea Carb. are frequently useful after *Sulphur,* but not before.

ANTIDOTES, *Aconitum Nap., Mercurius Sol., Nux Vom., Puls.*

Thuja Occidentalis

White Cedar—Vegetable—*Anti-Sycotic.*

Thuja bears the same relation to the sycosis of Hahnemann,—fig warts, condylomata and wart-like excrescences upon mucous and cutaneous surfaces—that *Sulphur* does to *Psora,* or *Merucry* to Syphilis. Acts well in lymphatic temperament, in very fleshy persons, dark complexion, black hair healthy skin. *Ailments from bad effects of vaccination (Antimonium Tart., Sil.),* from suppressed or maltreated gonorrhea (*Med.*). The *great anti-sycotic remedy* constitutionally indicated by the presence of cauliflower excrescences, fungoid growths, fig warts, "seed warts", polypi, where these are present. *Thuja* will prove constitutionally beneficial in any disease, also for ill-health dating from vaccination, or gonorrhea. Otorrhea, flow of foul smelling pus from the ears, with growths in ear. Nasal polypi, warts, and foul greenish mucus, nasal catarrh. Warts about anus. Rheumatism following gonorrhea. Fetid foot-sweat. Sycotic pains, *i.e.*, tearing in muscles and joints, worse at rest, better in dry weather, worse, damp, humid atmosphere, lameness. Complaints from moonlight. *Rapid exhaustion and emaciation. Left-sided and chilly medicine.*

SWEAT, *only on uncovered parts, or all over except the head* (rev, of *Sil.*), when he sleeps stops when he wakes (rev. of *Samb.*), profuse, sour smelling fetid at night. Sensation as if body, especially the limbs *were made of glass, and would break easily. Nails, deformed, brittle (Antimonium Crud.).*

WORSE, at night, from heat of bed, at 3 a.m. and 3 p.m., from cold, damp air, narcotics.

BETTER, left side, while drawing up a limb.

RELATIONS—COMPLEMENTARY, *Med., Sab., Sil., Natrium Sulph.*

COMPARE, *Sil., Natrium Sulph., Puls.*

Tuberculinum

Pus (with bacilli) from tubercular abscess—(A Nosode-Constitutional).

Adapted to persons of light complexion, tall, slim, flat, narrow chest, active and precocious mentally, weak physically, the tubercular diathesis. *When, with a family history of tubercular affections, the best selected remedy fails to relieve or permanently improve, without reference to name of disease.*

Lax fibre, low recuperative powers, and very susceptible to changes in the weather. Patient always tired, motion causes fatigue, aversion to work, wants constant changes.

Rapid emaciation. Of great value in epilepsy, neurasthenia, and in nervous children. Diarrhea in children running for weeks, extreme wasting, bluish pallor, exhaustion. Mentally deficient children. Enlarged tonsils. Skin affections, *acute particular rheumatism*. Very sensitive, mentally and physically. General exhaustion. Nervous weakness. Trembling. Epilepsy. Arthritis.

WORSE, motion, music, before a storm, standing, dampness, from draugh, early morning, and after sleep.

BETTER, open air.

RELATIONS—COMPLEMENTARY, *Psor., Sulph.,* when *Psor., Sulph.* or the best selected remedy fails to relieve or permanently improve, follow *Psor.* as a constitutional remedy in hay fever, asthma.

BELLADONNA, for acute attacks, congestive or inflammatory, occurring in tubercular diseases.

HYDRASTIS to fatten patients cured with *Tuber*.

Veratrum Album

White hellebore (Vegetable).

For children and old people, the *extremes of life*, persons who are habitually cold and deficient in vital reaction, young people of a nervous, sanguine temperament. A perfect picture of *collapse*, with *extreme coldness, blueness,* and *weakness,* is offered by this drug. Post-operative shock with cold sweat on forehead, pale face, rapid, feeble pulse. *Cold perspiration on the forehead, with nearly all complaints. Vomiting, purging and cramps in extremities. The profuse, violent retching and vomiting* is most characteristic. surgical shock. Face, *pale, blue, collapsed, features sunken, hippocratic,* red, while lying, becomes pale, on rising up, (*Aconitum Nap.*). *Thirst intense,* unquenchable, for large quantities of *very cold water* and *acid drinks, wants everything cold.*

Icy coldness, of face, tip of nose, feet, legs, hands, arms and many other parts. *Violent vomiting, with profuse diarrhea. Bad effects of opium eating, tobacco chewing. In congestive, or pernicious, intermittent fever, with extreme coldness, thirst, face cold and collapsed,* skin cold and clammy, great prostration, cold sweat on forehead and deathly pallor on face. Vertigo, bronchitis, dysuria, dysmenorrhea, rheumatism, etc., *when accompanied or followed by the cold sweats.* Mania with desire to cut and tear everything, especially clothes, with lewd and lascivious talk, amorous or religious.

WORSE, at night, wet cold weather, from least motion, after drinking, before and during menses, during stool, when perspiring, after fright.

BETTER, walking and warmth.

RELATIONS, after, *Arsenicum Alb., Arnica Mont., China off., Cup Met., Ipec.,* after *Camph.,* in cholera and cholera morbus. After *Amm Carb., Carbo Vom.,* in dysmenorrhea with vomiting and purging.

ANTIDOTES, *Ipec., Arsenicum Alb., Camph., Aconitum Nap., China off.*

Zincum Metallicum

Zinc—Metal—*Anti-Psoric.*

Persons suffering from cerebral and nervous exhaustion, *defective vitality, brain or nerve power wanting,* too weak to develop exanthemata or menstrual function, to expectorate, to comprehend, to memorise.

Incessant and violent fidgety feeling in feet or lower extremities, must move them constantly. Tissues are worn out faster than they are repaired. *The nervous symptoms of most importance.* Impending brain paralysis. *Period of depression in disease.* Spinal affections, *burning whole length of spine,* spinal irritation, great prostration of strength. Great relief from discharges. Chorea, from fright or suppressed eruption, *convulsions with pale face and no heat.* Marked anemia with profound prostration. *In chronic diseases with brain and spinal symptoms, trembling, convulsive, twitching and fidgety feet are guiding symptioms.* HUNGER, ravenous, about 11 or 12 a.m. (*Sulph.*), *great greediness when eating, cannot eat fast enough* (incipient brain disease in children).

WORSE, at menstrual period, from touch, between 5 to 7 p.m., after dinner, from wine.

BETTER, while eating, discharges, and appearance of eruptions, menstrual flow. Is followed well by *Ign.,* but not by *Nux Vom.* which disagrees.

RELATIONS, Compare, *Hell Nig., Tuberc.* in incipient brain diseases from suppressed eruptions.

INIMICAL, *Cham.,* and *Nux Vom.* should not be used before or after.

APPENDIX–III

GLOSSARY

Abdomen	—	The cavity between the thorax and pelvis, the belly.
Abnormal	—	Not natural, unhealthy.
Abrasion	—	Loss of skin or membrane by scraping, excoriation.
Acne punctata	—	Red pimples upon the face and nose of young people.
Adenoid	—	Resembling a gland.
Adipose	—	Pertaining to fat, fatty.
Adynamic	—	Attended with great debility, prostration.
Agglutination	—	Adhesion, joining together.
Ague	—	Malarial or Intermittent fever.
Alae nasi	—	Wings of the nose.
Alimentary tract	—	Includes mouth, tongue, gullet, stomach, intestines and rectum up to anus, the tracts associated with digestion.
Alopecia	—	Baldness.
Albumen	—	An organic element of the blood, etc., found almost pure in the white of an egg.
Alkaline	—	Substance which neutralises acids.
Alveoli (alveolar)	—	Bony sockets of the teeth.

Alvine	—	Pertaining to the stomach or intestines.
Amaurosis	—	Paralysis of the optic nerve, partial or total blindness.
Amblyopia	—	Dimness of sight.
Amenable	—	Governable.
Amenorrhea	—	Stoppage of menses.
Anemia	—	Deficiency of blood or red corpuscles.
Anamnesis	—	The past history of a disease.
Anesthesia	—	A state of insensibility.
Anasarca	—	Dropsy of the cellular tissue. A species of dropsy between the skin and the flesh.
Aneurism	—	Morbid enlargement of an artery.
Angina	—	Inflammation of the air passages of the throat.
Anorexia	—	Loss of appetite.
Anterior	—	Before, in front.
Anteversion	—	A bending forward
Antiphlogistic	—	Preventive of inflammation, cooling remedies.
Antipsoric	—	Opposed to psora, or a tendency to certain forms of disease, especially skin affections.
Antipyretic	—	Agent reducing temperature.
Anuria	—	Suppression of urine.
Anus	—	External opening of the rectum.

GLOSSARY

Aorta	—	The great artery of the body.
Apathy	—	Insensibility, indifference.
Aphonia	—	Loss of voice.
Aphthae	—	Roundish, whitish vesicles found in sore mouth.
Aponea	—	Temporary absence of respiration.
Apoplexy	—	Sudden rupture of blood vessels in the brain with paralysis and unconsciousness
Apyrexia	—	Interval between paroxysms of fever.
Arterio sclerosis	—	Thickening of coats of arteries promoting blood pressure.
Arteries	—	Vessels conveying the blood from the heart.
Arthritis	—	Inflammation of the joints.
Ascarides	—	Small intestinal worms, pin worms, threadworms.
Ascites	—	Dropsy (accumulation of watery fluid) of the abdomen.
Asphyxia	—	Suspended animation, as by suffocation, etc.
Assimilate	—	To convert into a similar substance, as food is assimilated by conversion into animal substances, flesh, chyle, blood, etc.
Asthenic	—	Debilitated, applied to disease, low.

Asthenopia	—	Weak or painful vision.
Asthma	—	Violent oppression of breathing
Astringents	—	Medicines used to contract muscular fibres and to constrict vessels to restrain discharge.
Atony	—	Relaxation, want of energy or tone.
Atrophy	—	Wasting away of the system from functional disturbances.
Auditory	—	Belonging to the sense of hearing.
Auscultation	—	A method of determining the condition of an organ by listening to the sounds produced by it.
Autopsy	—	A *post-mortem* examination.
Axilla	—	Arm-pit.
Belching	—	The throwing off, or ejecting, of wind from the stomach.
Biliary	—	Pertaining to the secretions of the liver.
Borborygmus	—	Rumbling of wind in the bowels.
Breech	—	The lower part of the body, from the middle down.
Bronchia	—	Air passages.
Bronchitis	—	Inflamation of the bronchial tubes.
Buccal	—	Belonging to the cheeks, pertaining to the mouth.

GLOSSARY

Bulimia	—	Excessive, morbid hunger.
Cachexia	—	Vitiated constitution, morbid condition of the body characterised by deficient digestion, nutrition and assimilation.
Cadaverous	—	Resembling a corpse.
Caecum	—	The blind pouch at the head of the large intestines.
Calcareous	—	Containing lime.
Calculus	—	Stone, gravel.
Callous	—	Hard.
Cancer	—	A scirrhous, livid tumour, intersected by firm whitish divergent bands.
Capillaries	—	Hair-like, minute vessels.
Capsule	—	Membranous sac.
Carcinoma	—	Cancer.
Cardiac	—	Pertaining to the heart.
Caries	—	Ulceration of the bone.
Carotids	—	Two large arteries of the neck.
Cartilage	—	An elastic and flexible substance found at the joints and at the extremities of the ribs.
Catamenia	—	Menses.
Catamenia	—	Purgative.
Catheter	—	A hollow tube, used to insert into the bladder to draw off urine.
Cell	—	A small cavity.

Cellular tissue	—	Netlike formation, composed of cells.
Cellulitis	—	Cellular inflammation.
Cephalalgia	—	Headache.
Cephalic	—	Pertaining to the head.
Cerebral	—	Pertaining to the brain.
Cerebrum	—	Upper and front part of the brain.
Cerumin	—	Ear-wax.
Cervicitis	—	Inflammation of the neck of the womb.
Cervix	—	The neck.
Change of life	—	See 'climacteric period.'
Chemosis	—	Inflammatory swelling of the Conjunctiva.
Cholesterin	—	A substance forming the crystalline part of certain biliary calculi.
Chlorosis	—	A disease affecting young females, more particularly those who have not menstruated. It is characterised by a pale, livid complexion. languor, depraved appetite and digestion.
Chorea	—	A nervous disease causing irregular, involuntary movements of the limbs or face.
Chronic	—	Of long standing.
Chyle	—	A nutritive fluid.

Cicatrix	—	Scar left after the healing of a wound.
Cilia	—	The hairs of the eyelids.
Cirrhosis	—	Hardening due to an increase in the connective tissue of an organ.
Clavicle	—	Collar-bone.
Climacteric period	—	Cessation of menstrual functions, usually occurring about the forty-fifth year.
Coagulum	—	Clot of blood.
Collapse	—	Failure of vital power.
Colon	—	A part of the large intestine from the caecum to the rectum.
Coma	—	Lethargy, stupor, collapse.
Conception	—	Impregnation of the ovum of the male sperm, whence results a new being.
Condylomata	—	Wartlike excrescences on the pudenda or anus, or on face.
Congenital	—	Hereditary, existing at birth.
Congestion	—	Over-fullness of the blood vessels.
Conjunctivitis	—	Inflammation of the mucous membrane of the eye.
Constipation (Costiveness)	—	When evacuation from the bowels do not take place as frequently as usual, or are unnaturally hard, and voided with difficulty.

Contagion	—	Propagation of disease by contact.
Contusion	—	Bruise.
Cornea	—	The transparent coat of front part of the eye-ball.
Corpuscle	—	A minute body, a cell.
Coryza	—	Discharge from the nose.
Cranium	—	Skull.
Croup	—	Inflammation of the larynx and trachea.
Crural	—	Belonging to the upper part of the inner side of the thigh.
Crypt or Follicle	—	A small hollow roundish body, situate in the substance of the skin, or mucous membranes.
Cutaneous	—	Belonging to the skin.
Cuticle	—	Outer skin.
Cyanosis	—	Blue discoloration of skin from nonoxidation of blood.
Cyst	—	A membranous sac containing fluid or semi-solid.
Cystitis	—	Inflammation of the bladder.
Cystocele	—	Hernia or ruptur of the bladder.
Defecation	—	Stool, alvine evacuation.
Deglutition	—	Act of swallowing.
Deltoid	—	Muscle of the shoulder.
Dementia	—	Insanity, Idiocy.
Dental	—	Pertaining to the teeth.
Dermis	—	True skin.

GLOSSARY

Desquamation	—	Peeling off of the skin.
Desiccation	—	Drying up.
Diagnosis	—	The discrimination of diseases.
Diaphragm	—	Muscular partition between the thorax and abdomen.
Diathesis	—	Constitutional tendency.
Dietetics	—	Pertaining to diet.
Digital	—	Belonging to the fingers.
Diplopia	—	Double vision.
Dislocation	—	Displacement, as of a joint.
Diuresis	—	An abundant secretion of urine.
Dorsum	—	The back, the posterior side of anything.
Dropsy	—	An unnatural collection of a watery fluid in any part of the body.
Duodenitis	—	Inflammation of the duodenum or upper part of the small intestine.
Dyscrasia	—	Abnormal state of the blood.
Dysentery	—	A disease of the intestines attended with frequent bloody and mucous stools.
Dysmenorrhea	—	Painful menstruation.
Dyspepsia	—	Weakness of digestion.
Dysphagia	—	Difficulty of swallowing.
Dyspnea	—	Difficult breathing.
Dystocia	—	Difficult labour.
Dysuria	—	Painful micturition, difficulty in making water.

Ecchymosis	—	Effusion of blood under the skin, as in bruises.
Eclampsia	—	puerperal convulsions.
Eczema	—	Eruption of small vesicles on various part of the skin, usually close, or crowded together, with little or no inflammation round their bases.
Efflorescence	—	Redness of the skin.
Emetic	—	Medicine to produce vomiting.
Empirical	—	Practice based on experience alone.
Encephalic	—	Pertaining to the brain.
Endemic	—	Peculiar to a circumscribed locality.
Endocarditis	—	Inflammation of the internal parts of the heart.
Endometritis	—	Inflammation of the lining membrane of the uterus.
Enema	—	A rectal injection of medicine or food.
Enuresis	—	Incontinence of urine.
Epidemic	—	A generally prevailling disease among human beings.
Epidermis	—	The true skin, the outside coat on the whole body.
Epigastrium	—	The region over the stomach.
Epilepsy	—	Disease of the brain characterised by unconsciousness convulsive fits, etc.

Epistaxis	—	Bleeding from the nose.
Erosion	—	Destruction by ulceration.
Eructation	—	Belching, rising of wind from the stomach.
Erysipelas	—	Inflammatory cutaneous disease characterised by extreme redness.
Etiology	—	History of the cause of disease.
Eustachian tube	—	The canal leading from the throat to the inner ear.
Exacerbation	—	Aggravation of a disease or symptom.
Exanthema	—	Cutaneous eruption.
Excrement	—	Everything which is discharged from the body as superfluous, such as urine, faecal matter, perspiration, etc.
Exfoliation	—	Peeling off in thin layers of dead tissue, as of the bones or nails.
Exostosis	—	A morbid enlargement, or tumour of a bone.
Expectoration	—	Expulsion of the secretion of the chest.
Extravasation	—	Effusion of blood into a structure.
Exudation	—	Passage of fluid through a membrane.
False pains	—	Pains like, or resembling labour pains.

Fauces	—	Throat.
Febrile	—	Pertining to fever, feverish condition.
Felon	—	Very painful tumour found on the fingers or toes.
Femur	—	Thign-bone.
Fissure	—	Crack, a chap, opening.
Fistula	—	An abnormal tube-like passage in the body.
Flatus	—	Gas in the alimentary canal.
Fontanelle	—	Aperture in the infant skull at the junction of the sutures.
Gall-stone	—	A stone formed in the gall-bladder.
Ganglion	—	A knot-like enlargement in a nerve.
Gangrene	—	The mortification or death of a soft tissue.
Gastralgia	—	Pain in the stomach.
Gastric	—	Pertaining to the stomach.
Gastro-enteric (gastro-intestinal	—	Relating to the stomach and intestines.
Genus Epidemicus	—	The prevailing type of a disease.
Glands	—	Small secretory bodies met with in various part of the system.
Globus hystericus	—	The sensation in hysteria of a ball in the throat.

Glottis	—	The opening into the windpipe at the larynx.
Gleet	—	Chronic stage of gonorrhea with muco-purulent discharge.
Heart-burn	—	Impaired appetite with gnawing or burning pains in the stomach.
Hectic, Hectic Fever	—	1. Habitual. 2. Pertaining to phthisis. 3. Debilitating and emaciating fever of phthisis.
Hematemesis	—	Vomiting of blood from the stomach.
Hematocele	—	Swelling of scrotum or spermatic cord containing blood.
Hematuria	—	Hemorrhage from the bladder, blood in the urine.
Hemoptysis	—	The spitting of blood.
Hemorrhage	—	A flow of blood.
Hemorrhoid (Piles)	—	Painful tumours around, or within the anus.
Hemicrania	—	Half side of the head.
Hepatic	—	Pertaining to the liver.
Hepatitis	—	Inflammation of the liver.
Hepatization	—	A conversion into a liver-like substance.
Hernia	—	Rupture.
Herpes	—	A skin disease with patches of distinct vesicles.

Hydrocele	—	Dropsy of the scrotum.
Hydrocephalus	—	Colection of water in the head, dropsy of the brain.
Hydrothorax	—	Dropsy of the chest.
Hyperesthesia	—	Excessive sensibility.
Hyperemesis	—	Excessive vomiting.
Hyperplasia	—	Excessive formation of tissue.
Hypertrophy	—	Abnormal enlargement of an organ.
Hypochondriac	—	One who is morbidly melancholy.
Hypogastrium	—	The lower anterior part of the abdomen.
Hypopyon	—	Effusion of pus in the anterior chamber of the eye.
Ichor	—	Fetid watery discharge from wounds, ulcers, etc.
Icterus	—	Jaundice.
Idiopatic, I. disease.	—	Primary, original disease.
Idiosyncrasy	—	Individual peculiarity of constitution.
Ileum	—	The lower half of the small intestine.
Impregnation	—	Fecundation of the ova.
Inanition	—	Exhaustion from want of nourishment.
Incarcerated	—	Imprisoned, strangulated, constricted.
Incontinence	—	Involuntary passage of urine, inability to retain semen, etc.

GLOSSARY

Incubation	—	The period that elapses between the introduction of a morbific principle into the system and the development of the disease.
Incubus	—	Nightmare.
Indigestion	—	Dyspepsia, impaired digestion.
Induration	—	Hardening.
Infection	—	Propagation of disease by *miasm or contact*.
Infiltration	—	Flowing of fluids into the cellular tissue.
Influenza	—	Epidemic catarrh.
Ingesta	—	Food.
Inguinal	—	Belonging to the groin.
Innervation	—	The nervous influence necessary for the maintenance of life and the functions of the various organs.
Innocuous	—	Harmless.
Insomnia	—	Sleeplessness.
Interstitial	—	Space between.
Integument	—	A covering, especially of the skin.
Intercostal	—	Between the ribs.
Intertrigo	—	An inflammation of the skin due to chafing or rubbing.
Intumescence	—	The swelling of a part or in the whole of the body.

Intussusception	—	A portion of the intestines falling into the adjoining part and choking up the opening, producing strangulation.
Ishuria	—	Retention or suppression of urine.
Jaundice	—	A bilious disease, inducing yellowness of the skin, etc.
Jugular	—	Large vein in the neck.
Labour	—	Parturition, childbirth.
Laceration	—	Tearing.
Lachrymation	—	Discharge of water from the eyes.
Lactation	—	Secretion of milk.
Larynx	—	Upper part of the windpipe.
Lesion	—	Hurt or injury caused by violence or diseae.
Leucophlegmatic	—	Torpid or sluggish temperament.
Leucorrhea	—	Whites. A discharge of a white, yellowish or greenish mucus from the vagina.
Lichen	—	A papular inflammation of the skin.
Lientery	—	Diarrhea consisting of undigested food.
Ligament	—	A band of fibrous tissue binding parts together.
Ligature	—	Cord tied around a bleeding vessel.
Lithotomy	—	The removal of stone from the bladder by surgical means.

GLOSSARY

Lochia	—	Vaginal discharge after labour.
Lumbar	—	Pertaining to the loins.
Lumbrici	—	Round worms in the intestines.
Luxation	—	Dislocation.
Lymph	—	A transparent fluid found in the lymphatic vessels and thoracic duct.
Malaise	—	Indisposition.
Malar	—	Pertaining to the cheek.
Malformation	—	Unnatural formation.
Malignant	—	Term used to denote great severity of a disease.
Malposition	—	Wrong position.
Mammae	—	The female breasts.
Mammary	—	Relating to the breasts.
Mania	—	Madness.
Marasmus	—	Wasting away of the body, emaciation.
Mastitis	—	Inflammation of the breasts.
Mastoid, M. Process	—	Shaped like a nipple, as the mastoid process: The protruding part of the temporal bone.
Meconium	—	Excrement discharged from the bowels of a newborn infant.
Medication	—	Treatment by medicine.
Medulla oblongata	—	Part of the brain within the cranium, nervous system of the senses.
Megrim-Migraine	—	One-sided headache.

Membrane	—	A thin, enveloping or lining substance.
Menopause	—	Cessation of the menstrual flow, change of life.
Menorrhagia	—	Excessive menstruation, excessive hemorrhage.
Menses or Catamenia	—	Monthly courses of women.
Mesentery	—	The investing and supporting membrane of the small intestines.
Metastasis	—	Transfer of a disease from one part to another.
Meteorism	—	Gas in the abdominal cavity.
Metritis	—	Inflammation of the womb.
Metrorrhagia	—	Discharge of blood from the womb, uterine hemorrhage.
Miasm	—	Poisonous influence from the atmosphere.
Micturition	—	Urination.
Miliary rash	—	Rash (eruption) like millet seed.
Mole	—	(1) A small brown cutaneous spot, (2) False conception.
Morbid	—	Diseased, unhealthy, unnatural.
Mucous membrane	—	The lining of the cavities communicating with the external air, as lining of the mouth, intestines, etc.
Mucus	—	Fluid discharged from the mucous membranes.

GLOSSARY

Muscular Asthenopia	—	Weak or painful vision due to strain of occular muscles.
Myalgia	—	Pain in the muscles, cramp.
Myocardium	—	The muscular mass of the heart.
Myopia	—	Short sight.
Nares	—	The nostrils.
Nates	—	Two projections of the body on which we sit, the buttocks.
Nausea	—	Sickness of stomach.
Nephritis	—	Inflammation of the kidneys.
Neuralgia	—	Pain of the nerves.
Nisus	—	The monthly courses of women.
Nosology	—	Classification of diseases by names.
Nucleus	—	Any body about which matter is collected, the germ of a new cell.
Nutriment	—	A substance capable of nourishing and repairing the losses of the system.
Nutrition	—	That function of which the nutritive matter already elaborated by the various organic actions assumes the nature of the different living tissues, to repair losses and maintain their strength.
Nymphomania	—	Excessive sexual desire in women.

Obesity	—	Abnormal accumulation of fat.
Occiput	—	Back part of the head.
Edema	—	Dropsical swelling, accumulation of serum in the cellular tissue.
Esophagus	—	Gullet, passage from the pharynx to the stomach.
Onanism	—	Masturbation.
Ophthalmia	—	Inflammation of the eye.
Opisthotonos	—	Spasmodic bending backward of the body.
Orbits	—	The circular cavities which contain the eyes.
Orgasm	—	A strong desire or impulse for something.
Orthopnea	—	Difficult respiration relieved only by upright position.
Osteomalacia	—	A morbid softening of bone.
Osseous	—	Bony.
Ossification	—	Conversion into bone.
Otorrhea	—	Running from the ear.
Otitis media	—	Inflammation of the middle ear.
Ovaritis	—	Inflammation of the Ovaries.
Ozoena	—	Fetid nasal ulceration and discharge.
Panaritium	—	Phlegmonous inflammation of a finger or toe, whitlow.
Pancreas	—	A gland in the abdomen, secreting a juice, the use of

GLOSSARY

		which is to emulsify fatty matters.
Papascent	—	Thin, paplike.
Papillae	—	Eminences on the tongue, skin, the inner coat of the bowels, etc.
Papular	—	Abounding in pimples.
Paraplegia	—	Paralysis of legs.
Parenchyma	—	The distinctive or functional elements of an organ in contradistinction to the sustentacular elements of an organ.
Parotitis	—	Inflammation of the parotids (the gland near the ear).
Parturition	—	The act of giving birth to a child.
Pathogenesis	—	The origin and development of disease.
Pathogenic (Pathogenetic)	—	Causing disease.
Pathognomonic	—	Characteristic, peculiar to.
Pathology	—	The science of diseases.
Pectoral	—	Pertaining to the chest.
Pelvis	—	The bony basin of the trunk, formed by the innominate bones and the sacrum.
Pemphigus	—	A skin disease with an eruption of bullas.
Pericardium	—	Sac containing the heart.
Pericarditis	—	Inflammation of the pericardium.

Periosteum	—	Membrane enveloping the bones.
Peristaltic motion	—	Alternate contraction and dilation.
Peritoneum	—	Serous membrane lining the abdomen and enveloping its contents.
Peruvian bark	—	Cinchona.
Pessary	—	An instrument placed in the vagina to support a displaced uterus.
Petechia	—	Purpel spots on the skin.
Phagedena	—	Corroding, ragged sore.
Pharynx	—	Throat, upper part of the gullet.
Phlebitis	—	Inflammation of a vein.
Photophobia	—	Intolerance of light.
Phlegmasia Alba Dolens	—	Milk leg, an acute edema especially of the leg from venous obstruction.
Phelgmonous	—	Pertaining to inflammation in the cellular tissue. Inflammation with swelling.
Phrenitis	—	Inflammation of the brain, Delirium.
Phthisical	—	Consumptive, pertaining to consumption.
Phthisis	—	Consumption.
Phthisis Pulmonalis	—	Consumption of the lungs.
Physiology	—	The science of the functions of the body.

GLOSSARY

Piles	—	Painful tumours around or within the anus.
Piles blind	—	Those which do not bleed.
Plethora	—	Overfulness of the blood vessels, repletion.
Pleura	—	Lining membrane of the thorax. Covering also the lungs.
Plexus	—	A network of nerves or vessels.
Plexus, celiac	—	Formed of numerous nervous filaments, and is situated in the abdomen.
Plexus, solar	—	Network of nerves lying upon the vertebral column, the aorta and the pillars of the diaphragm.
Plica Polonica	—	A disease characterised by interlacing, twisting and agglutination or matting of the hair.
Pneumogastric	—	Belonging to the lungs and the stomach.
Pneumonia	—	Inflammation of the lungs.
Pneumo-thorax	—	Air in the pleural cavity.
Polychrest	—	Having many virtues, medicine useful in many diseases.
Polypus	—	Soft tumour in the nose, uterus, etc.
Posterior	—	The back part of anything.

Postmortem	—	Occurring after death.
Postpartum	—	After child-birth, with special reference to hemorrhage.
Precursory	—	Forewarning.
Primipara	—	A woman about to bear her first child.
Prodromic	—	Immediately preceding the attack of a sickness.
Prognosis	—	Act of foretelling results in disease—how long it will last, what will be the end, etc.
Progressive Locomotor Ataxia	—	Inability to walk steadily.
Prolapsus	—	Falling, as of the womb or rectum.
Proliferous	—	Bearing many young.
Prophylactics	—	Means used as preventives against disease.
Prostate gland	—	Situated around the neck of the bladder in the male.
Prurigo	—	A chronic papular skin disease with intense itching.
Pruritus	—	Intense itching.
Psora	—	Itch.
Psoriasis	—	Cutaneous disease, with a rough and scaly state of skin.
Ptyalism	—	Excessive secretion of saliva.
Puberty	—	The period when childhood ends and adolescence begins.
Puerperal	—	Pertaining to or following childbirth.

GLOSSARY

Pulmonary	—	Pertaining to the lungs.
Purulent	—	Having the character of pus.
Pus	—	Creamlike matter produced in abscesses, etc.
Putrescence	—	Rottenness, decay.
Pylorus	—	Lower orifice of the stomach.
Pyemia	—	A condition in which pyogenic (developing or secreting pus) bacteria circulate in blood and form abscesses wherever they lodge.
Pyorrhea	—	A discharge of pus.
Pyrosis	—	Heartburn, waterbrash.
Rachitis (Rickets)	—	A constitutional disease of childhood marked by the increased cell growth of the bones, deficiency of earthy matter, deformities and changes in the liver and spleen. Said to be due to lack of Vitamin D.
Rale	—	A bubbling sound heard in the bronchi in diseases.
Ranula	—	A tumour under the tongue.
Rash	—	An exanthematous eruption on the skin.
Rectum	—	The lower part of the large intstine.
Regurgitation	—	Return of food or drink from the stomach.
Renal	—	Belonging to the Kidneys.

Respiration	—	The act of breathing.
Retina	—	A thin membrane of the eye.
Retention	—	Stopping of natural discharges. as of urine, etc.
Retrocession	—	A retrograde movement.
Retroflexion	—	A bending or flexing backward.
Retroversion	—	A turning back.
Rhagades	—	Chaps or cracks of the skin.
Rigor	—	Coldness, stiffness, rigidity.
Sac	—	Bag.
Sacrum	—	Posterior bone of the pelvis on which the spine rests.
Saliva	—	Spittle.
Salivary glands	—	Glands secreting saliva or spittle.
Sanguineous	—	Bloody.
Sanguinolent	—	Tinged with blood.
Sarcocele	—	A fleshy tumour of the testicle.
Sarcoma	—	A fleshy, malignant tumour or growth.
Scapula	—	Shoulder-blade.
Sciatic	—	Pertaining to the inferior part of the hip-bone.
Scirrhous	—	Indolent, hard tumour, a form of cancer.
Sclerotica	—	The hard coat of the eyelid, white of the eye.
Scrofula	—	A morbid state of the system characterised by indolent,

		glandular tumours, they suppurate slowly, heal with difficulty, leave scars, etc.
Scrotum	—	Bag holding the testicles.
Secretion	—	A flowing or discharge.
Septicemia	—	An unhealthy condition of the blood, blood poisoning.
Septum	—	A partition.
Serum	—	Fluid portion of the blood.
Similimum	—	The remedy that corresponds most nearly to the existing symptoms.
Sinciput	—	The fore and upper part of the head.
Sinus	—	A cavitvy or hollow.
Slough	—	The part which separates from a foul ulcer, decaying bone. etc.
Sordes	—	Fetid accumulations about the teeth.
Spasms	—	Severe morbid contractions of the muscles.
Spermatorrhea	—	An involuntary emision of semen.
Sporadic	—	Scattered, not epidemic.
Sputa	—	Spittle.
Sternum	—	The breast-bone.
Stasis	—	Stagnation of the blood-current.
Sthenic	—	Strong, active.
Strabismus	—	Squinting.

Strangury	—	Painful urination drop by drop.
Strumous	—	Scrofulous.
Stye	—	A small inflammatory pimple on the eyelid.
Stupor	—	Drowsiness, sleep.
Subcutaneous	—	Beneath the skin.
Sublingual	—	Beneath the tongue.
Subsultus Tendinum	—	Convulsive muscular twitching.
Suppuration	—	The formation of pus.
Suture (Surgery)	—	The sewing up of a wound.
Sycosis	—	Fig-wart, a venereal disease.
Symphysis	—	A union of bones.
Symptom	—	Any unnatural change perceptible to the senses in any organ or function.
Symptomatology	—	The science of symptoms.
Synchronous	—	Occurring at the same time.
Syncope	—	Fainting.
Synocha, synochus	—	A continued fever.
Synovia	—	Lubricating fluid of a synovial membrane (joints).
Syndrome	—	A complexus of symptoms.
Syphilis	—	A venereal disease communicated by sexual intercourse.
Taenia	—	Tapeworm.
Tendon	—	The white, tough extremity of the muscles.
Tenesmus	—	Painful, ineffectual urging to stool.

GLOSSARY

Testes-Testicles	—	Two glandular organs of the male contained in the scrotum whose function is to secrete semen.
Tetanus	—	Lock-jaw.
Tetter	—	Herpetic eruption.
Therapeutics-Therapia	—	Relating to the cure of diseases by remedial agents.
Thorax	—	The chest.
Thrush	—	Aphthae.
Thymus gland	—	A gland behind the sternum, usually disappearing in adult life.
Thyroid gland	—	A ductless glandular body at the upper part of the trachea consisting of two lateral lobes connected centrally by an isthmus.
Tonsils	—	Stands on each side of the fauces.
Torticollis	—	Twisted or wry neck.
Trachea	—	Windpipe.
Traumatic	—	Resulting from wounds or injuries.
Trigeminal	—	Pertaining to trigeminus, the trifacial nerve.
Trismus	—	Spasm of the muscles of mastication, lock-jaw.
Tubercle	—	A small nodule of granular cells constituting the specific lesion of the tubercle bacillus.

Tuberculosis	—	An infectious disease due to a specific bacillus, characterised by the formation of tubercles.
Tumefaction	—	A swelling of a part.
Tumour	—	A swelling bigger or smaller, developed by a morbific cause in some part of the body.
Tympanitis	—	Flatulent distension of the abdomen.
Ulcer	—	Suppuration upon a free surface, an open sore.
Ulceration	—	The process of ulcer formation.
Umbilicus	—	The navel.
Uremia	—	Auto-intoxication due to retention in the blood, of unknown substances, the cause is undetermined but it is ascribed to (1) renal impairment, (2) perverted metabolism.
Ureter	—	A tube carrying urine from kidney to bladder.
Urethra	—	The excretory canal of the bladder.
Urticaria	—	Nettle rash, an ephermeral skin eruption with itching.
Varicella	—	Chicken-pox.
Varices	—	Dilated veins with knotty livid tumours.

GLOSSARY

Varicocele	—	Enlargement of blood vessels of the scrotum.
Varicose	—	Swollen, knotted.
Variola	—	Small-pox
Vascular	—	Pertaining to vessels, particularly the blood-vessels.
Vaso-motor	—	The force which controls the circulation of the blood.
Veins	—	Vessels for the conveyance of impure blood from every part of the body to the heart.
Velum palati	—	Back part of the mouth, the soft palate.
Ventricles	—	Cavities in the brain or heart.
Vermicular	—	That which resembles a worm.
Vertebrae	—	Bones of the spine.
Vertex	—	The crown or top of the head.
Vertigo	—	Dizziness, giddiness.
Vesical	—	Pertaining to the bladder.
Vesication	—	The formation of blisters.
Viscera	—	The contents of the body cavities, entrails.
Vomiturition	—	Retching, an ineffectual effort to vomit.
Waterbrash	—	Regurgitation of watery fluid from the stomach.
Whitlow	—	Felon.
Zygoma	—	Cheek-bone.

Zymotic	—	A term used to characterise the entire class of epidemic, endemic and contagious diseases due to specific viruses.

INDEX

A

Abdomen, Affections of the Stomach and 191
Abortion, Threatening 342
　Preventives for 344
Abscesses 470
Acids, Poisons, Antidotes for, 515
Acidity of stomach 191
Acne 476
Administration of Medicines 19, 73
Affections of
　Ears 117
　Head 101
　Mouth 189
　Nose 122
　Stomach and abdomen 191
　Teeth 185
　Throat 174
　Tongue 189
After-pains 353
Aggravation, Medicina l77
Ague 288
Air sickness 193
Alkaline Poisons, Antidotes for, 516
Anterior Poliomyelitis 444
Alternating diseases 51

Antipsoric Prophylactics, during pregnancy 49, 341
　for infants 367
Antipsoric remedies 46
Antipsoric Treatment, possibilities of, 49
Appendicitis 92
Application of Homeopathy 57
Arsenic, Injurious effects of, 573
Asthma 133
　Leading indications for, 134

B

Back, Pains in the, 485
Back Pains during pregnancy 334
Bed sores 478
Bilious fever 301
Biliousness 192
Bites, of snakes 517
Bites, of mad dogs 518
Bites, of angry animals 517
Bleeding from nose 123
　Piles 202
Blood Pressure 155
Boils 472
Brain, Inflammation of the, 416
　Diseases of the, and Nervous system 416

Breast Cancer 269
Breasts, Preparation of the,
during pregnancy 347
Gathered, after delivery 359
    Swelling of, in infants 370
Bronchitis1 31
Burns and Scalds 504

C

Cancer-Carcinoma 255
Cancer of the,
    Tongue 256
    Lower lip 258
    Esophagus 260
    Stomach 260
    Intestine 266
    Rectum 266
    Breast 269
    Womb 272
Car sickness 193
Carbuncle 473
Case, Individualisation of,
    of disease 10
Castor oil, Use of, 512
Catarrh of the nose 124
Catarrh of the stomach 191
Cellular tissue, Hardening of
    the 370
Change of life 317
Change of life remedies 79
Chicken-pox 284
    Preventive for, 284
Chilblain 473
Chills and fever 278
Chloral, Hydrate of,
    Bad effects of, 510

Chlorosis 315
Cholera
    After-effects of,
        and Convalescence 225
    Proplylactics for, 220
    Proper 222
    Summary of treatment for, 224
Chlorine 221
Chorea 432
Chronic Diseases. Hahnemann's,
    (synopsis) 27-42
    Further explanation 42-44
    Skin phase of, 44
Coffee, Bad effects of, 508
Cold, Common 124
Colic in bowels 193
    Menstrual, 310
    of infants 374
Collapse 496
Complaints accompanying
    Intermittent fever 288
Complaint, Summer, of
    infants 379
Confinement, Duration of, 353
Consequences of spirituous
    liquors etc. 507
Constipation of Lying in
    women 199, 357
    Pregnant women 199, 330
    Nursing infants 199, 373
    Continual crying of
    infants 375
Convalescence 493
Convulsions. Epileptic 422
    during labour 351
    of infants 378

INDEX

Corns 475
Coryza 124
Cough, 126
    Whooping, 138
Cramps during cholera 222
Cramps during labour 351
Cramps during pregnancy 334
Croup 129
Crying of infants 375
Cyanosis of infants 368

D

Deformities of infants 368
Delayed menstruation 304
Delivery, Easy 247, 352
Delivery, Flooding at, 345
Delivery, treatment
    after, 352
    After-pains 353
    Child-bed fever 361
    Constipation 357
    Diarrhea 357
    Duration of confinement 353
    Excessive perspiration 365
    Excessive secretion of milk 357
    Falling off of the hair 366
    Flooding 353
    Gathered breasts 359
    Lochia 354
    Milk fever 355
    Milk leg 362
    Nursing sore mouth 363
    Perspiration 364
    Retention of urine 358
    Sore nipples 359
    Suppressed secretion of milk 356
    Weakness from nursing 366
Dentition of children 378
Derangements during pregnancy 325
Diarrhea 211
    After certain articles 216
    After certain diseases 217
    After confinement 357
    During pregnancy 330
    Of infants 374
    With certain conditions 217
Diabetes
    Mellitus 235
    Glycosuria 235
    Insipidus 238
    Polyuria 238
Diet and other restrictions 35, 85
    General instructions for particular diseases 87
Digestion, Derangements of, 194
Digitalis, Bad effects of, 571
Diphtheria 181
Directions for prescribing 11-19, 57-64
Diseases of children,
    Rickets-Rachitis 386
    Scurvy Rickets 388
    Mal-nutrition,
        Wasting, Marasmus 388
    Tuberculosis Disease 392
    Epidemic Diarrhea 396
    Severe urgent cases with collapse 397

Diseases, Classification of, 9, 42
Drug, 49
Diseases of,
  The Aged 411
  Brain & Nervous system 417
  Children 384
  Eyes1 13
  Heart1 47
  Kidneys 239
  Organs of Respiration1 24
  Skin 453
  Women 304
Dose,
  Historical Development of the Homeopathic, 66
  The Homeopathic, 67
  The Physiological, 67
Doses, Suitable, for adults & children 73
  Precautions to be observed regarding, 78
  Hahnemann's rules regarding, 80
  Repetition of, 20, 37, 76
Drugs, Effects of,
  injurious, in use 510
  Primary and after effects of, 9
Dynamizations, Homeopathic, 67
Dysentery 218
Dysmenorrhea 310
Dyspepsia 194
  Classification of, 194
  During pregnancy 328
Dysuria (Difficult urination) 233
  During pregnancy 340

E

Earache 117
Ears, Affections of, 117
  Discharge from, in infants, 381
  Inflammations of, 119
  Mumps 117
  Running of, 120
Eczema 455
Eczema
  Leading indications in 456
Eclampsia 352
Elongation of the head of infants 369
Emergencies 495
Enuresis (frequent urination) 234
Enlargement of the
  Tonsils 177
  Uvula 181
Epilepsy, Special indications in, 429
Epistaxis 122
Epsom salts, Bad effects of, 511
Eruptive Fevers–
  Measles 281
  Chicken-pox 284
  Small-pox 285
Erysipelas 465
Examination of the patient and record of symptoms 57
Excoriation of infants 373
External injuries
  Remedies for, 502

INDEX

Eyes,
    After operations on the, 116
    Sore, of infants 111, 369
    Inflammation of the, 114
Eyelids,
    Chronic inflammation of the, 115
    Stye on the, 115

F

Fainting, During pregnancy 331
Falling of the,
    Womb 319
    Palate 181
False Pains 347
Fear, Effects of, 429
Felon 469
Fevers
    Leading indications in,
        Ordinary, 278
        Bilious 301
        Chicken-pox 284
        Child-bed 361
        Filarial 302
        Gastric 301
        Influenza 279
        Intermittent 288
        measles 281
        Milk 355
        Rheumatic 299
        Small-pox 285
        Typhoid 295
Filariasis, Filarial fever 302
Fits 422
Flatulency 194
Flooding,
    at delivery 345
    after delilvery 353
    during pregnancy 345
Food, and other restrictions 85
Fractures 504
Fright, Consequences of, 429
Frostbite 43
Fruits, Diarrhea after, 216

G

Ganja, Bad effects of, 510
Gases, Poisonous, Antidotes for, 515
Gastric fever 301
Gathered Breasts 359
Gathering in ear 120
General Dyscrasias and Constitutional Treatment,
    Scrofulosis 399
    Tuberculosis 404
    Glandular Affections 406
    Diseases of the Bones 407
    Advantages of constitutional Treatment 408
Giddiness 101
Gout 484
Green sickness 315
Grief and sorrow 328
Gum, Red, of infants 373
Gums, Bleeding of, 189
Gumboil 189

H

Hemorrhage from piles 202
Hemorrhoids 202

During pregnancy 337
Hahnemann's Life and Works, 3
Hahnemann's 'Chronic-Diseases' (a synopsis) 27-42
    Latest method 68
    Law of Cure 4
    Nosology 42-50
    Organon (a synopsis) 7-42
    Philosophy 51-57
Hair, Falling out of the, 426
Hair, Falling after delivery 366
Hardness of Hearing 121
Head, Affections of the, 101
    Scald, 376
    Scurf on the, of infants 375
Headache,
    Bilious 105
    Catarrhal 104
    Congestive 103
    During pregnancy 326
    Leading indications in, 101
    Nervous 108
    Rheumatic 105
Hearing, Hardness of, 121
Heart, Palpitation of the,
    During pregnancy 333
Heartburn 191
    During pregnancy 328
Heat spots, of infants 381
Hernia 207
    Congenital, of infants 370
Herpes
    Circinatus (Ring-worm) 467
    Zoster (Shingles) 467
Hiccough, of infants 371

Hip-disease 486
Hoarseness 174
Homeopathy,
    Application of, 57
    Defined 3
Homeopathy,
    Fundamental Principles explained 7
    Law explained 4
    Points of advantages over other systems indicated 3
    Prophylsis 499
Hydrocephalus Acute 419
    Chronic 421
Hysteria 428
    During pregnancy 331

I

Incontinence of urine 233
    During pregnancy 339
Indigestion 194
Infants, Treatment Of,—
    Antipsoric Prophylactics 367
    Breasts, swelling of 370
    Colic 374
    Congenital hernia 370
    Constipation 373
    Crying 375
    Cyanosis 368
    Deformities 368
    Diarrhea 374
    Discharge from ears 381
    Ecchymosis 367
    Excoriation 373
    Gum 373

INDEX

    Hardening of the
        Cellular tissue 370
    Heat Spots 381
    Hiccough 371
    Jaundice 372
    Marks 368
    Meconium 369
    Milk-crust 376
    Restlessness 375
    Retention of urine 373
    Scald head 376
    Scurf on head 375
    Snuffles 371
Infants, Treatment
    of—
    Sore eyes 369
    Sore mouth 372
    Sore throat 372
    Spasms 378
    Stuttering 382
    Summer Complaint 379
    Swelling and Elongation
    of head 369
    Teething 378
    Wakefulness 375
    Weaning 382
    Wetting bed 382
    Whites 382
    Inflammation of brain 417
    of tongue 189
    of tonsils 177
    of kidney 239
Inflammatory
    Rheumatism 299
Influenza 279

Ingrowing toe nails 477
Injuries, External 502
Injurious Drugs, 50
    Effects of, 510
Insanity, Acute 50
Insects, Stings of, 517
Intermittent diseases 51
Intermittent fever 288
Intestine Cancer of 266
Intoxication, Effects of, 507
Iodine, Injurious
    Effects of, 512
Itch 453
Itching of
    Anus 204
    Private Parts 331
    the skin 453

J

Jaundice 229
    During pregnancy 339
    of infants 231

K

Knees, Rheumatism of the, 482

L

Labour 350
    Easy, 347
        Spasmodic pains,
        Cramps and convulsions
        during, 351
Lead, Injurious effects of, 513
Leucorrhea 321
    of children 382
Limbs, Cramps in, 223

Liver, Affections of the, 226
    Special indication in complaints of the, 228
Lochia, Excessive 354
    Protracted 354
    Suppression of the, The, 355
Loins, Pains in 485
Lower lip, cancer of, 258
Lumbago 485

M

Mad dogs, Bites of, 518
Magnesia salts,
    Injurious effects of, 511
Malaria 288
    After effects of, 294
Marks of infants 368
Measles, Leading
    indications for, 282
        After-effects of, 284
        Prophylactics for, 283
Meconium 369
Medicinal
    aggravation 37, 77, 78
Medicines, Preparation of, 23-27
Membranous Croup 129
Meningitis, Acute 419
    tubercular 421
Menorrhagia 308
Menstruation
    Delayed and obstructed 304
    Cessation of, 317
    Continued, during Pregnancy
    Painful 326
Menstruation
    Profuse 308
    Suppression of 306
    Tard and scanty 313
Mental Diseases,
    their treatment 50
Mercury, Injurious effects of, 512
Metallic Substances,
    poisoning, Antidotes for, 516
Milk, Excessive or involuntary secretion of, 357
    Fever 355
    Leg 362
    Suppression of 346
Milk-crust, of infants 376
Miscarriage, 342
    preventives of, 343
Morning sickness 328
Mouth,
    Nursing sore, 363
    sore, 189
    Sore, of infants 372
Mumps 117

N

Nails,
    Affections of 477
    Ingrowing toe 477
Nasal Catarrh1 24
Nausea, and Vomiting 192
    During pregnancy 328
    From riding in a carriage, Motor car or by Air 193
Navel, Rupture of the in infants 370
Nephritis 239
Nervous Headache 108
Nervous system,
    Diseases of the

INDEX

Brain and, 417
Nettle Rash 462
Neuralgia
   During Pregnancy 334
Neuralgic Headache 108
Neuritis 448
Nipples, sore 359
Nose, Affections of, 122
   Bleeding of, 122
   Catarrh of,
   Leading indications
     in, 124
   Obstruction of,
     in infants 371
Nursing, Falling off of hair
   while, 366
   Weakness from, 366
   Sore mouth 363

O

Esophagus, cancer of, 260
Ophthalmia 115
   of Infants 369
Opium, Poisoning by, 510
   Injurious effects of 510
Organon, Synopsis of the, 7-27
Overfeeding, Effects of, 193

P

Pains, After—, 353
   False labour, 347
   Griping, in bowels 193
   In the back and sides during
     pregnancy 334
Palpitation of the Heart, during
   Pregnancy 333
Perspiration after Delivery 364
Excessive, after Delivery 365

Paralysis 435
Phlebitis, crural
   (Milk-leg) 362
Piles 202
   During pregnancy 357
Pimples on the face 470
Pleurisy, Pleuritis 141
Pneumonia1 43
Poisoned wounds
   Bites of mad dogs 518
   Bites of snakes 517
   Stings of bees, & etc. 517
Poisons. Treatment of, 515
   Antidotes for—
   Acids 575
   Alkaline 516
   Gases 515
   Metallic substances 516
   Vegetable 516
Posology (potencies) 66
Post Diphtheric
   paralysis 184
Potassium, Iodide of,
   Injurious effects of, 512
Pregnancy
   Derangements during— 326
   Constipation 330
   Continued Menstruation 326
   Cramps 334
   Depression of Spirits 340
   Diarrhea 330
   Dyspepsia 328
   Dysury and Strangury 340
   Easy delivery 347
   False pains 347
   Flooding 345
   Headache and Vertigo 326

Heartburn 328
Hemorrhoids or Piles 351
Hysterical fits 331
Incontinence of urine 339
Itching 331
Jaundice 339
   Miscarriage or Abortion 342
Morning sickness 328
Neuralgia 334
Pains in the back and sides 334
Palpitation of the heart 333
Preparation of the breasts 347
Prophylactics 341
Toothache 333
Varicose veins 335
Prescribing,
   Direction for 57
Prickly heat 381
Prolapsus of the
   anus 206
   uterus 319
Prophylactic (Preventive) medicines for—
   Abortion 343
   Chicken-pox 284
   Cholera 220
   Infants 367
   Measles 282
   Pregnant women 341
   Small-pox 288
Pruritis 331
Psora 30
Psoric theory,
   Underlying facts of the, 45

Q

Quinine, Antidotes for,
   Injurious effects of, 294, 510
Quinsy (Tonsillitis) 177

R

Rash, Nettle 462
Raw surface of infants 373
Rectum (Anus),
   Prolapsus of the, 206
Rectum, cancer of 266
Red Gum 373
Remedies, External 505
   Mode of Administration of, 19-22, 73-76
   Repetition of, 19-22, 77-80
   Selection of the Similar, 10-19, 64-66
Respiration, Diseases of Organs of, 124
Restlessness of Infants 375
Rheumatism, Chronic 480
   Headache from 105
   Inflammatory (acute) 299
Ringworm on Scalp 467
Ringworm of infants 376
Running of the ears 120
Rupture 207

S

Scabies 453
Scalds and Burns 504
Scalp, Ringworm on, 467
Sciatica 486
scurf on the Head 375
Sea-sickness 193
Shingles 467

INDEX

Sick headache 105
Sides pain in the during Pregnancy 334
Similar Remedy,
    Selection on the 64-66
Skin, Diseases of the, 453
    Itching of the on the, 453
Skull, Ecchymosis on the 367
Sleeplessness
    of infants 375
Small-pox 285
    Preventives for 286
    Summary of treatment for 288
Snakes, Bites of, 517
Snuffles 371
Sore eyes of infants 369
    mouth 189
    mouth of infants 372
    Nipples 359
    Throat 174
Sore disposition to 177
Sore from cold1 74
Sore of infants 372
Sour stomach 191
    things, Bad effects of, 508
Spasms 422
Spasmodic pains
    during labour 351
Spices, Bad effects of, 508
Spirits, Depression of,
    during Pregnancy 340
Spirituous liquors,
    Effects of, 507
Spleen, Affections of the, 231
Sprains 503

Stings 505, 577
Stomach, Affections of the, and Abdomen 191
    Cancer of 260
    Catarrh of the 191
    Diarrhea from disordered, 211
    Headache from over-loaded, 103
Strangury 233
Stuttering of children 382
Styes on eyelids 115
Sulphur, Injurious effects of, 512
Summer Complaint 379
Sun-stroke 490
Suppression of the,
    Menses 306
    Suppression urine 232
Sycosis 31-32, 47-48
symptoms, totality of, 58-64
Syphilis 32-33, 48
Swelling of the head of infants 369
    Swelling of the Tongue 189
    Swelling of the Veins during Pregnancy 335

T

Tape worms 204
Tea, Bad effects of, 508
Teeth, Affections of, 185
Teeth Leading
    indications for, 185
Teething of infants 378
Throat, Affections of the, 174
Throat, Affections Disposition to 176

Throat, Affections sore 174
Throat, Affections from cold 174
Throat, Affections of infants 372
Thrush of infants 372
Tobacco, Bad effects of 508
Tongue, Inflammation of, 189
    Cancer of, 256
Tonsillitis, Causes of, 177
    Acute 179
Tonsils, Inflammation of the, 177
Tonsils, Chronic 180
Tonsils, Use of the, 177
Toothache, Leading indications
    for, 185
    During Pregnancy, 333
Treatment after Delivery 352
Treatment of Infants 367
Tubercular Meningitis 421
Tumours 472
Typhlitis, Perityphlitis and
    Appendicitis 248
Typhoid fever 295
Typhoid for difficult
cases 298

U

Umbilical Hernia of infants 370
Urination, Difficult 233
    Frequent 234
    Involuntary 234
    Painful 233
Urine, Incontinence of,
    During Pregnancy 339
    Retention of, after
    Delivery 358
Retention in infants 232
Suppression of 232
Urticaria 462

Uterus, Prolapsus of the, 319
Uvula, enlargement of the, 181

V

Vaccination 500
Vaccination, Diarrhea
    after, 217
Varicose veins during
    Pregnancy 335
Vegetable poisons,
    Antidotes for, 576
Vertigo 101
    During Pregnancy 326
Vomiting from travelling in a car
    or by air 193

W

Wakefulness of infants 375
Warts 475
Waterbrash 191
Weaning 382
Wetting the bed 234
Wetting of children 234
Whites 321
Whites of children 382
Whitlow 469
Whooping cough 138
Womb, Cancer of 272
    falling of the, 319
Women, Diseases of, 304
Worms 204
    Tape 205
Wounds, Contused, 502, 503
    Lacerated 502, 503
    Poisoned 515

Z

Zoster, Herpes 467